S A N F O R D   G U I D E ®

®

Thirty-sixth Edition

THE SANFORD GUIDE
TO ANTIMICROBIAL
THERAPY
2006

David N. Gilbert, M.D.
Director of Medical Education & Earl A. Chiles Research Institute
Providence Portland Medical Center
Professor of Medicine
Oregon Health Sciences University
Portland, Oregon

Robert C. Moellering, Jr., M.D.
Shields Warrren-Mallinckrodt Professor of Medicine
Harvard Medical School
Boston, Massachusetts

George M. Eliopoulos, M.D.
Chief, James L. Tullis Firm, Beth Israel Deaconess Hospital
Professor of Medicine
Harvard Medical School
Boston, Massachusetts

Merle A. Sande, M.D.
Professor of Medicine
University of Washington School of Medicine
Seattle, Washington

THE SANFORD GUIDE TO ANTIMICROBIAL THERAPY 2006
36TH EDITION

JAY P. SANFORD, M.D.
1928-1996

EDITORS

DAVID N. GILBERT, M.D.
ROBERT C. MOELLERING, JR., M.D.
GEORGE M. ELIOPOULOS, M.D.
MERLE A. SANDE, M.D.

The Sanford Guide to Antimicrobial Therapy is published annually by:

ANTIMICROBIAL THERAPY, INC.
P.O. Box 276, 11771 Lee Highway
Sperryville, VA 22740-0276 USA
Tel 540-987-9480 Fax 540-987-9486
Email: info@sanfordguide.com

www.sanfordguide.com

Printed in the United States of America
ISBN 978-1-930808-31-3
Spiral Edition

PUBLISHER'S PREFACE

This edition marks the 36th revision of the Sanford Guide to Antimicrobial Therapy. The manuscript for the first edition in 1969 was prepared by Carolyn Wickwire who was then Jay Sanford's administrative assistant. Carolyn has prepared the manuscript for every new edition that followed including this one. She retires from her service to the SANFORD GUIDE with this edition. Carolyn's remarkable tenure is not likely to be repeated. We wish her all the best in her future endeavors.

NOTE TO READER

Every effort is made to ensure the accuracy of the content of this guide. However, current full prescribing information available in the package insert of each drug should be consulted before prescribing any product. The editors and publisher are not responsible for errors or omissions or for any consequences from application of the information in this book and make no warranty, express or implied, with respect to the currency, accuracy, or completeness of the contents of the publication. Application of this information in a particular situation remains the professional responsibility of the practitioner.

—TABLE OF CONTENTS—

SUMMARY OF ABBREVIATIONS

DRUG NAME ABBREVIATIONS

Antibacterial & Antimycobacterial Drugs
AG = aminoglycoside
AMK = amikacin
AM-CL = amoxicillin-clavulanate
AM-CL-ER = amoxicillin-clavulanate extended release
Amox = amoxicillin
AMP = ampicillin
AM-SB = ampicillin-sulbactam
AP Pen = antipseudomonal penicillins
APAG = antipseudomonal aminoglycoside (tobra, gent, amikacin)
Azithro = azithromycin
BL/BLI = beta-lactam/beta-lactamase inhibitor
CARB = carbapenems (ERTA, IMP, MER)
Cefpodox = cefpodoxime proxetil
Ceftaz = ceftazidime
CFP = cefepime
Chloro = chloramphenicol
CIP = ciprofloxacin; **CIP-ER** = CIP extended release
Clarithro = clarithromycin; **ER** = extended release
Clav = clavulanate
Clinda = clindamycin
CLO = clofazimine
Dapto = daptomycin
Dirithro = dirithromycin
Doxy = doxycycline
EES = erythromycin ethyl succinate
ERTA = ertapenem
Erythro = erythromycin
ETB = ethambutol
FQ = fluoroquinolone (CIP, Oflox, Lome, Peflox, Levo, Gati, Moxi, Gemi)
Gati = gatifloxacin
Gemi = gemifloxacin
Gent = gentamicin
GNB = gram-negative bacilli
IMP = imipenem-cilastatin
INH = isoniazid
IVIG = intravenous immune globulin
Levo = levofloxacin
Lome = lomefloxacin
Macrolides = azithro, clarithro, dirithro, erythro, roxithro
MER = meropenem
Metro = metronidazole
Mino = minocycline
Moxi = moxifloxacin
NF = nitrofurantoin
O Ceph 1,2,3 = oral cephalosporins—*see Table 10B*
Oflox = ofloxacin
P Ceph 1,2,3,4 = parenteral cephalosporins—*see Table 10B*
P Ceph 3 AP = parenteral cephalosporins with antipseudomonal activity—*see Table 10B*
Peflox = pefloxacin
PIP-TZ = piperacillin-tazobactam
PZA = pyrazinamide
Quinu-dalfo = Q-D = quinupristin-dalfopristin
RFB = rifabutin
RFP = rifapentine
RIF = rifampin
Roxi = roxithromycin
SM = streptomycin
Sulb = sulbactam
Tazo = tazobactam
TC-CL = ticarcillin-clavulanate
Teico = teicoplanin
Telithro = telithromycin
Tetra = tetracycline
Ticar = ticarcillin
TMP-SMX = trimethoprim-sulfamethoxazole
Tobra = tobramycin
Vanco = vancomycin

Antifungal Drugs
Ampho B = amphotericin B
ABCC = ampho B cholesteryl complex
ABLC = ampho B lipid complex
LAB = liposomal ampho B
Clot = clotrimazole
Flu = fluconazole
Flucyt = flucytosine
Griseo = griseofulvin
Itra = itraconazole
Keto = ketoconazole
Vori = voriconazole

Antiparasitic Drugs
AP = atovaquone proguanil
CQ = chloroquine phosphate
MQ = mefloquine
PQ = primaquine
Pyrt = pyrimethamine
QS = quinine sulfate

Antivirals; Anti-HIV Drugs
3TC = lamivudine
d4T = stavudine
ddC = zalcitabine
ddI = didanosine
FTC = emtricitabine
TDF = tenofovir
DLV = delavirdine
ADF = adefovir
ZDV = zidovudine
EFZ = efavirenz
NVP = nevirapine
ATV = atazanavir
FOS-APV = fos-amprenavir
IDV = indinavir
IFN = interferon
LP/R = lopinavir/ritonavir
NFR = nelfinavir
RTV = ritonavir
SQV = saquinavir
TPV = Tipranavir
ENT = entecavir

DRUG DOSAGE & DRUG ADMINISTRATION
mcg = microgram
mg = milligram
AD = after dialysis
div = divided
gm = gram
DS = double strength
bid = twice a day
tid = 3 times a day
qid = 4 times a day
BW = body weight
DOT = directly observed therapy
IP = intraperitoneal
IT = intrathecal
po = per os (by mouth)
subcut = subcutaneous
dc = discontinue
rx = treatment

DRUG-RELATED
G = generic
I = investigational
IA = injectable agent
NB = name brand
NFDA-I = not FDA-approved indication
NUS = not available in the U.S.
ASA = aspirin
NSAIDs = non-steroidal anti-inflammatory drugs

DISEASE-ASSOCIATED
ARDS = acute respiratory distress syndrome
ARF = acute rheumatic fever
CAPD = continuous ambulatory peritoneal dialysis
CAVH = continuous arteriovenous hemofiltration
CSD = cat-scratch disease
DIC = disseminated intravascular coagulation
ESRD = endstage renal disease
HEMO = hemodialysis
PEP = post-exposure prophylaxis
PTLD = post-transplant lymphoproliferative disease
RTI = respiratory tract infection
STD = sexually transmitted disease
TBc = tuberculosis
UTI = urinary tract infection

ORGANISMS
CMV = cytomegalovirus
DOT group = B. distasonis, B. ovatus, B. thetaiotaomicron
DRSP = drug-resistant S. pneumoniae
EBV = Epstein-Barr virus
GC = gonorrhea
HHV = human herpesvirus
HIV = human immunodeficiency virus
HSV = herpes simplex virus
LCM = lymphocytic choriomeningitis virus
MSSA/MRSA = methicillin-sensitive/resistant S. aureus
M. Tbc = Mycobacterium tuberculosis
Rick = Rickettsia
RSV = respiratory syncytial virus
VISA = vancomycin intermediately resistant S. aureus
VZV = varicella-zoster virus

MISCELLANEOUS

Diagnosis
C&S = culture & sensitivity
CXR = chest x-ray
ESBLs = extended spectrum β-lactamases
ESR = erythrocyte sedimentation rate
HLR = high-level resistance
LCR = ligase chain reaction
PCR = polymerase chain reaction
TEE = transesophageal echocardiography
VL = viral load

Organizations
ATS = American Thoracic Society
CDC = Centers for Disease Control
ICAAC = International Conference on Antimicrobial Agents & Chemotherapy
IDSA = Infectious Diseases Society of America
WHO = World Health Organization

Other
AUC = area under the curve
DBPCT = double-blind placebo-controlled trial
EDC = expected date of confinement
PRCT = Prospective randomized controlled trials
Pts = patients
R = resistant
S = potential synergy in combination with penicillin, AMP, vanco, teico
Sens = sensitive (susceptible)
VR = very rare

ABBREVIATIONS OF JOURNAL TITLES

AAC: Antimicrobial Agents & Chemotherapy
Adv PID: Advances in Pediatric Infectious Diseases
AIDS Res Hum Retrovir: AIDS Research & Human Retroviruses
AJM: American Journal of Medicine
AJRCCM: American Journal of Respiratory Critical Care Medicine
AJTMH: American Journal of Tropical Medicine & Hygiene
Aliment Pharmacol Ther: Alimentary Pharmacology & Therapeutics
Am J Hlth Pharm: American Journal of Health-System Pharmacy
AnEM: Annals of Emergency Medicine
AnIM: Annals of Internal Medicine
AnPharmacother: Annals of Pharmacotherapy
AnSurg: Annals of Surgery
Antivir Ther: Antiviral Therapy
ArDerm: Archives of Dermatology
ArIM: Archives of Internal Medicine
ARRD: American Review of Respiratory Disease
BMJ: British Medical Journal
Brit J Derm: British Journal of Dermatology
Can JID: Canadian Journal of Infectious Diseases
CCM: Critical Care Medicine
CCTID: Current Clinical Topics in Infectious Disease
CID: Clinical Infectious Diseases
Clin Micro Inf: Clinical Microbiology and Infection
Clin Micro Rev: Clinical Microbiology Reviews
COID: Current Opinion in Infectious Disease
Curr Med Res Opin: Current Medical Research and Opinion
Derm Ther: Dermatologic Therapy

Dig Dis Sci: Digestive Diseases and Sciences
DMID: Diagnostic Microbiology and Infectious Disease
EID: Emerging Infectious Diseases
EJCMID: European Journal of Clin. Micro. & Infectious Diseases
Eur J Neurol: European Journal of Neurology
Exp Mol Path: Experimental & Molecular Pathology
Gastro: Gastroenterology
Hpt: Hepatology
ICHE: Infection Control and Hospital Epidemiology
IDC No. Amer: Infectious Disease Clinics of North America
IDCP: Infectious Diseases in Clinical Practice
IJAA: International Journal of Antimicrobial Agents
Inf Med: Infections in Medicine
JAIDS: JAIDS Journal of Acquired Immune Deficiency Syndromes
JAIDS & HR: Journal of AIDS and Human Retrovirology
JAll Clin Immun: Journal of Allergy and Clinical Immunology
J Am Ger Soc: Journal of the American Geriatrics Society
J Chemother: Journal of Chemotherapy
JCI: Journal of Clinical Investigation
J Clin Micro: Journal of Clinical Microbiology
J Clin Virol: Journal of Clinical Virology
J Derm Treat: Journal of Dermatological Treatment
J Hpt: Journal of Hepatology
J Inf: Journal of Infection
J Med Micro: Journal of Medical Microbiology
J Micro Immunol Inf: Journal of Microbiology, Immunology, & Infection
J Ped: Journal of Pediatrics

JAC: Journal of Antimicrobial Chemotherapy
JAMA: Journal of the American Medical Association
JAVMA: Journal of the Veterinary Medicine Association
JID: Journal of Infectious Diseases
JNS: Journal of Neurosurgery
JTMH: Journal of Tropical Medicine and Hygiene
J Viral Hep: Journal of Viral Hepatitis
Ln: Lancet
LnID: Lancet Infectious Disease
Mayo Clin Proc: Mayo Clinic Proceedings
Med Lett: Medical Letter
Med Mycol: Medical Mycology
MMWR: Morbidity & Mortality Weekly Report
NEJM: New England Journal of Medicine
Neph Dial Transpl: Nephrology Dialysis Transplantation
Ped Ann: Pediatric Annals
Peds: Pediatrics
Pharmacother: Pharmacotherapy
PIDJ: Pediatric Infectious Disease Journal
QJM: Quarterly Journal of Medicine
Scand J Inf Dis: Scandinavian Journal of Infectious Diseases
Sem Resp Inf: Seminars in Respiratory Infections
SMJ: Southern Medical Journal
Surg Neurol: Surgical Neurology
Transpl: Transplantation
Transpl Inf Dis: Transplant Infectious Diseases
TRSM: Transactions of the Royal Society of Medicine
West J Med: Western Journal of Medicine

TABLE 1*
CLINICAL APPROACH TO INITIAL CHOICE OF ANTIMICROBIAL THERAPY (Abbreviations on page 2)
Treatment based on presumed site or type of infection. In selected instances, treatment and prophylaxis based on identification of pathogens

ANATOMIC SITE/DIAGNOSIS/ MODIFYING CIRCUMSTANCES	ETIOLOGIES (usual)	SUGGESTED REGIMENS*		ADJUNCT DIAGNOSTIC OR THERAPEUTIC MEASURES AND COMMENTS
		PRIMARY	ALTERNATIVE§	
ABDOMEN: See Peritoneum, pages 34–35, Gallbladder, page 13, and Pelvic Inflammatory Disease, page 19				
BONE: Osteomyelitis. Microbiologic diagnosis is essential. If blood culture negative, need culture of bone. Culture of sinus tract drainage not predictive of bone culture. Review: Ln 364:369, 2004				
Hematogenous Osteomyelitis				
Empiric therapy—Collect bone and blood cultures before empiric therapy				
Newborn (<4 mos.) See Table 16 for dose	S. aureus, Gm-neg. bacilli, Group B strep.	**MRSA possible:** **Vanco+ P Ceph 3**	**MRSA unlikely: (Nafcillin or oxacillin) + P Ceph 3**	Table 16 for dose. Severe allergy or toxicity: (**Linezolid**NFDA1 10 mg per kg IV/po q8h + **aztreonam**). Could substitute **clindamycin** for linezolid
Children (>4 mos.)—Adult: Osteo of extremity	S. aureus, Group A strep, Gm-neg. bacilli rare	**MRSA possible: Vanco**	**MRSA unlikely: Nafcillin or oxacillin**	Severe allergy or toxicity: **Clinda** or **TMP-SMX** or **linezolid**NFDA1. Dosages in Table 16. See Table 10 for adverse reactions to drugs.
		Add **P Ceph 3** if Gm-neg. bacilli on Gram stain. Doses: Table 16		
Adult (>21 yrs) **Vertebral osteo ± epidural abscess.** other sites	S. aureus most common but variety other organisms. **Blood & bone cultures essential.**	**MRSA possible: Vanco** 1 gm IV q12h	**MRSA unlikely: Nafcillin** or oxacillin 2 gm IV q4h	**Dx: MRI early to look for epidural abscess.** Allergy or toxicity: **TMP-SMX** 8–10 mg per kg per day div. IV q8h or **linezolid** 600 mg IV/po q12h (AnIM 138:135, 2003)NFDA1. See Table 10 for adverse drug reactions. Epidural abscess ref.: AnIM 164:2409, 2004.
Specific therapy—Culture and in vitro susceptibility results known				
	MSSA	Nafcillin or oxacillin 2 gm IV q4h or cefazolin 2 gm IV q8h	Vanco 1 gm q12h IV	Severe allergy or toxicity: **Clinda** 600–900 mg IV q8h or **TMP-SMX** 8–10 mg per kg per day div IV q8h. **If no response to clinda, check for "inducible" resistance** (CID 40:280, 2005). If susceptible in vitro, **CIP** 750 mg po bid or **Levo** 750 mg po q24h) + **RIF** 300 mg po bid. See Table 10 for adverse drug reactions.
	MRSA—See Table 6, page 57		Linezolid 600 mg q12h IV/po + RIF 300 mg po/IV bid	Severe allergy or toxicity: **Clinda** 600–900 mg IV q8h (check for inducible resistance (CID 40:280, 2005)); **TMP-SMX** 8–10 mg per kg per day div q8h IV. **Linezolid** rapidly penetrates & accumulates in bone (JAC 50:73 & 747, 2002).
Hemoglobinopathy: Sickle cell/thalassemia	Salmonella; other Gm-neg. bacilli	CIP 400 mg IV q12h	Levo 750 mg IV q24h	Thalassemia: transfusion and iron chelation risk factors.
Contiguous Osteomyelitis Without Vascular Insufficiency				
Empiric therapy: Get cultures!				
Foot bone osteo due to nail through tennis shoe	P. aeruginosa	CIP 750 mg po bid or Levo 750 mg po q24h	Ceftaz 2 gm IV q8h or CFP 2 gm IV q12h	See Skin—Nail puncture, page 41. Need debridement to remove foreign body.
Long bone, post-internal fixation of fracture	S. aureus, Gm-neg. bacilli, P. aeruginosa	Vanco 1 gm IV q12h + [ceftaz or CFP (see footnote¹)]. See Comment	Linezolid 600 mg IV/po bidNFDA1 + (ceftaz or CFP). See Comment	Often necessary to remove hardware to allow bone union. May need revascularization. Regimens listed are empiric. Adjust after culture data available. If susceptible Gm-neg. bacillus, **CIP** 750 mg po bid or **Levo** 750 mg po q24h.
Prosthetic joint	See Prosthetic joint, page 25			
Sternum, post-op	S. aureus, S. epidermidis	Vanco 1 gm IV q12h	Linezolid 600 mg po/IVNFDA1 bid	Sternal debridement for cultures & removal of necrotic bone.
Contiguous Osteomyelitis With Vascular Insufficiency. Ref.: CID S115–22, 2004				
Most pts are **diabetics** with peripheral neuropathy & infected skin ulcers (see Diabetic foot, page 12)	Polymicrobic (Gm+ cocci (to include MRSA), (aerobic & anaerobic) and Gm-neg. bacilli (aerobic & anaerobic)	Debride overlying ulcer & submit bone for histology & culture. Select antibiotic based on culture results & treat for 6 weeks. **No empiric therapy unless acutely ill**, see suggestions, Diabetic foot, page 12. Revascularize if possible. Full contact cast.		**Diagnosis of osteo:** Culture of biopsied bone gold standard. Marrow edema on MRI best imaging. Probe to bone has high predictive value. **Treatment:** (1) Revascularize if possible. (2) Culture bone. (3) Specific antimicrobial(s). (4) Full contact cast.

* **DOSAGES SUGGESTED** are for adults (unless otherwise indicated) with clinically severe (often life-threatening) infections. **Dosages also assume normal renal function, and not severe hepatic dysfunction.** § **ALTERNATIVE THERAPY INCLUDES these considerations:** allergy, pharmacology/pharmacokinetics, compliance, costs, local resistance profiles.

¹ Drug dosage: **IMP** 0.5 gm IV q6h; **MER** 1 gm IV q8h (not licensed indication but should be effective), **ERTA** 1 gm q24h, **TC-CL** 3.1 gm IV q6h, **PIP-TZ** 3.375 gm IV q6h or 4.5 gm q8h, **AM-SB** 3 gm IV q6h; **ceftazidime** 2 gm IV q8h, **CFP** 2 gm IV q12h, **metro** 1 gm loading dose and then 0.5 gm IV/po q6h or 1 gm IV q12h, **aztreonam** 2 gm IV q8h, **vanco** 1 gm IV q12h.

TABLE 1 (2)

ANATOMIC SITE/DIAGNOSIS/ MODIFYING CIRCUMSTANCES	ETIOLOGIES (usual)	SUGGESTED REGIMENS*		ADJUNCT DIAGNOSTIC OR THERAPEUTIC MEASURES AND COMMENTS
		PRIMARY	ALTERNATIVE§	
BONE *(continued)*				
Chronic Osteomyelitis: Specific therapy By definition, implies presence of dead bone. **Need valid cultures**	S. aureus, Enterobacteriaceae, P. aeruginosa	**Empiric rx not indicated.** Base systemic rx on results of culture, sensitivity testing. If acute exacerbation of chronic osteo, rx as acute hematogenous osteo.		Important adjuncts: removal of orthopedic hardware, surgical debridement, vascularized muscle flaps, distraction osteogenesis (Ilizarov) techniques. Antibiotic-impregnated cement & hyperbaric oxygen adjunctive. **NOTE: RIF + (vanco or β-lactam)** effective in animal model and in a clinical trial of S. aureus chronic osteo *(SMJ 79:947, 1986)*.
BREAST: Mastitis—Obtain culture; need to know if MRSA present. Review with definitions: *Ob & Gyn Clin No Amer 29:89, 2002*				
Postpartum mastitis Mastitis without abscess Ref.: *JAMA 289:1609, 2003*	S. aureus; less often S. pyogenes (Gp A or B), E. coli, bacteroides species, maybe Corynebacterium sp. & selected coagulase-neg. staphylococci (e.g., S. lugdunensis)	**NO MRSA: Outpatient: Dicloxacillin** 500 mg po qid or **cephalexin** 500 mg po qid.	**MRSA Possible: Outpatient: TMP-SMX-DS** po bid	If no abscess, increased frequency of nursing may hasten response; no risk to infant. Corynebacterium sp. assoc. with chronic granulomatous mastitis *(CID 35:1434, 2002)*. Bartonella henselae infection reported *(Ob & Gyn 95:1027, 2000)*.
Mastitis with abscess		**Inpatient: Nafcillin/oxacillin** 2 gm IV q4h	**Inpatient: Vanco** 1 gm IV q12h	With abscess, d/c nursing. (&D standard; needle aspiration reported successful *(Am J Surg 182:117, 2001)*. Resume breast feeding from affected breast as soon as pain allows.
Non-puerperal mastitis with abscess	S. aureus; less often Bacteroides sp., peptostreptococcus, & selected coagulase-neg. staphylococci			**If subareolar & odoriferous**, most likely anaerobes; need to **add metro** 500 mg IV/po tid. If not subareolar, staph. Need pretreatment aerobic/anaerobic cultures. Surgical drainage for abscess.
CENTRAL NERVOUS SYSTEM				
Brain abscess Primary or contiguous source Ref.: *CID 25:763, 1997*	Streptococci (60–70%), bacteroides (20–40%), Enterobacteriaceae (25–33%), S. aureus (10–15%). Rare: Nocardia *(Table 11A, page 82)*	**P Ceph 3 (cefotaxime** 2 gm IV q4h or **ceftriaxone** 2 gm IV q12h) + **metro** 7.5 mg per kg q6h or 15 mg per kg IV q12h	**Pen G** 3-4 million units IV q4h + **metro** 7.5 mg per kg q6h or 15 mg per kg IV q12h	If CT scan suggests cerebritis *(JNS 59:972, 1983)*, abscesses <2.5 cm and pt neurologically stable and conscious, start antibiotics and observe. Otherwise, surgical drainage necessary. Neurologic deterioration usually mandates surgery. Experience with Pen G (HD) + metro without P Ceph 3 or nafcillin/oxacillin has been good. We use P Ceph 3 because of frequency of isolation of Enterobacteriaceae.
		Duration of rx unclear; rx until response by neuroimaging (CT/MRI)		**S. aureus rare without positive blood culture; if S. aureus, include vanco until susceptibility known.** Strep. milleri group esp. prone to produce abscess.
Post-surgical, post-traumatic	S. aureus, Enterobacteriaceae	**(Nafcillin** or **oxacillin)** 2 gm IV q4h + **P Ceph 3**	**Vanco** 1 gm IV q12h + **P Ceph 3**	**If MRSA a consideration, substitute vanco for nafcillin or oxacillin.** P Ceph 3 dose as for brain abscess, primary.
HIV-1 infected (AIDS)	Toxoplasma gondii	See Table 13, page 99		
Subdural empyema: In adult 60–90% are extension of sinusitis or otitis media. Rx same as primary brain abscess. Surgical emergency: must drain *(CID 20:372, 1995)*.				
Encephalitis/encephalopathy Ref.: *Ln 359:507, 2002 (See Table 14, page 109, and for rabies, page 20C, page 144)*	Herpes simplex, arboviruses, rabies, West Nile virus. Rarely: listeria, cat-scratch disease	Start IV **acyclovir** while awaiting results of CSF PCR for H. simplex.		Newly recognized strain of bat rabies. May not require a break in the skin. Eastern equine encephalitis causes focal MRI changes in basal ganglia and thalamus *(NEJM 336:1867, 1997)*. Cat-scratch ref.: *PIDJ 14:866, 1995)*. Ref. on West Nile & related viruses *NEJM 351:370, 2004*
Meningitis, "Aseptic": Pleocytosis of 100s of cells, CSF glucose normal, neg. culture for bacteria *(see Table 14, page 106)*	Enteroviruses, HSV-2, LCM, HIV, other viruses, drugs (NSAIDs, metronidazole, carbamazepine, TMP-SMX, IVIG), rarely leptospirosis	For all but leptospirosis, IV fluids and analgesics. D/C drugs that may be etiologic. For lepto **(doxy** 100 mg IV/po q12h) or **(Pen G** 5 million units IV q6h) or **(AMP** 0.5–1 gm IV q6h). Repeat LP if suspect partially-treated bacterial meningitis.		If available, PCR of CSF for enterovirus. HSV-2 unusual without concomitant genital herpes. Drug-induced aseptic meningitis: *ArIM 159:1185, 1999.* For lepto, positive epidemiologic history and concomitant hepatitis, conjunctivitis, dermatitis, nephritis.

NOTE: All dosage recommendations are for adults (unless otherwise indicated) and assume normal renal function.

6

TABLE 1 (3)

ANATOMIC SITE/DIAGNOSIS/ MODIFYING CIRCUMSTANCES	ETIOLOGIES (usual)	SUGGESTED REGIMENS*		ADJUNCT DIAGNOSTIC OR THERAPEUTIC MEASURES AND COMMENTS
		PRIMARY	ALTERNATIVE§	
CENTRAL NERVOUS SYSTEM (continued)				
Meningitis, Bacterial, Acute: Goal is empiric therapy, then CSF exam within 30 min. If focal neurologic deficit, give empiric rx, then do head CT, then do LP. (CID 39:1267, 2004) NOTE: In children, treatment caused CSF cultures to turn neg. in 2 hrs with meningococci & partial response with pneumococci in 4 hrs (Peds 108:1169, 2001)				
Empiric Therapy—CSF Gram stain is negative—immunocompetent				
Age: Preterm to <1 month Ln 361:2139, 2003	Group B strep 49%, E. coli 18%, listeria 7%; misc. Gm-neg. 10%, misc. Gm-pos. 10%	**AMP + cefotaxime** Intraventricular rx not recommended. Repeat CSF exam/culture 24–36 hrs after start of rx For dosage, see Table 16	**AMP + gentamicin**	Primary & alternative regimens active vs Group B strep, most coliforms, & listeria. If premature infant with long nursery stay, S. aureus, enterococci, and resistant coliforms potential pathogens. Optional empiric regimens: [nafcillin + (ceftazidime or cefotaxime)]. If high risk of MRSA, use vanco + cefotaxime. Alter regimen after culture/sensitivity data available.
Age: 1 mo.– 50 yrs See footnote[1] for empiric treatment rationale.	S. pneumo, meningococci, H. influenzae now very rare, **listeria unlikely if young & immunocompetent** (add ampicillin if suspect listeria. 2 gm IV q4h)	Adult dosage: [(**Cefotax-ime** 2 gm IV q4-6h OR **ceftriaxone** 2 gm IV q12h)] + (**dexametha-sone**) + **vanco** (see footnote[3]). Peds: see footnote[3] **Dexamethasone:** 0.15 mg per kg IV q6h times 2–4 days. **Give with or just before 1st dose of antibiotic to block TNF production** (see Comment). See footnote[3] for rest of ped. dosage	[(**MER** 2 gm IV q8h) (Peds: 40 mg per kg IV q8h)] + IV **dexamethasone** + **vanco** (see footnote[3]) Peds: see footnote[3]	**For pts with severe pen. allergy: Chloro** 12.5 mg per kg IV q6h (max. 4 gm per day) (for meningococcus) + **TMP-SMX** 5 mg per kg q6-8h (for listeria if immunocompromised) + **vanco.** Rare meningococcal isolates chloro-resistant (NEJM 339:868, 1998). The standard alternative for pts with severe pen. allergy was chloro. However, high failure rate in pts with DRSP (Ln 339: 405, 1992; Ln 342:240, 1993). **So far, no vanco-resistant S. pneumo.** **Value of dexamethasone** documented in children with H. influenzae & now confirmed in adults with S. pneumo & N. meningitidis (NEJM 347:1549 & 1613, 2002; LnID 4:139, 2004). **Give 1st dose 15–20 min. prior to or concomittant with 1st dose of antibiotic. Dose: 0.15 mg per kg IV q6h times 2–4 days.** **For meningococcal immunization, see Table 20, page 142.**
Age: >50 yrs or alcohol-ism or other debilitating associated diseases or impaired cellular immunity	S. pneumo, listeria, Gm-neg. bacilli. Note absence of meningo-coccus	[**AMP** 2 gm IV q4h) + (**ceftriaxone** 2 gm IV q12h or **cefotaxime** 2 gm IV q8h)] + **vanco** + IV **dexamethasone** For vanco dose, see footnote[3]. Dexamethasone: 0.15 mg per kg IV q6h times 2–4 days; 1st dose before or concomitant with 1st dose of antibiotic.	**MER** 2 gm IV q8h + **vanco** + IV **dexamethasone** **For severe pen. Allergy, see Comment**	**Severe penicillin allergy: Vanco** 500–750 mg per kg q6-8h + **TMP-SMX** 5 mg per kg q6-8h pending culture results. Chloro has failed vs DRSP (Ln 342:240, 1993).
Post-neurosurgery, post-head trauma, or post-cochlear implant (NEJM 349:435, 2003)	S. pneumoniae most common, esp. if CSF leak. Other: S. aureus, coliforms, P. aeruginosa	**Vanco** (until known not MRSA) 500–750 mg IV q6h[2] + (**cefepime** or **cef-tazidime** 2 gm IV q8h)(see Comment)	**MER** 2 gm IV q8h + 1 gm IV q6-12h	**Vanco** alone not optimal for S. pneumo. If/when suscept. S. pneumo identified, quickly switch to **ceftriaxone** or **cefotaxime.** If coliform or pseudomonas meningitis, some add intrathecal gentamicin (4 mg q12h into lateral ventricles). Cure of acinetobacter meningitis with intrathecal colistin (JAC 53:290, 2004).
Ventriculitis/meningitis due to infected ventriculo-peritoneal (atrial) shunt	S. epidermidis, S. aureus, coliforms, diphtheroids (rare), P. acnes	**Vanco** 500–750 mg IV q6h + (**cefepime** or **cef-tazidime** 2 gm IV q8h). If unable to remove shunt, consider intraventricular therapy; for dosages, see footnote[4]	**Vanco** 500–750 mg IV q6h + **MER** 2 gm IV q8h	Usual care: 1st, remove infected shunt & culture; external ventricular catheter for drainage/pressure control; antimicrobic times10–14 days. For timing of new shunt, see CID 39:1267, 2004.

[1] **Rationale**: Hard to get adequate CSF concentrations of anti-infectives, hence MIC criteria for in vitro susceptibility are lower for CSF isolates (AnM 161:2538, 2001).
[2] Low and erratic penetration of **vanco** into the CSF (PIDJ 16:895, 1997). Recommended **dosage in children** is 15 mg per kg IV q6h (double the standard adult dose). **In adults,** a maximum dose of 2–3 gm/day is suggested: **500–750 mg IV q6h.**
[3] **Dosage of drugs used to rx children ≥1 mo. of age:** Cefotaxime 200 mg per kg per day IV div. q6-8h; ceftriaxone 100 mg per kg per day IV div. q12h; vanco 15 mg per kg IV q6h.
[4] Dosages for intraventricular therapy. The following are daily adult doses in mg: amikacin 30, gentamicin 4–8, polymyxin E (Colistin) 10, tobramycin 5–20, vanco 10–20. Ref.: CID 39:1267, 2004.
 NOTE: All dosage recommendations are for adults (unless otherwise indicated) and assume normal/renal function.
 Abbreviations on page 2.

TABLE 1 (4)

ANATOMIC SITE/DIAGNOSIS/ MODIFYING CIRCUMSTANCES	ETIOLOGIES (usual)	SUGGESTED REGIMENS*		ADJUNCT DIAGNOSTIC OR THERAPEUTIC MEASURES AND COMMENTS
		PRIMARY	ALTERNATIVE§	
CENTRAL NERVOUS SYSTEM *(continued)*				
Meningitis, Bacterial, Acute *(continued) (CID 39:1267, 2004)*				
Empiric Therapy—Positive CSF Gram stain				
Gram-positive diplococci	S. pneumoniae	Either **(ceftriaxone** 2 gm IV q12h or **cefotaxime** 2 gm IV q4–6h) + **vanco** 500–750 mg IV q6h + timed **dexamethasone** 0.15 mg per kg q6h IV times 2–4 days.		Alternatives: **MER** 2 gm IV q8h or **Moxi** 400 mg IV q24h or **Gati** 400 mg IV q24h. All + **dexamethasone.**
Gram-negative diplococci	N. meningitidis	**(Cefotaxime** 2 gm IV q4–6h or **ceftriaxone** 2 gm IV q12h) + timed **dexamethasone** *(dose above)*		Alternatives: **Pen G** 4 mill. units IV q4h or **AMP** 2 gm IV q4h or **Gati/Moxi** 400 mg IV q24h or **chloro** 1 gm IV q6h
Gram-positive bacilli or coccobacilli	Listeria monocytogenes	**AMP** 2 gm IV q4h ± **gentamicin** 2 mg per kg loading dose then 1.7 mg per kg q8h		If pen-allergic, use TMP-SMX 5 mg per kg q6-8h or **MER 2 gm IV q8h**
Gram-negative bacilli	H. influenzae, coliforms, P. aeruginosa	**(Ceftazidime** or **cefepime** 2 gm IV q8h) + **gentamicin** 2 mg per kg 1st dose then 1.7 mg per kg q8h		Alternatives: **CIP** 400 mg IV q8-12h; **MER** 2 gm IV q8h
Specific Therapy—Positive culture of CSF with in vitro susceptibility results available. Interest in monitoring/reducing intracranial pressure: *CID 38:384, 2004*				
H. influenzae	β-lactamase +	**Ceftriaxone** (peds): 50 mg per kg IV q12h		Pen. allergic: **Chloro** 12.5 mg per kg IV q6h (max. 4 gm per day.)
Listeria monocytogenes		**AMP** 2 gm IV q4h ± **gentamicin** 2 mg per kg loading dose, then 1.7 mg per kg q8h		Pen. allergic: **TMP-SMX** 20 mg per kg per day div. q6–12h. One report of greater efficacy of AMP + TMP-SMX as compared to AMP + gentamicin *(JID 33:79, 1996)*. Alternative: **MER** 2 gm IV q8h. Success reported with **linezolid** + **RIF** *(CID 40:908, 2005).*
N. meningitidis	MIC 0.1–1 mcg per mL	**Ceftriaxone** 2 gm IV q12h times 7 days *(see Comment)*; if pen. allergic, **chloro** 12.5 mg per kg (up to 1 gm) IV q6h		Rare isolates chloro-resistant *(NEJM 339:368 & 917, 1998)*. Alternatives: **MER** 2 gm IV q8h or **Gati/Moxi** 400 mg q24h.
S. pneumoniae	Pen G MIC	**Pen G** 4 million units IV q4h or **AMP** 2 gm IV q4h		
NOTES:	< 0.1 mcg per mL			Alternatives: **Ceftriaxone** 2 gm IV q12h, **chloro** 1 gm IV q6h
1. Assumes dexamethasone just prior to 1st dose & x4 days.	0.1–1 mcg per mL	**Ceftriaxone** 2 gm IV q12h or **cefotaxime** 2 gm IV q4–6h		Alternatives: **Cefepime** 2 gm IV q8h or **MER** 2 gm IV q8h
2. If MIC ≥1, repeat CSF exam after 24–48h.	≥2 mcg per mL	**Vanco** 500–750 mg IV q6h + (**ceftriaxone** or **cefotaxime** as above)		Alternatives: **Gati** or **Moxi** 400 mg IV q24h
3. Treat for 10–14 days	Ceftriaxone MIC ≥1 mcg per mL	**Vanco** 500–750 mg IV q6h + (**ceftriaxone** or **cefotaxime** as above)		Alternatives: **Gati** or **Moxi** 400 mg IV q24h If MIC to ceftriaxone >2 mcg per mL, add **RIF** 600 mg once daily.
E. coli, other coliforms, or P. aeruginosa	Consultation advised—need susceptibility results	**(Ceftazidime** or **cefepime** 2 gm IV q8h) ± **gentamicin**		Alternatives: **CIP** 400 mg IV q8–12h; **MER** 2 gm IV q8h. For discussion of intraventricular therapy: *CID 39:1267, 2004*
Prophylaxis for H. influenzae and N. meningitidis				
Haemophilus influenzae type b *(Neisseria next page)* Household and/or day care contact: residing with index case or ≥4 hrs. Day care contact: same day care as index case for 5–7 days before onset		**RIF** 20 mg per kg po (not to exceed 600 mg) q24h times 4 doses. **Adults: RIF** 600 mg q24h times 4 days		**Household:** If there is one unvaccinated contact ≤4 yrs in the household, RIF recommended for all household contacts except pregnant women. **Child Care Facilities:** With 1 case, if attended by unvaccinated children ≤2 yrs, consider prophylaxis + vaccinate susceptibles. If all contacts >2 yrs: no prophylaxis. If ≥2 cases in 60 days & unvaccinated children attend, prophylaxis recommended for children & personnel *(Am Acad Ped Red Book 2003, page 297).*

Abbreviations on page 2.   NOTE: All dosage recommendations are for adults (unless otherwise indicated) and assume normal renal function.

TABLE 1 (5)

ANATOMIC SITE/DIAGNOSIS/ MODIFYING CIRCUMSTANCES	ETIOLOGIES (usual)	SUGGESTED REGIMENS*		ADJUNCT DIAGNOSTIC OR THERAPEUTIC MEASURES AND COMMENTS
		PRIMARY	ALTERNATIVE§	
CENTRAL NERVOUS SYSTEM/Meningitis, Bacterial/Prophylaxis (continued)				
Neisseria meningitidis exposure (close contact) [MMWR 46(RR-5):1, 1997] CDC recommends informing college freshmen living in dormitories & residence halls of available vaccine [MMWR 46(RR-7):1, 2000 & 50/23:487, 2001]		**RIF** 600 mg po q12h times 4 doses. (Children >1 mo. age 10 mg per kg po q12h times 4 doses, <1 mo. age 5 mg per kg q12h times 4 doses)] or **CIP** (adults) 500 mg po single dose] or [**Ceftriaxone** 250 mg IM times 1 dose (child <15 yrs 125 mg IM times 1)]	**Spiramycin** 500 mg po q6h times 5 days. Children 10 mg per kg po q6h times 5 days.	N. meningitidis spread by respiratory droplets, not aerosols, hence close contact required. ↑ risk if close contact for at least 4 hrs during week before illness onset (e.g., housemates, day care contacts, cellmates) or exposure to pt's naso-pharyngeal secretions (e.g., via kissing, mouth-to-mouth resuscitation, intubation, nasotracheal suctioning). RIF-resistant N. meningitidis documented but rare (EID 11:977, 2005). Primary prophylactic regimen in many European countries.
Meningitis, chronic Defined as symptoms + CSF pleocytosis for ≥4 wks	M. tbc 40%, cryptococcosis 7%, neoplastic 8%, Lyme, syphilis, Whipple's disease	Treatment depends on etiology. No urgent need for empiric therapy.		Long list of possibilities: bacteria, parasites, fungi, viruses, neoplasms, vasculitis, and other miscellaneous etiologies—see chapter on chronic meningitis in latest edition of Harrison's Textbook of Internal Medicine. Whipple's: JID 188:797 & 801, 2003.
Meningitis, eosinophilic AJM 114:217, 2003 (See Table 13A, page 100)	Angiostrongyliasis, gnatho-stomiasis, rarely others	Corticosteroids	Not sure antihelminthic rx works	1/3 lack peripheral eosinophilia. Need serology to confirm dx. Steroid ref.: CID 31:660, 2001. Recent outbreak: NEJM 346:668, 2002.
Meningitis, HIV-1 infected (AIDS) See Table 11, SANFORD GUIDE TO HIV/AIDS THERAPY	As in adults, >50 yrs: also consider cryptococci, M. tuberculosis, syphilis, HIV aseptic meningitis, Listeria monocytogenes	If etiology not identified: rx as adult >50 yrs + obtain CSF/serum cryp-tococcal antigen (see Comments)	For crypto rx, see Table 11A, pages 79–80	C. neoformans most common etiology in AIDS pt. H. influenzae, pneumococci, Tbc, syphilis, viral, histoplasma & coccidioides also need to be considered. Obtain blood cultures. L. monocytogenes risk >60x ↑, ¾ present as meningitis (CID 17:224, 1993).
EAR				
External otitis "Swimmer's ear" PIDJ 22:299, 2003	Pseudomonas sp., Entero-bacteriaceae, Proteus sp. (Fungi rare.) Acute infection usually 2° S. aureus	Eardrops: **Oflox 0.3% soln bid** or [(**polymyxin B + neomycin + hydrocortisone**) qid] or (**CIP + hydrocortisone bid**) For acute disease: **dicloxacillin** 500 mg po 4 times per day.		Rx should include gentle cleaning. Recurrences prevented (or decreased) by drying with alcohol drops, 2/3 rubbing alcohol) after swimming, then antibiotic drops or 2% acetic acid solution. Ointments should not be used in ear. Do not use neomycin if tympanic membrane punctured.
Chronic	Usually 2° to seborrhea	Eardrops: [(**polymyxin B + neomycin + hydrocorti-sone** qid) + **selenium sulfide**]		Control seborrhea with dandruff shampoo containing selenium sulfide (Selsun) or [(ketoconazole shampoo) + (medium potency steroid solution, triamcinolone 0.1%)].
"Malignant otitis externa" Risk groups: Diabetes mellitus, AIDS, chemotherapy	Pseudomonas aeruginosa in >90%	(**IMP** 0.5 gm IV q6h) or (**MER** 1 gm IV q8h) or [**CIP** 400 mg IV q12h or 750 mg po q12h)] or (**ceftaz** 2 gm IV q8h) or (**CFP** 2 gm q12h) or (**PIP** 4–6 gm IV q4–6h + **tobra**) or (**TC** 3 gm IV q4h + **tobra**)		CIP po especially useful for outpatient rx with early disease. Surgical debridement usually required, but not radical excision. R/O osteomyelitis. CT or MRI scan more sensitive than X-ray. If bone involved, rx for 4–6 wks. Ref.: LnID 4:34, 2004

Abbreviations on page 2. NOTE: All dosage recommendations are for adults (unless otherwise indicated) and assume normal renal function.

TABLE 1 (6)

ANATOMIC SITE/DIAGNOSIS/ MODIFYING CIRCUMSTANCES	ETIOLOGIES (usual)	SUGGESTED REGIMENS*		ADJUNCT DIAGNOSTIC OR THERAPEUTIC MEASURES AND COMMENTS
		PRIMARY	ALTERNATIVE§	
EAR (continued)				
Otitis media—infants, children, adults				
Acute (NEJM 347:1169, 2002; Peds 113:1451, 2004). For correlation of bacterial eradication from middle ear & clinical outcome, see LnID 2:593, 2002.				
Initial empiric therapy of acute otitis media (AOM) NOTE: Pending new data, **rx children <2 yrs old**. If >2 yrs old, afebrile, no ear pain, neg./questionable exam—consider analgesic treatment without anti-microbials	Overall detection in middle ear fluid: No pathogen 25% Virus 5–48% Bact. + virus 15% Bacteria only 55% Role of viruses: Clin Micro Rev 16:230, 2003 Pathogens from middle ear, 2000–2003: S. pneumo 31%, H. influenzae 56%, M. catarrhalis 11% (PIDJ 23:829, 2004)	**If NO antibiotics in prior month:** Amox po HD[1]	**Received antibiotics in prior month:** Amox HD[1] or **AM-CL** HD[1] or cefdinir or cefpodoxime or cefprozil or cefuroxime axetil For dosage, see footnotes[1] and[2] **All doses are pediatric** **Duration of rx:** <2 yrs old times10 days; ≥2 yrs old times 5–7 days. Appropriate duration unclear. 5 days may be inadequate for severe disease (NEJM 347:1169, 2002) For adult dosages, see Sinusitis, pages 36–37, and Table 10	**If allergic to β-lactam drugs?** If history unclear or rash, effective oral ceph OK; avoid ceph if IgE-mediated allergy, e.g., anaphylaxis. High failure rate with **TMP-SMX** if etiology is DRSP or H. influenzae (PIDJ 20:260, 2001); **azithro times 5 days or clarithro times 10 days** (both have ↓ activity vs DRSP). **Up to 50% S. pneumo resistant to macrolides**. AM-CL superior to azithro in recent controlled trial (ICAAC Abst. 2324, 2003). Rationale & data for single dose azithro, 30 mg per kg: PIDJ 23:S102 & S108, 2004. **Spontaneous resolution:** 90% pts infected with M. catarrhalis, 50% with H. influenzae, and 10% with S. pneumoniae; overall 80% resolve within 2–14 days (Ln 363:465, 2004). Risk of DRSP ↑ if age <2 yrs, antibiotics last 3 mos., and/or daycare attendance. Selection of drug based on (1) effectiveness against β-lactamase producing H. influenzae & M. catarrhalis and (2) effectiveness against S. pneumo, including DRSP. **Cefaclor, loracarbef, & ceftibuten less active vs DRSP** than other agents listed. Variable acceptance of drug taste/smell by children 4–8 y.o. [PIDJ 19 (Suppl.2):S174, 2000].
Treatment for clinical failure after 3 days rx	Drug-resistant S. pneumoniae main concern	**NO antibiotics in month prior to last 3 days:** **AM-CL** HD[1] or cefdinir or cefpodoxime or cefprozil or cefuroxime axetil or IM ceftriaxone times 3 days.	**Antibiotics in month prior to last 3 days:** (IM ceftriaxone) or (clindamycin) and/or (tympanocentesis) See clindamycin Comments For dosage, see footnotes[1] and[2] **All doses are pediatric** Duration of rx as above	**Clindamycin** not active vs H. influenzae or M. catarrhalis. S. pneumo resistant to macrolides are usually also resistant to clinda. Definition of failure: no change in ear pain, fever, bulging TM or otorrhea after 3 days of rx. Tympanocentesis will allow culture. **Newer FQs active vs DRSP, but not approved for use in children** (PIDJ 23:390, 2004), **Vanco is active vs DRSP.** Ceftriaxone for 1-day treatment vs DRSP (PIDJ 19:1040, 2000). AM-CL HD reported successful for pen-resistant S. pneumo AOM (PIDJ 20:829, 2001).
After >48 hrs of nasotracheal intubation.	Pseudomonas sp., klebsiella, enterobacter	**Ceftazidime** or **CFP** or **IMP** or **MER** or **TC-CL** or **CIP** (For therapy, see Ear, malignant otitis externa, page 8)		With nasotracheal intubation >48 hrs, about ½ pts will have otitis media with effusion.
Prophylaxis: acute otitis media PIDJ 22:10, 2003	Pneumococci, H. influenzae, M. catarrhalis, Staph. aureus, Group A strep (see **Comments**)	Sulfisoxazole 50 mg per kg po at bedtime or **amoxicillin** 20 mg per kg po q24h	**Use of antibiotics to prevent otitis media is a major contributor to emergence of antibiotic-resistant S. pneumo** Pneumococcal protein conjugate vaccine decreases freq. AOM in general & due to vaccine serotypes Adenoidectomy at time of tympanostomy tubes ↓ need for future hospitalization for AOM (NEJM 344:1188, 2001).

---

[1] **Amoxicillin UD or HD = amoxicillin usual dose or high dose; AM-CL HD** = amoxicillin-clavulanate high dose.

[2] **Drugs and peds dosage (all po unless specified) for acute otitis media: Amoxicillin UD** = 40 mg per kg per day div q12h or q8h. **Amoxicillin HD** = 90 mg per kg per day div q12h or q8h. **AM-CL HD** = 90 mg per kg per day of amox component (Augmentin ES-600) available with 600 mg AM & 42.9 mg CL per 5 mL—dose 90/6.4 mg per kg per day bid. **Cefuroxime axetil** 30 mg per kg per day div q12h. **Ceftriaxone** 50 mg per kg IM times 3 days. **Clindamycin** 20–30 mg per kg per day div qid (may be effective vs DRSP but no activity vs H. influenzae)

Other drugs suitable for drug (e.g., penicillin)-sensitive S. pneumo: TMP-SMX 4 mg per kg of TMP q12h. **Erythro-sulfisoxazole** 50 mg per kg per day of erythro div q6–8h. **Clarithro** 15 mg per kg per day div q12h; **azithro** 10 mg per kg per day times 1 and then 5 mg per kg q24h on days 2–5. Other FDA-approved regimens: 10 mg per kg q24h times 3 days & 30 mg per kg times 1. **Cefprozil** 15 mg per kg q12h; **cefpodoxime proxetil** 10 mg per kg per day as single dose; **cefaclor** 40 mg per kg per day div q8h; **loracarbef** 15 mg per kg q12h. **Cefdinir** 7 mg per kg q12h or 14 mg per kg q24h.

Abbreviations on page 2. NOTE: All dosage recommendations are for adults (unless otherwise indicated) and assume normal renal function.

TABLE 1 (7)

ANATOMIC SITE/DIAGNOSIS/ MODIFYING CIRCUMSTANCES	ETIOLOGIES (usual)	SUGGESTED REGIMENS* PRIMARY	ALTERNATIVE§	ADJUNCT DIAGNOSTIC OR THERAPEUTIC MEASURES AND COMMENTS
EAR (continued) **Mastoiditis**				
Acute				
Outpatient	Strep. pneumoniae 22%, S. pyogenes 16%, Staph. aureus 7%, H. influenzae 4%, P. aeruginosa 4%; others <1%	Empirically, same as Acute otitis media, above: need **vanco** or **nafcillin/oxacillin** if culture + for S. aureus.		Has become a rare entity, presumably as result of the aggressive rx of acute otitis media.
Hospitalized		**Cefotaxime** 1–2 gm IV q4–8h (depends on severity) or (**cef-triaxone** 2 gm IV q24h < age 60; 1 gm IV q24h > age 60).		Small ↑ in incidence in Netherlands where use of antibiotics limited to children with complicated course or high risk (PIDJ 20:140, 2001).
Chronic	Often polymicrobic: anaerobes, S. aureus, Enterobacteriaceae, P. aeruginosa	Treatment for acute exacerbations or perioperatively. Ideally, no treatment until surgical cultures obtained. Examples of empiric regimens: **IMP** 0.5 gm IV q6h, **TC-CL** 3.1 gm IV q6h, **PIP-TZ** 3.375 gm IV q4–6h or 4.5 gm q8h.		May or may not be associated with chronic otitis media with drainage via ruptured tympanic membrane. Antimicrobials given in association with surgery. Mastoidectomy indications: chronic drainage and evidence of osteomyelitis by MRI or CT, evidence of spread to CNS (epidural abscess, suppurative phlebitis, brain abscess).
EYE—General Reviews: CID 21:479, 1995; IDCP 7:447, 1998				
Eyelid				
Blepharitis	Etiol. unclear. Factors include Staph. aureus & Staph. epidermidis, seborrhea, rosacea, & dry eye	Lid margin care with baby shampoo & warm compresses q24h. Artificial tears if assoc. dry eye (see Comment).		Usually topical ointments of no benefit. If associated rosacea, add doxy 100 mg po bid times2 wks and then q24h.
Hordeolum (Stye)				
External (gland of Zeis)	Staph. aureus	Hot packs only. Will drain spontaneously.		Infection of superficial sebaceous gland.
Internal (Meibomian glands)	Staph. aureus	Oral **nafcillin/oxacillin** + hot packs		Also called acute meibomianitis. Rarely drain spontaneously.
Conjunctiva: NEJM 343:345, 2000				
Conjunctivitis of the newborn (**ophthalmia neonatorum**): by day of onset post-delivery—all doses pediatric				
Onset 1st day	Chemical (due to AgNO₃ prophylaxis)	None		Usual prophylaxis is erythro ointment; hence, AgNO₃ irritation rare.
Onset 2–4 days	N. gonorrhoeae	**Ceftriaxone** 25–50 mg per kg IV times 1 dose (not to exceed 125 mg		Treat mother and her sexual partners. Hyperpurulent. Topical rx inadequate. **Treat neonate for concomitant Chlamydia trachomatis.**
Onset 3–10 days	Chlamydia trachomatis	**Erythro syrup** 12.5 mg per kg q6h times 14 days). No topical rx needed.		Diagnosis by antigen detection. Azithro susp 20 mg per kg po q24h times 3 days reported efficacious (PIDJ 17:1049, 1998). Treat mother & sexual partner.
Onset 2–16 days	Herpes simplex types 1, 2	See keratitis, next page		Consider IV acyclovir if concomitant systemic disease.
Ophthalmia neonatorum prophylaxis: **Silver nitrate** 1% times 1 or **erythro** 0.5% ointment times 1 or **tetra** 1% ointment times 1 application				
Pink eye (viral conjunctivitis) Usually unilateral	Adenovirus (types 3 & 7 in children, 8, 11 & 19 in adults)	No treatment. If symptomatic, cold artificial tears may help.		Highly contagious. Onset of ocular pain and photophobia in an adult suggests associated keratitis—rare.
Inclusion conjunctivitis (**adult**) Usually unilateral	Chlamydia trachomatis	**Doxy** 100 mg bid po times 1–3 weeks	**Erythro** 250 mg po qid times 1–3 weeks	Oculogenital disease. Diagnosis by culture or antigen detection or PCR—availability varies by region and institution. Treat sexual partner.
Trachoma	Chlamydia trachomatis	**Azithro** 20 mg per kg po single dose—78% effective in children	**Doxy** 100 mg po bid times14 days or **tetra-cline** 250 mg po qid times 14 days.	Starts in childhood and can persist for years with subsequent damage to cornea. Topical therapy of marginal benefit. Avoid doxy/tetracycline in young children. Mass treatment works (JAMA 292:721, 2004).
Suppurative conjunctivitis				
Non-gonococcal; non-chlamydial Med Lett 46:25, 2004	Staph. aureus, S. pneumoniae, H. influenzae, et al. Outbreak due to atypical S. pneumo. NEJM 348:1112, 2003	Ophthalmic solution: Gati 0.3%, Levo 0.5%, or Moxi 0.5%. All 1–2 gtts q2h while awake 1st 2 days, then q4–8h up to 7 days.	Polymyxin B + trimethoprim solution 1–2 gtts q3–6h times 7–10 days.	FQs best spectrum for empiric therapy but expensive: $40–50 for 5 mL. High concentrations ↑likelihood of activity vs S. aureus—even MRSA. TMP spectrum only includes MRSA. Polymyxin B spectrum only Gm–neg. bacilli but no ophthal. prep of only TMP. Most S. pneumo resistant to gent & tobra.
Gonococcal (peds/adults)	N. gonorrhoeae	**Ceftriaxone** 125 mg IM/IV as one dose in children; 1 gm IM/IV as one dose in adults		

Abbreviations on page 2   NOTE: All dosage recommendations are for adults (unless otherwise indicated) and assume normal renal function

TABLE 1 (8)

ANATOMIC SITE/DIAGNOSIS/ MODIFYING CIRCUMSTANCES	ETIOLOGIES (usual)	SUGGESTED REGIMENS* PRIMARY	SUGGESTED REGIMENS* ALTERNATIVE§	ADJUNCT DIAGNOSTIC OR THERAPEUTIC MEASURES AND COMMENTS
EYE (continued) **Cornea (keratitis):**	**Usually serious and often sight-threatening. Prompt ophthalmologic consultation essential! Herpes simplex most common etiology in developed countries; bacterial and fungal infections more common in underdeveloped countries.**			
Viral H. simplex	H. simplex, types 1 & 2	Trifluridine, one drop q1h, 9 times per day for up to 21 days.	Vidarabine ointment— useful in children. Use 5 times per day for up to 21 days. If child fails vidarabine, try trifluridine.	Fluorescein staining shows topical dendritic figures. 30–50% rate of recurrence within 2 years. 400 mg acyclovir po bid ↓ recurrences, p 0.005 (NEJM 339:300, 1998).
Varicella-zoster ophthalmicus	Varicella-zoster virus	Famciclovir 500 mg po tid or valacyclovir 1 gm po tid times 10 days	Acyclovir 800 mg po 5 times per day times 10 days	Clinical diagnosis most common: dendritic figures with fluorescein staining in patient with varicella-zoster of ophthalmic branch of trigeminal nerve.
Bacterial		**All rx listed for bacterial, fungal, & protozoan is topical**		
Contact lens users	P. aeruginosa	Tobra or gentamicin (14 mg per mL) + piperacillin or ticarcillin eye drops (6–12 mg per mL) q15–60 min. around clock times 24–72 hrs, then slow reduction	CIP 0.3% or Levo 0.5% drops q15–60 min. around clock times 24–72 hrs	Pain, photophobia, impaired vision. Recommend alginate swab for culture and sensitivity testing.
Dry cornea, diabetes, immunosuppression	Staph. aureus, S. epidermidis, S. pneumoniae, S. pyogenes, Enterobacteriaceae, listeria	Cefazolin (50 mg per mL) + gentamicin or tobra (14 mg per mL) q15–60 min. around clock times 24–72 hrs, then slow reduction	Vanco (50 mg/mL) + ceftazidime (50 mg/mL) q15–60 min. around clock times 24–72 hrs, then slow reduction. See Comment.	Specific therapy guided by results of alginate swab culture + sensitivity. CIP 0.3% found clinically equivalent to cefazolin + tobra; only concern was efficacy of CIP vs S. pneumoniae (Ophthalmology 163:1854, 1996).
Fungal	Aspergillus, fusarium, candida. No empiric therapy—see Comment	Natamycin (5%) drops q3–4 hrs with subsequent slow reduction	Ampho B (0.05–0.15%) q3–4 hrs with subsequent slow reduction	No empiric therapy. Wait for results of Gram stain or culture in Sabouraud's medium.
Protozoan Soft contact lens users (over-night use ↑ risk 10–15 fold)	Acanthamoeba, hartmannella	Propamidine 0.1% + neomycin/gramicidin/ polymyxin Eyedrops q waking hour for 1 week and then slow taper	Polyhexamethylene biguanide (PHMB) 0.02% or chlorhexidine 0.02%	Uncommon. Trauma and soft contact lenses are risk factors. Corneal scrapings stained with calcofluor white show characteristic cysts with fluorescent microscopy. PHMB source: Leiter's Park Ave. Pharm., 800-292-6773. Ref.: CID 35:434, 2002
Lacrimal apparatus Canaliculitis	Actinomyces most common. Rarely, Arachnia, fusobacterium, nocardia, candida	Remove granules & irri-gate with pen G (100,000 mcg per mL)	If fungi: irrigate with nystatin approx. 5 mcg per mL + 1 gtt tid	Digital pressure produces exudate at punctum; Gram stain confirms diagnosis. Hot packs to punctal area qid.
Dacryocystitis (lacrimal sac)	S. pneumo, S. aureus, H. influenzae, S. pyogenes, P. aeruginosa	Child: AM-CL or O Ceph 2 Often consequence of obstruction of lacrimal duct. Empiric rx based on Gram stain of aspirate—see Comment.		Need ophthalmologic consultation. Can be acute or chronic. Culture to detect MRSA.

Endophthalmitis. For post-op endophthalmitis, see CID 38:542, 2004

Bacterial: Haziness of vitreous key to diagnosis. Needle aspirate of both vitreous and aqueous humor for culture prior to therapy. Intravitreal administration of antimicrobials essential.				
Postocular surgery (cataracts) Early, acute onset (incidence 0.05%)	S. epidermidis 60%, Staph. aureus, streptococci, & enterococci each 5-10%, Gm-neg. bacilli 6%	Immediate ophthal. consult. If only light perception or worse, immediate vitrectomy + intravitreal vanco 1 mg & intravitreal ceftazidime 2.25 mg. No clear data on intravitreal steroid. May need to repeat intravitreal antibiotics in 2–3 days. Can usually leave lens in.		
Low grade, chronic	Propionibacterium acnes, S epidermidis, S. aureus (rare)	May require removal of lens material. Intraocular vanco ± vitrectomy.		

Abbreviations on page 2.   NOTE: All dosage recommendations are for adults (unless otherwise indicated) and assume normal renal function.

TABLE 1 (9)

ANATOMIC SITE/DIAGNOSIS/ MODIFYING CIRCUMSTANCES	ETIOLOGIES (usual)	SUGGESTED REGIMENS* PRIMARY	ALTERNATIVE§	ADJUNCT DIAGNOSTIC OR THERAPEUTIC MEASURES AND COMMENTS
EYE/Endophthalmitis/Bacterial (continued)				
Post filtering blebs for glaucoma	Strep. species (viridans & others), H. influenzae	[Intravitreal and topical agent and consider systemic **AM-CL, AM-SB** or **P Ceph 2**]		
Post-penetrating trauma	Bacillus sp., S. epiderm.	[Intravitreal agent as above + systemic **clinda** or **vanco**. Use topical antibiotics post-surgery (tobra & cefazolin drops).]		
None, suspect hematogenous	S. pneumoniae, N. meningitidis, Staph. aureus	**P Ceph 3** (**cefotaxime** 2 gm IV q4h or **ceftriaxone** 2 gm IV q24h) + **vanco** 1 gm IV q12h pending cultures. Intravitreal antibiotics as with early post-operative.		
IV heroin abuse	Bacillus cereus, Candida sp.	[Intravitreal agent + (systemic **clinda** or **vanco**)]		
Mycotic (fungal) Broad-spectrum antibiotics, often corticosteroids, indwelling venous catheters	Candida sp., Aspergillus sp.	Intravitreal **ampho B** 0.005–0.01 mg in 0.1 mL. Also *see Table 11, pages 76–78 for concomitant systemic therapy. See Comment.*		With ampho/marked vitritis, options include systemic rx + vitrectomy ± intravitreal ampho B (*CID 27:1130 & 1134, 1998*). Report of failure of ampho B lipid complex (*CID 28:1177, 1999*).
Retinitis				
Acute retinal necrosis	Varicella zoster, Herpes simplex	IV **acyclovir** 10–12 mg per kg IV q8h times 5–7 days, then 800 mg po 5 times per day times 6 wks.		Strong association of VZ virus with atypical necrotizing herpetic retinopathy (*CID 24:603, 1997*).
HIV+ (AIDS) CD4 usually <100 per mm³	Cytomegalovirus	See Table 14, page 108		Occurs in 5–10% of AIDS patients
Orbital cellulitis (*see page 39 for erysipelas, facial*)	S. pneumoniae, H. influenzae, M. catarrhalis, S. aureus, anaerobes, group A strep. occ. Gm-neg. bacilli post-trauma	**Nafcillin** 2 gm IV q24h (or if MRSA-**vanco** 1 gm IV q12h) + **ceftriaxone** 2 gm IV q24h + **metro** 1 gm IV q12h		**If penicillin/ceph allergy: Vanco + levo** 750 mg IV once daily + **metro** IV. Problem is frequent inability to make microbiologic diagnosis. Image orbit (CT or MRI). Risk of cavernous sinus thrombosis.
FOOT				
"Diabetic"—Empiric therapy. Refs.: *CID 39:885, 2004; NEJM 351:48, 2004*				
Ulcer without inflammation	Colonizing skin flora	No antibacterial therapy		
Ulcer with <2 cm of superficial inflammation	S. aureus (assume MRSA), S. agalactiae (Gp B), S. pyogenes predominate	**Oral therapy:** (**TMP-SMX-DS** or **minocycline**) plus (**Pen VK** or selected **O Ceph 2, 3,** or **FQ**) *Dosages in footnote²*		**General:** 1. Glucose control, no weight-bearing 2. Assess for peripheral vascular disease—very common (*CID 39:437, 2004*) **Principles of empiric antibacterial therapy:**
Ulcer with ≥2 cm of inflammation with extension to fascia	As above, plus coliforms	**Oral therapy:** (**AM-CL-ER** plus **TMP-SMX-DS**) or [(**CIP** or **Levo**) plus **linezolid**] *Dosages in footnote²*		1. Include drug empirically active vs MRSA. If outpatient, can assume community-acquired MRSA (CA-MRSA) until culture results available. 2. As culture results dominated by S. aureus & Streptococcus species, empiric drug regimens should include strep & staph. Role of enterococci uncertain.
Extensive local inflammation plus systemic toxicity	As above, plus anaerobic bacteria	**Parenteral therapy:** (**Vanco** plus **β-lactam/β-lactamase inhibitor**) or (**vanco** plus **carbapenem**). Other alternatives: 1. **Dapto** or **linezolid** for vanco 2. (**CIP** or **Levo** or **aztreonam**) plus **metronidazole** for β-lactam/β-lactamase inhibitor *Dosages in footnote¹*		3. Severe limb and/or life-threatening infections require initial parenteral therapy with predictable activity vs Gm-positive cocci, coliforms & other aerobic Gm-neg. rods, & anaerobic Gm-neg. bacilli. 4. **NOTE:** The regimens listed are suggestions consistent with above principles. Other alternatives exist & may be appropriate for individual patients.
Onychomycosis: See Table 11, page 80, fungal infections				
Puncture wound: Nail/Toothpick	P. aeruginosa	Cleanse. Tetanus booster. Observe.	See page 4.	1–2% evolve to osteomyelitis. Other organisms if toothpick injury (*PIDJ 23:80, 2004*).

[1] **Vanco** 1 gm IV q12h, **parenteral β-lactam/β-lactamase inhibitors: AM-SB** 3 gm IV q6h, **PIP-TZ** 3.375 gm IV q6h or 4.5 gm IV q8h; **TC-CL** 3.1 gm IV q6h; **carbapenems: ERTA** 1 gm IV q24h, **IMP** 0.5 gm IV q6h, **MER** 1 gm IV q8h; **daptomycin** 6 mg per kg IV q24h, **linezolid** 600 mg IV q12h, **aztreonam** 2 gm IV q8h. **CIP** and **Levo** dosages in footnotes 2 and 3, **metro** 1 gm IV loading dose & then 0.5 gm IV q6h or 1 gm IV q12h

[2] **TMP-SMX-DS** 2 tabs po bid, **minocycline** 100 mg po bid, **Pen VK** 500 mg po qid, **cefprozil** 500 mg po q12h, **cefuroxime axetil** 500 mg po q12h, **cefdinir** 300 mg po q12h, **cefpodoxime** 200 mg po q12h, **CIP** 750 mg po q12h, **Levo** 750 mg po q24h.

[3] **AM-CL-ER** 2000/125 po bid, **TMP-SMX-DS** 2 tabs po bid, **Levo** 750 mg po q24h, **linezolid** 600 mg po bid

Abbreviations on page 2. NOTE: *All dosage recommendations are for adults (unless otherwise indicated) and assume normal renal function.*

ANATOMIC SITE/DIAGNOSIS/ MODIFYING CIRCUMSTANCES	ETIOLOGIES (usual)	SUGGESTED REGIMENS*		ADJUNCT DIAGNOSTIC OR THERAPEUTIC MEASURES AND COMMENTS
		PRIMARY	ALTERNATIVE§	

GALLBLADDER

Cholecystitis, cholangitis, biliary sepsis, or common duct obstruction (partial: 2° to tumor, stones, stricture)	Enterobacteriaceae 68%, enterococci 14%, bacteroides 10%, Clostridium sp. 7%, rarely candida	PIP-TZ or AM-SB or TC-CL or ERTA or MER If life-threatening: IMP *Dosages in footnote 1, previous page*	P Ceph 3 + metro OR Aztreonam + metro OR CIP + metro	For severely ill pts, antibiotic rx is complementary to adequate biliary drainage. 15–30% pts will require decompression: surgical, percutaneous or ERCP-placed stent. Whether empirical rx should always cover pseudomonas & anaerobes is uncertain (*CID 19:279, 1994*). Ceftriaxone associated with biliary sludge (by ultrasound 50%, symptomatic 9%, *NEJM 322:1821, 1990*); clinical relevance still unclear but has led to surgery (*MMWR 42:39, 1993*).

GASTROINTESTINAL

Gastroenteritis—Empiric Therapy (laboratory studies not performed or culture, microscopy, toxin results NOT AVAILABLE) (Ref.: *NEJM 350:38, 2004*)

Premature infant with necrotizing enterocolitis	Associated with intestinal flora	Treatment and rationale as for diverticulitis/peritonitis, *pages 16–17. See Table 16, page 133 for pediatric dosages.*		Pneumatosis intestinalis on x-ray confirms dx. Bacteremia-peritonitis in 30–50%. If Staph. epidermidis isolated, add vanco (IV).
Mild diarrhea (≤3 unformed stools per day, minimal associated symptomatology)	Bacterial (*see Severe, below*), viral, parasitic. Viral usually causes mild to moderate disease. For traveler's diarrhea, *see page 15*	Fluids only + lactose-free diet, avoid caffeine		**Rehydration: For po fluid replacement, see Cholera, page 15.** **Antimotility:** Loperamide (Imodium) 4 mg po, then 2 mg after each loose stool to max. of 16 mg per day. Bismuth subsalicylate (Pepto-Bismol) 2 tablets (262 mg) po qid. Do not use if suspect hemolytic uremic syndrome.
Moderate diarrhea (≥4 unformed stools per day and/or systemic symptoms)		Antimotility agents (*see Comments*) + fluids		**Hemolytic uremic syndrome (HUS):** Risk in **children** infected with E. coli 0157:H7 is 8–10%. Early treatment with TMP-SMX or FQs ↑ risk of HUS (*NEJM 342:1930 & 1990, 2000*). Controversial meta-analysis: *JAMA 288:996 & 3111, 2002.*
Severe diarrhea (≥6 unformed stools per day, and/or temperature ≥101°F, tenesmus, blood, or fecal leukocytes) NOTE: **Severe afebrile bloody diarrhea should ↑ suspicion of E. coli 0157:H7 infection**—causes only 1–3% all cases diarrhea in U.S.—but causes up to 36% cases of bloody diarrhea (*CID 32:573, 2001*)	Shigella, salmonella, C. jejuni, E. coli 0157:H7 toxin-positive C. difficile. E. histolytica. *For typhoid fever, see page 44*	FQ (CIP 500 mg po q12h or Levo 500 mg q24h) times 3–5 days If recent antibiotic therapy possible: **add:** Metro 500 mg po tid times 10–14 days	TMP-SMX-DS po bid times 3–5 days. Campylobacter resistance to TMP-SMX common in tropics. (C. difficile toxin colitis Vanco 125 mg po qid times 10–14 days	**Other potential etiologies:** Cryptosporidia—no treatment in immunocompetent host (*see Table 13A & JID 170:272, 1994*). Cyclospora—usually chronic diarrhea, responds to TMP-SMX (*see Table 12A & AIM 123:409, 1995*). **Severe diarrhea** treated with CIP 500 mg po bid decreases duration of diarrhea and other symptoms without changing duration of fecal carriage. Increasing resistance of campylobacter to FQs.

Gastroenteritis—Specific Therapy (results of culture, microscopy, toxin assay AVAILABLE). Ref.: *NEJM 350:38, 2004*

If culture negative, probably Norovirus (Norwalk) or rarely (in adults) Rotavirus— *see Table 14A, page 112* NOTE: **In 60 hospital pts with unexplained WBCs ≥15,000, 35% had C. difficile toxin present** (*AJM 115:543, 2003; CID 34:1585, 2002*)	Aeromonas/Plesiomonas	CIP 500 mg po bid times 3 days	TMP-SMX-DS po bid times 3 days	Although no absolute proof, increasing evidence as cause of diarrheal illness.
	Amebiasis (Entamoeba histolytica, Cyclospora, Cryptosporidia and Giardia), *see Table 13A*			
	Campylobacter jejuni CAUTION: *See Comment on FQ resistance.* Fever in 53–83%, H/O¹ bloody stools 37%	Azithro 500 mg po q24h times 3 days or CIP 500 mg po bid (*See Comment*)	Erythro stearate 500 mg po qid times 5 days	↑ **worldwide resistance to FQs** varies by region from 10% (USA) to 84% (Thailand) (*AAC 47:2358, 2003*). Erythro resistance rarely reported (*CID 37:131, 2003*). **Post-Campylobacter Guillain-Barré**: assoc. 15% of cases (*CID 37:307, 2003*). Assoc. with small bowel lymphoproliferative disease; may respond to antimicrobials (*NEJM 350:239, 2003*). **Reactive arthritis** another potential sequelae.

¹ **H/O** = history of
Abbreviations on page 2.   NOTE: *All dosage recommendations are for adults (unless otherwise indicated) and assume normal renal function.*

TABLE 1 (11)

ANATOMIC SITE/DIAGNOSIS/ MODIFYING CIRCUMSTANCES	ETIOLOGIES (usual)	SUGGESTED REGIMENS* PRIMARY	SUGGESTED REGIMENS* ALTERNATIVE§	ADJUNCT DIAGNOSTIC OR THERAPEUTIC MEASURES AND COMMENTS
Gastrointestinal/Gastroenteritis *(continued)* *(continued from above)*	Specific Therapy *(continued)*			
	C. difficile toxin positive antibiotic-associated colitis (Ref.: *LnID* 5:549, 2005) **Remember: Contact isolation indicated** Fever in 28%. **Diagnosis:** Tissue culture—detects toxin A&B, most sensitive. Takes 48 hrs. Rapid immunoassays: Less sens., detect toxin A, B, or both. 10–20% false-neg. rate.	**Metro** 500 mg po tid or 250 mg qid times 10–14 days. If severe, use vanco (*AAC* 46:1647, 2002; *CID* 40:1586 & 1591 & 1598, 2005).	(**Vanco** 125 mg po qid) or (**bacitracin** 25,000 units po qid) or (**cholestyramine** 4 gm po tid) times 10–14 days. **Teicoplanin**ᴺᵁˢ 400 mg po bid times 10 days.	**DC antibiotic if possible; avoid antimotility agents; hydration; enteric isolation.** **Relapse occurs in 10–20%:** First, re-treat with **metro**. For refractory disease, **vanco** po + **RIF** po reported effective (*ICHE* 16:459, 1995); **metro** + **RIF** should work but no published data. **Other relapse rx regimens: Metro** times 10 days, then (**cholestyramine** 4 gm po tid + **lactobacillus** 1 gm qid) times 4 wks **OR vanco** 125 mg po every other day times 4 wks **OR vanco taper**, all doses 125 mg po: week 1—qid, week 2—bid, week 3—q24h, week 4—every other day, weeks 5 and 6 q3 days. **When po rx not possible**, use IV **metro** + **vanco**. 500 mg per L saline via small bowel tube and/or via pigtail catheter in cecum (in severe typhilitis pts). Perfuse at 1-3 mL per min. to q24h max. of 2 gm (*CID* 35:690, 2002). **NOTE: IV vanco not effective.** Unclear how much IV metro gets to colonic mucosa & colonic content; hence combination of IV metro and po (or via tube) vanco.
	E. coli O157:H7 H/O¹ bloody stools 63%	**NO TREATMENT** with antimicrobials or anti-motility drugs, may enhance toxin release and ↑ risk of hemolytic uremic syndrome (HUS) (*NEJM* 342:1930 & 1990, 2000). Hydration important (*Ln* 365:1073, 2005).		NOTE: 5–10% of pts develop HUS (approx. 10% with HUS die or have permanent renal failure; 50% HUS pts have some degree of renal impairment (*CID* 38:1298, 2004).
	Listeria monocytogenes	**AMP** 50 mg per kg IV q6h	**TMP-SMX** 20 mg per kg po per day IV div. q6-8h	Recently recognized cause of food poisoning, manifest as febrile gastroenteritis. Percentage with complicating bacteremia/meningitis unknown. Not detected in standard stool culture (*NEJM* 336:100 & 130, 1997).
	Salmonella, non-typhi— For typhoid fever, see page 44 Fever in 71–91%, H/O¹ bloody stools in 34%	If pt asymptomatic or illness mild, antimicrobial therapy not indicated. Treat if <1 yr old or >50 yrs old, if immunocompromised, if vascular grafts or prosthetic joints (see *typhoid fever, page 44*). **CIP** 500 mg po bid times 5–7 days. Resistance ↑ (*Ln* 353:1590, 1999)	**Azithro** 1 gm po once, then 500 mg q24h times 6 days (*AAC* 43:1441, 1999)	↑ resistance to TMP-SMX and chloro. Ceftriaxone, cefotaxime usually active (see *footnote, page 19, for dosage*); ceftriaxone & FQ resistance in SE Asia (*CID* 40:315, 2005; *Ln* 363:1285, 2004). Primary treatment of enteritis is fluid and electrolyte replacement. No adverse effects from FQs in children (*Ln* 348:547, 1996). If immunocompromised, rx 14 days.
	Shigella Fever in 58%, H/O¹ bloody stools 51%	**FQs** po: (**CIP** 500 mg bid) or (**Levo** 500 mg q24h)—times 3 days. *See Comment for peds rx per dose*	(**TMP-SMX-DS** po bid times 3 days) or (**azithro** 500 mg po x1, then 250 mg q24h times 4 days)	**Peds doses:** TMP-SMX 5/25 mg per kg po times 3 days. For severe disease, ceftriaxone 50–75 mg per kg per day times 2–5 days. CIP suspension 10 mg per kg bid times 5 days. (*Ln* 352:522, 1998) CIP superior to ceftriaxone in children (*LnID* 3:537, 2003). **Immunocompromised children & adults: Treat for 7–10 days.** Azithro superior to cefixime in trial in children (*PIDJ* 22:374, 2003).
	Staphylococcus aureus *See Comment*	**Vanco** 1 gm IV q12h + 125 mg po qid reasonable		Case reports of toxin-mediated pseudomembranous enteritis/colitis (pseudomembranes in small bowel) (*CID* 39:747, 2004). **Clinda** to stop toxin production reasonable if organism susceptible.
	Spirochetosis (Brachyspira pilosicoli)	Benefit of treatment unclear. Susceptible to **metro**, **ceftriaxone**, and **Moxi** (*AAC* 47:2354, 2003).		Anaerobic intestinal spirochete that colonizes colon of domestic & wild animals plus humans. Case reports of diarrhea with large numbers of the organism (*AAC* 39:347, 2001; *Am J Clin Path* 120:828, 2003).

¹ **H/O** = history of

ANATOMIC SITE/DIAGNOSIS/ MODIFYING CIRCUMSTANCES	ETIOLOGIES (usual)	SUGGESTED REGIMENS*		ADJUNCT DIAGNOSTIC OR THERAPEUTIC MEASURES AND COMMENTS
		PRIMARY	ALTERNATIVE§	
Gastrointestinal/Gastroenteritis—Specific Therapy *(continued)*				
Vibrio cholerae Treatment decreases duration of disease, vol. losses, and duration of excretion *CID 37:272, 2003; Ln 363:223, 2004*		**CIP** 1 gm po times 1 + fluids. **Primary rx is hydration** *(see Comment)*	**Doxy** 300 mg po times 1 + fluids *(see Comment)*. For children—<8 yrs & in pregnancy; **TMP-SMX-DS**, one bid po times 3 days or for Peds alternative: **azithro** or CIP times 1—*see doses in Comment*	Primary rx is fluid. **IV** use (per liter): 4 gm NaCl, 1 gm KCl, 5.4 gm Na lactate, 8 gm glucose. **PO** use (per liter potable water): 1 level teaspoon table salt + 4 heaping teaspoons sugar *(JTMH 84:73, 1981)*. Add orange juice or 2 bananas for K⁺. Volume given = fluid loss. Mild dehydration, give 5% body weight; for moderate, 7% body weight. (Refs.: *CID 20:1485, 1995; TRSM 89:103, 1995*). Peds azithro 20 mg per kg (to 1 gm max.) times 1 *(Ln 360:1722, 2002)*; CIP 20 mg per kg *(Ln 366:1085, 2005)*.
Vibrio parahaemolyticus		Antimicrobial rx does not shorten course. Hydration.		Shellfish exposure common. Treat severe disease: **FQ, doxy, P Ceph 3**
Vibrio vulnificus		Usual presentation is skin lesions & bacteremia; life-threatening; treat early: **ceftaz + doxy**—*see page 40*		
Yersinia enterocolitica Fever in 68%, bloody stools in 26%		No treatment unless severe. If severe, combine **doxy** 100 mg IV bid + (**tobra** or **genta** 5 mg per kg per day once q24h). **TMP-SMX** or **FQs** are alternatives.		Mesenteric adenitis pain can mimic acute appendicitis. Lab diagnosis difficult: requires "cold enrichment" and/or yersinia selective agar. Desferrioxamine rx ↑ severity, discontinue if pt on it. Iron overload states predispose to yersinia *(CID 27:1362 & 1367, 1998)*
Gastroenteritis—Specific Risk Groups—Empiric Therapy				
Anorectal—Intercourse				
Proctitis (distal 15 cm only)	Herpes viruses, gonococci, chlamydia, syphilis. *See Genital Tract, page 18*			
Colitis	Shigella, salmonella, campylobacter, E. histolytica *(see Table 13A)*		**FQ** (e.g., **CIP** 500 mg po) q12h times 3 days.	
HIV-1 infected (AIDS); >10 days diarrhea				
Acid-fast organisms:	Cryptosporidium parvum, Cyclospora cayetanensis	See Table 13A	For influence of highly active antiretroviral therapy, see *CID 28:701, 1999*	
	Isospora belli, microsporidia (Enterocytozoon bieneusi, Septata intestinalis)	See Table 13A		
Other:		See Table 13A		
	G. lamblia			
Neutropenic enterocolitis or "typhlitis" *(CID 27:695 & 700, 1998)*	Mucosal invasion by **Clostridium septicum**. Occasionally caused by C. sordelli or P. aeruginosa	As for perirectal abscess. Ensure empiric regimen includes drug active vs Clostridia species; e.g., **pen G**, **AMP**, or **clinda** *(see Comment re: resistance)*. Empiric regimen should have predictive activity vs P. aeruginosa also.		Tender right lower quadrant. Surgical resection controversial but may be necessary. **NOTE:** Resistance of clostridia to clindamycin reported.
Traveler's diarrhea, self-medication. Patient usually afebrile *(LnID 5:349, 2005)*	**Acute:** 60% due to toxigenic E. coli, shigella, salmonella, or campylobacter. C. difficile, amebiasis *(see Table 13)*. **If chronic:** cyclospora, cryptosporidia, giardia, isospora	**Levo** 500 mg po times 1 dose. Alternative: **CIP** or **other FQ** bid times 3 days *(see footnote¹)*. **Imodium** optional: 4 mg times 1, then 2 mg after each loose stool to max.16 mg per day.	**Azithro** 1 gm po times 1 dose or **rifaximin** 200 mg po tid times 3 days.	Treatment based on randomized trial *(CID 37:1165, 2003)*. Peds & pregnancy: Avoid FQs. Azithro peds dose: 5–10 mg per kg times 1 dose. Rifaximin approved for age 12 or older. Adverse effects similar to placebo. No loperamide if fever or blood in stool.
Prevention		Not routinely indicated. Current recommendation is to take **FQ** + **Imodium** with 1st loose stool.	Alternative during 1st 3 weeks & only if activities are essential: **Rifaximin** 200 mg po bid *(AnIM 142:805 & 861, 2005)*.	
Gastrointestinal Infections by Anatomic Site: Esophagus to Rectum				
Esophagitis	Candida albicans, HSV, CMV	See SANFORD GUIDE TO HIV/AIDS THERAPY		

¹ **FQ** dosage po for self-rx traveler's diarrhea—mild disease: **CIP** 750 mg times 1; severe: 500 mg bid times 3 days. **Oflox** 300 mg bid times 3 days. Once q24h times 3 days: **Levo** 500 mg; **Gati** or **Moxi** 400 mg probably would work but not FDA-approved indication.
Abbreviations on page 2.　　*NOTE: All dosage recommendations are for adults (unless otherwise indicated) and assume normal renal function.*

TABLE 1 (13)

ANATOMIC SITE/DIAGNOSIS/ MODIFYING CIRCUMSTANCES	ETIOLOGIES (usual)	SUGGESTED REGIMENS*		ADJUNCT DIAGNOSTIC OR THERAPEUTIC MEASURES AND COMMENTS
		PRIMARY	ALTERNATIVE§	
Gastrointestinal Infections by Anatomic Site: Esophagus to Rectum *(continued)*				
Duodenal/Gastric ulcer; gastric cancer, MALT lymphomas (not 2° NSAIDs) (*NEJM 347:1175, 2002; Can J Gastro 17:25B, 2003*)	**Helicobacter pylori** See Comment Prevalence of pre-treatment resistance increasing	**Rx q12h po for 14 days: (Omeprazole or rabeprazole 20 mg)** [1] + **amox** 1 gm + **clarithro** 500 mg. Efficacy 80-95%	**Rx po for 14 days: Bismuth** (see *footnote*[2]), bismuth subsalicylate 2 tabs qid + **tetracycline** 500 mg qid + **metro** 500 mg tid + **omeprazole**[1] 20 mg bid. Efficacy 90-99%	**Dx: Stool antigen**—>90% sens. & specific. Cheap & practical. Rare false-pos. due to other Helicobacter species (*BMJ 320:148, 2000*). Other tests: Urea breath test; if endoscoped, rapid urease &/or histology &/or culture. **Antimicrobial resistance: Predicts rx failure** (*AnIM 139:463, 2003*). Geographic differences but overall resistance: amox & tetra uncommon, clarithro 10%, metro 30-50%. **Treatment success:** Correlates with active drugs & pt compliance. Suggested **rx duration** varies between 7-14 days; we suggest bid regimen times 14 days to ↑ compliance & hopefully efficacy (7-9% ↑ cures with 14 days) (*Aliment Pharmacol Ther 14:603, 2000*). **Test of cure:** Repeat stool antigen >8 wks post-treatment.
Small intestine: Whipple's disease (*CID 32:457, 2001; Ln 363:654, 2004*) See *Infective endocarditis, culture-negative, page 23*	Tropheryma whipplei	**Initial 10-14 days** (**Pen G** 6-24 million units IV q4h + **streptomycin** 1 gm IM/IV q24h) OR **ceftriaxone** 2 gm IV q24h **Then, for approx. 1 year** **TMP-SMX-DS** 1 tab po bid	**TMP-SMX-DS** 1 tab po bid (**Doxy** 100 mg po bid) or (**cefixime** 400 mg po bid) or (**Pen VK** 500 mg po qid)	Rx regimen based on empiricism and retrospective analyses. TMP-SMX: CNS relapses during TMP-SMX rx reported. Interesting in vitro susceptibility study: combination of doxy & hydroxychloroquine bactericidal (*AAC 48:747, 2004*). Cultivated from CSF in pts with intestinal disease and no neurologic findings (*JID 188:797 & 801, 2003*).
Inflammatory bowel disease: Ulcerative colitis, Crohn's disease Mild to moderate Ref. *Ln 359:331, 2002*	Unknown	**Sulfasalazine** 1 gm po q6h **or mesalamine (5ASA)** 1 gm po q6h	**Coated mesalamine** (Asacol) 800 mg bid or qid equally effective. Corticosteroid enemas (*Gastro 123:33, 2002*).	Check stool for E. histolytica. Try aminosalicylates 1st in mild/mod. disease. See review article for more aggressive therapy.
Severe Crohn's	Unknown	In randomized controlled trial, CIP + metro had no benefit		Screen for latent TBc before blocking TNF (*MMWR 53:683, 2004*). Delay anti-TNF drugs until TBc prophylaxis complete. For other anti-TNF risks: *NEJM 351:42, 2004.*
Severe Crohn's		Etanercept	Infliximab/adalimumab	
Diverticulitis, perirectal abscess, peritonitis Also see *Peritonitis, page 34* CID (in press)	Enterobacteriaceae, occ. P. aeruginosa, Bacteroides sp., enterococci	**Outpatient rx—mild diverticulitis, drained perirectal abscess:** (**TMP-SMX-DS** bid) or (**CIP** 750 mg bid or **Levo** 750 mg q24h)] + **metro** 500 mg q6h. All po times 7-10 days.	**AM-CL-ER** 1000/62.5 mg 2 tabs po bid times 7-10 days	Must "cover" both Gm-neg. aerobic and Gm-neg. anaerobic bacteria. **Drugs active only vs anaerobic Gm-neg. bacilli:** clinda, metro. **Drugs active only vs aerobic Gm-neg. bacilli:** APAG[3], P Ceph 2/3/4, aztreonam, AP Pen, CIP, Levo, Gati. **Drugs active vs both aerobic/anaerobic Gm-neg. bacteria:** cefoxitin, cefotetan, TC-CL, PIP-TZ, AM-SB, ERTA, IMP, MER, & Moxi, tigecycline. Increasing resistance of Bacteroides species:

	Cefoxitin	Cefotetan	Clindamycin
% Resistant:	4-25	17-87	16-44

Resistance to metro, PIP-TZ rare (*CID 35(Suppl.1):S126, 2002*). Few case (continued on next page)

---

[1] Can substitute other **proton pump inhibitors** for omeprazole or rabeprazole—all bid: esomeprazole 20 mg (*FDA-approved*), lansoprazole 30 mg (*FDA-approved*), pantoprazole 40 mg (*not FDA-approved for this indication*)

[2] **3 bismuth preparations:** (1) In U.S., **bismuth subsalicylate (Pepto-Bismol)** 262 mg tabs; adult dose for helicobacter is 2 tabs (524 mg) qid. (2) Outside U.S., colloidal bismuth subcitrate (De-Nol) 120 mg chewable tablets; dose is 1 tablet qid. (3) Another treatment option: Ranitidine bismuth citrate 400 mg: give with metro 500 mg and clarithro 500 mg—all bid times 7 days. Worked despite metro/clarithro resistance (*Gastro 114:A323, 1998*).

[3] **APAG = antipseudomonal aminoglycoside,** e.g., **amikacin, gentamicin, tobramycin**

TABLE 1 (14)

ANATOMIC SITE/DIAGNOSIS/ MODIFYING CIRCUMSTANCES	ETIOLOGIES (usual)	SUGGESTED REGIMENS*		ADJUNCT DIAGNOSTIC OR THERAPEUTIC MEASURES AND COMMENTS
		PRIMARY	ALTERNATIVE$	
Gastrointestinal Infections by Anatomic Site: Esophagus to Rectum (continued)				
Diverticulitis, perirectal abscess, peritonitis (continued)		**Mild–moderate disease—Inpatient—Parenteral Rx:** (e.g., focal peri-appendiceal peritonitis, peri-diverticular abscess, endomyometritis) **PIP-TZ** 3.375 gm IV q6h or 4.5 gm IV q8h **or AM-SB** 3 gm IV q6h, **or TC-CL** 3.1 gm IV q6h **or ERTA** 1 gm IV q24h	**CIP** 400 mg IV q12h) or (**Levo** 750 mg IV q24h)] + **metro** 500 mg IV q6h or 1 gm IV q12h **OR tigecycline** 100 mg IV 1st dose & then 50 mg IV q12h	(continued from previous page) reports of metro resistance (CID 40:e67, 2005; J Clin Micro 42:4127, 2004). Resistance mechanisms reviewed: CID 39:92, 2004). **Ertapenem** less active vs P. aeruginosa/Acinetobacter sp. than IMP or MER. **Concomitant surgical management important.** esp. with moderate-severe disease. **Role of enterococci remains debatable.** Probably pathogenic in infections of biliary tract. Probably need drugs active vs enterococci in pts with valvular heart disease.
		Severe life-threatening disease, ICU patient: **IMP** 0.5 gm IV q6h or **MER** 1 gm IV q8h	**AMP + metro + CIP** 400 mg IV q12h or **Levo** 750 mg IV q24h) **OR [AMP** 2 gm IV q6h + **metro** 500 mg IV q6h + **APAG** (see Table 10D, page 74)	**Severe penicillin/cephalosporin allergy: (aztreonam** 2 gm IV q6h) + [**metro** (500 mg IV q6h) or (1 gm IV q12h)] **OR** [(**CIP** 400 mg IV q12h) or (**Levo** 750 mg IV q24h) + **metro**]. Based on in vitro data, could sub **Gati/Moxi** for **CIP/Levo**, but insufficient clinical data.
GENITAL TRACT: Mixture of empiric & specific treatment. Divided by sex of the patient. For sexual assault (rape), see Table 15A, page 124. See Guidelines for Dx of Sexually Transmitted Diseases, MMWR 51(RR-6), 2002 or CID 35(Suppl.2):S135, 2002 or www.cdc.gov/std/treatment/toc2002tg.htm				
Both Women & Men: **Chancroid** Ref.: CID 28(Suppl. 1):S14, 1999	H. ducreyi	**Ceftriaxone** 250 mg IM single dose OR azithro 1 gm po single dose	**CIP** 500 mg bid po times 3 days OR **erythro base** 500 mg qid po times 7 days.	In HIV+ pts, failures reported with single dose azithro (CID 21:409, 1995).
Chlamydia, et al. non-gonococcal or post-gonococcal urethritis, cervicitis NOTE: Assume concomitant N. gonorrhoeae Chlamydia conjunctivitis, see page 10	Chlamydia 50%. Myco-plasma hominis. Other known etiologies (10–15%): Ureaplasma, trichomonas, herpes simplex virus, Myco-plasma genitalium. Chlamydia ref.: NEJM 349: 2424, 2003	**(Doxy** 100 mg bid po times 7 days) or (**azithro** 1 gm po as single dose). Evaluate & rx sex partner **In pregnancy: erythro base** 500 mg po qid times 7 days OR **amox** 500 mg po tid times 7 days.	(**Erythro base** 500 mg qid po times 7 days) or (**Oflox** 300 mg q12h po times 7 days) or (**Levo** 500 mg qd x24h times 7 days). **In pregnancy: azithro** 1 gm po times 1 **Doxy & Oflox** contra-indicated	**Diagnosis:** Nucleic acid amplification tests for C. trachomatis & N. gonorrhoeae on urine specimens equivalent to cervix or urethra specimens (AnIM 142:914, 2005). **For recurrent or persistent disease:** either metro 2 gm IV q1 + either erythro base 500 mg qid times 7 days or erythro ethylsuccinate 800 mg po qid times 7 days. **Evaluate & treat sex partners.**
Recurrent/persistent urethritis	**Occult trichomonas**, tetra-resistant U. urealyticum	**Metro** 2 gm po x1 + **erythro base** 500 mg po qid times 7 days.	**Erythro ethylsuccinate** 800 mg po qid times 7 days	In men with NGU, 20% infected with trichomonas (JID 188:465, 2003).
Gonorrhea [MMWR 51(RR-6), 2002 or CID 35(Suppl.2), 2002 or CID 35(Suppl.2):S135, 2002]				
Conjunctivitis (adult)	N. gonorrhoeae	**Ceftriaxone** 1 gm IM, IV or IV times one dose	**Spectinomycin** 2 gm IM times 1	Consider saline lavage of eye times 1
Disseminated gonococcal infection (DGI, dermatitis-arthritis syndrome)	N. gonorrhoeae	**(Ceftriaxone** 1 gm IV q24h) or **(cefotaxime** 1 gm q8h IV), or **(ceftizox-ime** 1 gm q8h IV)—see Comment	**Spectinomycin** 2 gm IM q12h or **CIP** 400 mg IV q12h or **Oflox** 400 mg IV q12h or **Levo** 250 mg IV q24h—see Comment	Continue IM or IV regimen for 24 hrs after symptoms ↓; reliable pts may be dis-charged 24 hrs after sx resolve to complete 7 days rx with **cefixime 400 mg po bid** or **CIP 500 mg po bid** or **Oflox 400 mg po bid** or **Levo 500 mg po q24h.** R/O meningitis/ endocarditis. **Treat presumptively for concomitant C. trachomatis.**
Endocarditis	N. gonorrhoeae	**Ceftriaxone** 1–2 gm IV q12h times 4 wks	**CIP** 500 mg po times 1 or **Levo** 250 mg po times 1	If chlamydia not ruled out: Azithro 1 gm po times 1 or doxy 100 mg po bid times 7 days. Some suggest test of cure culture after 1 week. Spectinomycin not effective
Pharyngitis	N. gonorrhoeae	**Ceftriaxone** 125 mg IM times 1		

Abbreviations on page 2.   NOTE: All dosage recommendations are for adults (unless otherwise indicated) and assume normal renal function.

TABLE 1 (15)

ANATOMIC SITE/DIAGNOSIS/ MODIFYING CIRCUMSTANCES	ETIOLOGIES (usual)	SUGGESTED REGIMENS* PRIMARY	SUGGESTED REGIMENS* ALTERNATIVE§	ADJUNCT DIAGNOSTIC OR THERAPEUTIC MEASURES AND COMMENTS
GENITAL TRACT/Both Women & Men/Gonorrhea *[MMWR 51(RR-6), 2002] (continued)*				
Urethritis, cervicitis, proctitis (uncomplicated) For prostatitis, see page 20. **Diagnosis**: Nucleic acid amplification test on urine or urethral swab—see *MMWR 51 (RR-15), 2002*	N. gonorrhoeae (50% of pts with urethritis, cervicitis have concomitant C. trachomatis —**treat for both**)	[(**Ceftriaxone** 125 mg IM times 1) or (**cefixime** 400 mg po times 1) or (**cefpodoxime** 400 mg po times 1) or (**CIP** 500 mg po times 1) or (**Oflox** 400 mg po times 1) or (**Levo** 250 mg po times 1) or (**Gati** 400 mg po times 1)] **PLUS** [(**Azithro** 1 gm po times 1) or (**doxy** 100 mg po times 7 days)] **NOTE**: Due to resistance of approx. 5%, do not use FQs to treat (1) men who have sex with men or (2) GC acquired in Hawaii, other Pacific Islands, West Coast of U.S., or England.		**Treat for both GC and C. trachomatis.** Screen for syphilis. Other alternatives for **GC**: Spectinomycin 2 gm IM times 1 Other single-dose cephalosporins: ceftizoxime 500 mg IM, cefotaxime 500 mg IM, cefoxitin 2 gm IM + probenecid 1 gm po. Azithro 1 gm po x1 effective for chlamydia but need 2 gm po for GC; not recommended for GC due to GI side-effects and expense. FQ resistance refs.: *MMWR 53:335, 2004; CID 38:649, 2004; EID 11:1009, 2005*
Granuloma inguinale (Donovanosis)	Calymmatobacterium granulomatis	**Doxy** 100 mg po bid times 3-4 wks OR **TMP-SMX-DS** q12h times 3 weeks	**Erythro** 500 mg po qid times 3 weeks OR **CIP** 750 mg po bid times 3 weeks OR **azithro** 1 gm po q wk times 3 weeks	Clinical response usually seen in 1 week. Rx until all lesions healed, may take 4 weeks. Treatment failures & recurrence seen with doxy and TMP-SMX. Report of efficacy with FQ and chloro. Ref.: *CID 25:24, 1997*
Herpes simplex virus	*See Table 14, page 110*			
Lymphogranuloma venereum	Chlamydia trachomatis, serovars. L1, L2, L3	**Doxy** 100 mg po bid times 21 days	**Erythro** 0.5 gm po qid times 21 days	Dx based on serology; biopsy contraindicated because sinus tracts develop. Nucleic acid ampli tests in development.
Phthirus pubis (pubic lice, "crabs")	*[Phthirus pubis & Sarcoptes scabiei See Table 13, page 103*			
Syphilis *(JAMA 290:1510, 2003); Syphilis & HIV: LnID 4:456, 2004; MMWR 53:RR-15, 2004*				
Early: primary, secondary, or latent <1 year	T. pallidum	**Benzathine pen G (Bicillin L-A)** 2.4 million units IM times 1	**Doxy** 100 mg po bid times 14 days) or (**tetracycline** 500 mg po qid times14 days) or (**ceftriaxone** 1 gm IM/IV q24h times 8-10 days). Follow-up mandatory.	If early or congenital syphilis, **quantitate VDRL at 0**, 3, 6, 12 & 24 months after rx. If 1° or 2° syphilis, VDRL should ↓ 2 tubes at 6 months, 3 tubes 12 months, & 4 tubes 24 months. Early latent 2 tubes ↓ at 12 months. With 1°, 50% will be RPR seronegative at 12 months, 24% neg. FTA/ABS at 2-3 yrs *(AnIM 114:1005, 1991)*. **Azithro-resistant syphilis** documented in California, Ireland, & elsewhere *(NEJM 351:122 & 154,2004)*.
More than 1 yr's duration (latent of indeterminate duration, cardiovascular, late benign)		**Benzathine pen G (Bicillin L-A)** 2.4 million units IM q week times 3 = 7.2 million units total	**Doxy** 100 mg po bid times 28 days or **tetracycline** 500 mg po qid times 28 days	No published data on efficacy of alternatives. The value of routine lumbar puncture in asymptomatic late syphilis is being questioned in the U.S. i.e.: no LP, rx all patients as primary recommendation. *ArIM 145:465, 1985.* **Indications for LP (CDC): neurologic symptoms, treatment failure, serum non-treponemal antibody titer ≥1:32, other evidence of active syphilis (aortitis, gumma, iritis), non-penicillin rx, + HIV test.**
Neurosyphilis—Very difficult to treat. Includes ocular (retrobulbar neuritis) syphilis		**Pen G** 3-4 million units IV q4h times 10-14 days.	(**Procaine pen G** 2.4 million units IM q24h + **probenecid** 0.5 gm po qid) both times 10-14 days—See Comment	**Ceftriaxone** 2 gm (IV or IM) q24h times 14 days. 23% failure rate reported *(AJM 93:481, 1992)*. For penicillin allergy: either desensitize to penicillin or obtain infectious diseases consultation. **Serologic criteria for response to rx: 4-fold or greater ↓ in VDRL titer over 6-12 mos.** *CID 28 (Suppl. 1):S21, 1999.*
HIV infection (AIDS) *(See SANFORD GUIDE TO HIV/AIDS THERAPY & refs. in Comments)*		Treatment same as HIV uninfected with closer follow-up Recommend CSF exam of all HIV+ pts regardless of stage of syphilis.		HIV+ plus RPR ≥1:32 plus CD4 count ≤350 per mcL increases risk of neurosyphilis nearly 19-fold—examine CSF *(JID 189:369, 2004)*; also, CSF changes less likely to normalize *(CID 38:1001, 2004)*. Reviews of syphilis & HIV: *LnID 4:456, 2004; MMWR 53:RR-15, 2004.*
Pregnancy and syphilis		Same as for non-pregnant, some recommend 2nd dose (2.4 million units) **benzathine pen G** 1 wk after initial dose esp. in 3rd trimester or with 2° syphilis	[Skin test for penicillin allergy. Desensitize if necessary.	Monthly quantitative VDRL or equivalent. If 4-fold ↑, re-treat. Doxy, tetracycline contraindicated. Erythro not recommended because of high risk of failure to cure fetus.

Abbreviations on page 2   NOTE: All dosage recommendations are for adults (unless otherwise indicated) and assume normal renal function

TABLE 1 (16)

ANATOMIC SITE/DIAGNOSIS/ MODIFYING CIRCUMSTANCES	ETIOLOGIES (usual)	SUGGESTED REGIMENS* PRIMARY	ALTERNATIVE§	ADJUNCT DIAGNOSTIC OR THERAPEUTIC MEASURES AND COMMENTS
GENITAL TRACT/Both Women & Men/Syphilis (continued)				
Congenital syphilis	T. pallidum	**Aqueous crystalline pen G** 50,000 units per kg per dose IV q8–12h times10–14 days	**Procaine pen G** 50,000 units per kg IM q24h for 10 days	Another alternative: Ceftriaxone ≤30 days old, 75 mg per kg IV/IM q24h or >30 days old 100 mg per kg IV/IM q24h. Treat 10–14 days. If symptomatic, ophthalmologic exam indicated. If more than 1 day of rx missed, restart entire course. **Need serologic follow-up!**
Warts, anogenital	See Table 14, page 112			
Women: Amnionitis, septic abortion	Bacteroides, esp. Prevotella bivius; Group B, A strepto-cocci; Enterobacteriaceae; C. trachomatis	**[Cefoxitin** or **TC-CL** or **IMP** or **MER** or **AM-SB** or **ERTA** or **PIP-TZ) + doxy]** OR **[Clinda + (APAG** or **P Ceph 3)]** Dosage: see footnote[1]		D&C of uterus. **In septic abortion,** Clostridium perfringens may cause fulminant intravascular hemolysis. **In postpartum patients** with enigmatic fever and/or pulmonary emboli, **consider septic pelvic vein thrombophlebitis** (see Vascular, septic pelvic vein thrombophlebitis, page 47). After discharge: doxy or continue clinda. **NOTE:** IV clinda effective for C. trachomatis. No data on po clinda (CID 19:720, 1994).
Cervicitis, mucopurulent	N. gonorrhoeae / Chlamydia trachomatis	Treat for gonorrhea, page 18 / Treat for non-gonococcal urethritis, page 17		Criteria for dx: yellow or green pus on cervical swab. >10 WBC/oil field. Gram stain for dx; if negative rx for C. trachomatis. If in doubt, send swab or urine for culture, EIA or nucleic acid amplification test and rx for both.
Endomyometritis/septic pelvic phlebitis				
Early postpartum (1st 48 hrs) (usually after C-section)	Bacteroides, esp. Prevotella bivius; Group B, A strepto-cocci; Enterobacteriaceae; C. trachomatis	**[Cefoxitin** or **TC-CL** or **ERTA** or **IMP** or **MER** or **AM-SB** or **PIP-TZ) + doxy]** OR **[Clinda + (APAG** or **P Ceph 3)]** Dosage: see footnote[1]	See Comments under Amnionitis, septic abortion, above	
Late postpartum (48 hrs to 6 wks) (usually after vaginal delivery)	Chlamydia trachomatis, M. hominis	**Doxy** 100 mg IV or po q12h times 14 days		Tetracyclines not recommended in nursing mothers; discontinue nursing. M. hominis sensitive to tetra, clinda, not erythro (CCTID 17:5200, 1993).
Fitzhugh-Curtis syndrome	C. trachomatis, N. gonorrhoeae	Treat as for pelvic inflammatory disease		Perihepatitis (violin-string adhesions)
Pelvic inflammatory disease (PID), salpingitis, tubo-ovarian abscess Outpatient rx: limit to pts with temp <38°C, WBC <11,000 per mm³, minimal evidence of peritonitis, active bowel sounds & able to tolerate oral nourishment See Table 11A, page 78	N. gonorrhoeae, chlamydia, bacteroides, Enterobacteria-ceae, streptococci	**Outpatient rx: [(Oflox** 400 mg po bid or **Levo** 500 mg po q24h) ± **metro** 500 mg po bid times 14 days] **OR [(ceftriaxone** 250 mg IM or IV times 1) ± **metro** 500 mg po bid times 14 days] + (**doxy** 100 mg po bid times 14 days)]	**Inpatient regimens: [(Cefotetan** 2 gm IV q12h or **cefoxitin** 2 gm IV q6h) ± (**doxy** 100 mg IV/po q12h)] OR **[Clinda** 900 mg IV q8h) + (**gentamicin** 2 mg per kg loading dose, then 1.5 mg per kg q8h or 4.5 mg per kg once per day), then **doxy** 100 mg po bid times 14 days	Alternative parenteral regimens: 1. (Oflox 400 mg IV q12h or Levo 500 mg IV q24h) + metro 500 mg IV q8h 2. AM-SB 3 gm IV q6h + doxy 100 mg IV/po q12h + Levo Remember: Evaluate and treat sex partner.
Vaginitis—MMWR 51 (RR-6), 2002 or CID 35 (Suppl.2):S135, 2002				
Candidiasis Pruritus, thick cheesy discharge, pH <4.5 See Table 11A, page 78	Candida albicans 80–90%. C. glabrata, C. tropicalis may be increasing—they are less susceptible to azoles.	**Oral azoles: Fluconazole** 150 mg po times 1; **itraconazole** 200 mg po bid times 1 day	**Intravaginal azoles:** variety of strengths—from 1 dose to 7–14 days. Drugs available (all end in -azole): butocon, clotrim, micon, tiocon, tercon (doses: Table 11A, footnote[1], page 78)	Nystatin vag. tabs times 14 days less effective. Other rx for azole-resistant strains: gentian violet, boric acid. If recurrent candidiasis (4 or more episodes per yr): 6 mos. suppression with: fluconazole 150 mg po q week or itraconazole 100 mg po q24h or clotrimazole vag. suppositories 500 mg q week.

[1] **P Ceph 2 (cefoxitin** 2 gm IV q6–8h; **cefotetan** 2 gm IV q12h; **cefuroxime** 750 mg IV q8h); **TC-CL** 3.1 gm IV q4–6h; **AM-SB** 3 gm IV q6h; **PIP-TZ** 3.375 gm IV q6h; **P Ceph 3 (cefotaxime** 2 gm IV q8h; **ceftriaxone** 2 gm IV q24h); **ertapenem** 1 gm IV q24h; **doxy** 100 mg IV/po q12h; **clinda** 450–900 mg IV q8h; **APAG (gentamicin,** see Table 10D, page 74); **P Ceph 3 (cefotaxime** 2 gm IV q8h; **ceftriaxone** 2 gm IV q24h; **cefotaxime** 2 gm IV q8h; **vanco** 1 gm IV q12h; **IMP** 0.5 gm IV q6h; **MER** 1 gm IV q8h; **azithro** 500 mg IV/po q12h; **vanco** 1 gm IV q12h; **linezolid** 600 mg IV/po q12h
Abbreviations on page 2. NOTE: All dosage recommendations are for adults (unless otherwise indicated) and assume normal renal function.

TABLE 1 (17)

ANATOMIC SITE/DIAGNOSIS/ MODIFYING CIRCUMSTANCES	ETIOLOGIES (usual)	SUGGESTED REGIMENS*		ADJUNCT DIAGNOSTIC OR THERAPEUTIC MEASURES AND COMMENTS
		PRIMARY	ALTERNATIVE§	
GENITAL TRACT, Women/Vaginitis *(continued)*				
Trichomoniasis Copious foamy discharge, pH >4.5 Treat sexual partners—see *Comment*	Trichomonas vaginalis	**Metro** 2 gm as single dose or 500 mg po bid times 7 days OR **Tinidazole** 2 gm po single dose **Pregnancy:** See *Comment*	**For rx failure:** Re-treat with metro 500 mg po bid times 7 days; if 2nd failure: metro 2 gm po q24h times 3–5 days. If still failure, suggest ID consultation and/or contact CDC: 770-488-4115 or www.cdc.gov/std.	**Treat male sexual partners (2 gm metronidazole as single dose).** Nearly 20% men with NGU are infected with trichomonas *(IJID 188:465, 2003).* Another option if metro-resistant: **Tinidazole** 500 mg po qid + intravaginal 500 mg po bid times 14 days. Ref.: *C/D 33:1341, 2001.* **Pregnancy:** No data indicating metro teratogenic or mutagenic *[MMWR 51(RR-6), 2002]*.
Bacterial vaginosis Malodorous vaginal discharge, pH >4.5	Polymicrobic: associated with Gardnerella vaginalis, bacteroides non-fragilis, mobiluncus, peptococci, Mycoplasma hominis	**Metro** 0.5 gm po bid times 7 days or **metro vaginal gel¹** (1 applicator intravaginally) 1 time per day times 5 days.	**Clinda** 0.3 gm po bid times 7 days or **2% clinda vaginal cream** 5 gm intravaginally at bedtime times 7 days or **clinda ovules** 100 mg intravaginally at bedtime times 3 days.	Rx of male sex partner **not** indicated unless balanitis present. **Metro 2 gm po times 1 not as effective as 5–7 day course** *(JAMA 268:92, 1992).* Metro extended release tabs 750 mg po q24h times 7 days available: no published data. **Pregnancy:** Rx same as non-pregnancy, except avoid clindamycin cream (↑ risk premature birth). Treatment of asymptomatic pts with oral clinda ↓ premature birth *(Ln 361:983, 2003).*
Men:				
Balanitis	Candida 40%, Group B strep, gardnerella	Oral **azoles** as for vaginitis		Occurs in ¼ of male sex partners of women infected with candida. Exclude circinate balanitis (Reiter's syndrome). Plasma cell balanitis (non-infectious) responds to hydrocortisone cream.
Epididymo-orchitis Age <35 years	N. gonorrhoeae, Chlamydia trachomatis	**Ceftriaxone** 250 mg IM times 1 + **doxy** 100 mg po bid times 10 days or **Oflox** 300 mg po bid times 10 days.		Also: bedrest, scrotal elevation, and analgesics.
Age >35 years or homosexual men (insertive partners in anal intercourse)	Enterobacteriaceae (coliforms)	**FQ: (CIP:** **CIP-ER** 500 mg po 1 time per day or **CIP** 400 mg IV bid or **Levo** 750 mg IV/po 1 time per day) times 10–14 days	**AM-SB, P Ceph 3, TC-CL, PIP-TZ** *(Dosage: see footnote page 19)*	Midstream pyuria and scrotal pain and edema. Also: bedrest, scrotal elevation, and analgesics.
Prostatitis—Review: *AJM 106:327, 1999*				
Acute ≤35 years of age	N. gonorrhoeae, C. trachomatis	**Oflox** 400 mg po times 1 then 300 mg po bid times 10 days or **ceftriaxone** 250 mg IM times 1 then **doxy** 100 mg po bid times 10 days.		Oflox effective vs gonococci & C. trachomatis and penetrates prostate. In AIDS pts, prostate may be focus of Cryptococcus neoformans.
≥35 years of age	Enterobacteriaceae (coliforms)	**FQ** *(dosage: see Epididymo-orchitis, >35 yrs, above)* or **TMP-SMX** 1 DS tablet (160 mg TMP) po bid times 10–14 days		Treat as acute urinary infection, 14 days (not single dose regimen). Some authorities recommend 3–4 week rx *(IDCP 4:325, 1995).*
Chronic bacterial	Enterobacteriaceae 80%, enterococci 15%, P. aeruginosa	**FQ (CIP** 500 mg po bid times 4 weeks, **Levo** 500 mg po q24h times 4 weeks—see *Comment*	**TMP-SMX-DS** 1 tab po bid times 1–3 mos.	With rx failures consider infected prostatic calculi.
Chronic prostatitis/chronic pain syndrome (New NIH classification, *JAMA 282:236, 1999*)	The most common prostatitis syndrome. Etiology is unknown, molecular probe data suggest infectious etiology *(Clin Micro Rev 11: 604, 1998).*	**(α-adrenergic blocking agents are controversial** *(AnIM 133:367, 2000).*		Pt has sx of prostatitis but negative cultures and no cells in prostatic secretions. Rev. *JAC 46:157, 2000.* In randomized double-blind study, CIP and an alpha-blocker of no benefit *(AnIM 141:581 & 639, 2004).*

¹ 1 applicator contains 5 gm of gel with 37.5 mg metronidazole
Abbreviations on page 2
NOTE: All dosage recommendations are for adults (unless otherwise indicated) and assume normal renal function

TABLE 1 (18)

ANATOMIC SITE/DIAGNOSIS/ MODIFYING CIRCUMSTANCES	ETIOLOGIES (usual)	SUGGESTED REGIMENS* PRIMARY	ALTERNATIVE§	ADJUNCT DIAGNOSTIC OR THERAPEUTIC MEASURES AND COMMENTS
HAND (*Bites: See Skin*)				
Paronychia				
Nail biting, manicuring	Staph. aureus (maybe MRSA)	I&D; do culture	**TMP-SMX-DS** 2 tabs po bid while waiting for culture result.	*See Table 6 for alternatives*
Contact with oral mucosa—dentists, anesthesiologists, wrestlers	Herpes simplex (Whitlow)	**Acyclovir** 400 mg tid po times 10 days	**Famciclovir** or **valacyclovir** should work; see *Comment*	Gram stain and routine culture negative. Famciclovir/valacyclovir doses used for primary genital herpes should work; see *Table 14, page 110*
Dishwasher (prolonged water immersion)	Candida sp.	**Clotrimazole** (topical)		Avoid immersion of hands in water as much as possible.
HEART				
Atherosclerotic coronary artery disease	Chlamydia pneumoniae—under study	New name: Chlamydophila pneumoniae. Ref.: *JAMA 290:1459 & 1515, 2003*		
Infective endocarditis—Native valve—empirical rx awaiting cultures—No IV illicit drugs		NOTE: Diagnostic criteria include evidence of continuous bacteremia (multiple positive blood cultures), new murmur (worsening of old murmur) of valvular insufficiency, definite emboli, and echocardiographic (transthoracic or transesophageal) evidence of valvular vegetations. Refs.: *Circulation 111:3167, 2005; Ln 363:139, 2004*		
Valvular or congenital heart disease including mitral valve prolapse but no modifying circumstances *See Table 15C, page 127 for prophylaxis*	Viridans strep 30–40%, "other" strep 15–25%, enterococci 5–18%, staphylococci 20–35%	[(**Pen G** 20 million units IV q24h, continuous or div. q4h) or (**AMP** 12 gm IV q24h, continuous or div. q4h)] + (**nafcillin** or **oxacillin** 2 gm IV q4h) + **gentamicin** 1 mg per kg IM or IV q8h (*see Comment*)]	**Vanco** 15 mg per kg¹ IV q12h (not to exceed 2 gm q24h unless serum levels monitored) + **gentamicin** 1 mg per kg IM or IV q8h.	If patient not acutely ill and not in heart failure, we prefer to wait for blood culture results. If initial 3 blood cultures neg. after 24–48 hrs, obtain 2–3 more blood cultures before empiric rx started. Nafcillin/oxacillin + gentamicin may not be adequate coverage of enterococci, hence addition of penicillin G pending cultures. When blood cultures +, modify regimen from empiric to specific based on organism, in vitro susceptibilities, clinical experience. **Gentamicin** used for synergy, peak levels need not exceed 4 mcg per mL.
Infective endocarditis—Native valve—IV illicit drug use ± evidence rt-sided endocarditis—empiric rx	S. aureus. All others rare	**Vanco** 1 gm IV q12h	**Dapto** 6 mg per kg q24h (*not FDA-approved indication, 9/04*)	Dapto clinical trials for bacteremia/endocarditis in progress. Quinupristin-dalfopristin cidal vs S. aureus if both constituents active.
Infective endocarditis—Native valve—culture positive (*JAMA 274:1706, 1995; NEJM 345:1318, 2001; CID 36:615, 2003; JAC 54:971, 2004²*)				
Viridans strep, S. bovis with penicillin G MIC ≤0.1 mcg per mL	Viridans strep, S. bovis	[(**Pen G** 12–18 million units per day IV, continuous or q4h times 2 wks) PLUS (**gentamicin** IV 1 mg per kg q8h IV times 2 wks)] **OR** (**Pen G** 12–18 million units IV, continuous or q4h times 4 wks) **OR** (**ceftriaxone** 2 gm IV q24h times 4 wks)	(**Ceftriaxone** 2 gm IV q24h + **gentamicin** 1 mg per kg IV q8h both times 2 wks). If allergy pen G or ceftriax, use **vanco** 15 mg per kg IV q12h to 2 gm per day max unless serum levels measured times 4 wks	Also effective: (ceftriaxone 2 gm IV q24h) + (netilmicin^NUS 4 mg per kg q24h) times 2 wks (*CID 21:1406, 1995*). Target gent levels: peak 3 mcg per mL, trough <1 mcg per mL. If very obese pt, recommend consultation for dosage adjustment. Infuse vanco over ≥1 hr to avoid "red man" syndrome. S. bovis suggests occult bowel pathology (new name: S. gallolyticus). Since relapse rate may be greater in pts ill for >3 mos. prior to start of rx, the penicillin-gentamicin synergism theoretically may be advantageous in this group.
Viridans strep, S. bovis (S. gallolyticus) with penicillin G MIC >0.1 to <0.5 mcg per mL	Viridans strep, S. bovis, nutritionally variant streptococci, tolerant strep³	**Pen G** 18 million units per day IV (continuous or q4h) times 4 wks PLUS **gentamicin** 1 mg per kg IV q8h times 2 wks NOTE: Low dose of gentamicin	**Vanco** 15 mg per kg IV q12h to max. 2 gm per day unless serum levels documented times 4 wks	Can use cefazolin for pen G in pt with allergy that is not IgE-mediated (e.g., anaphylaxis). Alternatively, can use vanco. (*See Comment above on gent and vanco*) NOTE: **If necessary to remove infected valve & valve culture neg., 2 weeks antibiotic treatment post-op sufficient** (*CID 41:187, 2005*).

---

¹ Assumes estimated creatinine clearance ≥80 mL per min., *see Table 17*
² Ref. for Guidelines of British Soc. for Antimicrob. Chemother. Includes drugs not available in U.S.: flucloxacillin IV, teicoplanin IV
³ Tolerant streptococci = MBC 32-fold greater than MIC

Abbreviations on page 2.   NOTE: *All dosage recommendations are for adults (unless otherwise indicated) and assume normal renal function.*

TABLE 1 (19)

ANATOMIC SITE/DIAGNOSIS/ MODIFYING CIRCUMSTANCES	ETIOLOGIES (usual)	SUGGESTED REGIMENS*		ADJUNCT DIAGNOSTIC OR THERAPEUTIC MEASURES AND COMMENTS
		PRIMARY	ALTERNATIVE§	
HEART/Infective endocarditis—Native valve—culture positive (continued)				
For viridans strep or S. bovis with **pen G MIC ≥0.5 and** enterococci susceptible to AMP/pen G, vanco, gentamicin NOTE: Inf. Dis. consultation suggested	**"Susceptible" entero-cocci, viridans strep, S. bovis, nutritionally variant streptococci** (new names are: Abiotrophia sp. & Granulicatella sp.)	[(Pen G 18–30 million units per 24h IV, continuous or q4h **times 4–6 wks) PLUS gentamicin** 1–1.5 mg per kg q8h IV **times 4–6 wks)]** OR (AMP 12 gm per day IV, continuous or q4h + **gent** as above **times 4–6 wks)**	**Vanco** 15 mg per kg IV q12h to max. of 2 gm per day unless serum levels measured **PLUS gentamicin** 1–1.5 mg per kg q8h IV **times 4–6 wks** NOTE: **Low dose of gent**	**4 wks of rx if symptoms <3 mos.; 6 wks of rx if symptoms >3 mos.** Vanco for pen-allergic pts; do not use cephalosporins. Do **not** give gent once-q24h for enterococcal endocarditis. Target gent levels: peak 3 mcg per mL, trough <1 mcg per mL. Vanco target serum levels: peak 20–50 mcg per mL, trough 5–12 mcg per mL. **NOTE:** Because of ↑ frequency of resistance (see below), all enterococci causing endocarditis should be tested in vitro for susceptibility to penicillin, β-lactamase production, gent susceptibility and vanco susceptibility.
Enterococci: MIC streptomycin >2000 mcg per mL; MIC gentamicin >500–2000 mcg per mL; no resistance to penicillin	**Enterococci, high-level aminoglycoside resist-ance**	**Pen G or AMP** IV as above **times 8–12** wks (approx. 50% cure)	If prolonged pen G/AMP fails, consider surgical removal of infected valve. See Comment	10–25% E. faecalis and 45–50% E. faecium resistant to high gent levels. May be sensitive to streptomycin, check MIC. Case report of success with combination of AMP, IMP, and vanco (Scand J Inf Dis 29:628, 1997).
Enterococci: β-lactamase production test is **positive** and **no gentamicin resistance**	**Enterococci, penicillin resistance**	**AM-SB** 3 gm IV q6h **PLUS gentamicin** 1–1.5 mg per kg q8h IV **times 4–6 wks. Low dose of gent**	**AM-SB** 3 gm IV q6h PLUS **vanco** 15 mg per kg IV q12h (check levels if >2 gm) **times 4–6 wks**	β-lactamase **not** detected by MIC tests with standard inocula. Detection requires testing with the chromogenic cephalosporin nitrocefin. **Once-q24h gentamicin rx not** efficacious in animal model of E. faecalis endocarditis (JAC 49:437, 2002).
Enterococci: β-lactamase test neg.; pen G MIC >16 mcg per mL; no gentamicin resistance	**Enterococci, intrinsic pen G/AMP resistance**	**Vanco** 15 mg per kg IV q12h (check levels if >2 gm) **PLUS gent** 1–1.5 mg per kg q8h IV **times 4–6 wks** (see Comment)		Desired vanco serum levels: peak 20–50 mcg per mL, trough 5–12 mcg per mL. **Gentamicin** used for synergy; peak levels need not exceed 4 mcg per mL.
Enterococci: Pen/AMP resistant + high-level gent/strep resistant + vanco resistant; usually VRE **Consultation suggested**	**Enterococci, vanco-resistant, usually E. faecium**	No reliable effective rx. Can try quinupristin-dalfopristin (Synercid) or linezolid—see Comment, footnote¹, and Table 5.	Teicoplanin active against a subset of vanco-resistant enterococci. Teicoplanin is not available in U.S.	Synercid activity limited to E. faecium and is usually bacteriostatic, therefore expect high relapse rate. Dose: 7.5 mg per kg IV (via central line) q8h. **Linezolid** active most enterococci, but bacteriostatic. Dose: 600 mg IV or po q12h. Linezolid failed in pt with E. faecalis endocarditis (CID 37:e29, 2003).
Staphylococcal endocarditis Aortic and/or mitral valve infection—MSSA	**Staph. aureus, methicillin-sensitive**	**Nafcillin** (oxacillin) 2 gm IV q4h **times 4–6 wks PLUS gentamicin** 1 mg per kg IV q8h **times 3–5 days NOTE: Low dose of gent for only 3–5 days.**	[(Cefazolin 2 gm IV q8h **times 4–6 wks) PLUS** (**gentamicin** 1 mg per kg IV q8h **times 3–5 days)]. Low dose of gent** OR **Vanco** 15 mg per kg IV q12h (check levels if >2 gm per day) **times 4–6 wks**	If IgE-mediated penicillin allergy, 10% cross-reactivity to cephalosporins (AnIM 141:16, 2004). Cefazolin failures reported (CID 37:1194, 2003). No definitive data, pro or con, on once-q24h gentamicin for S. aureus endocar-ditis. At present, favor q8h dosing times 3–5 days. ↑ recognition of IV catheter-associated S. aureus endocarditis. May need TEE to detect endocarditis. 23% of S. aureus bacteremia in association with IV catheter had endocarditis (CID 115:106 & 115, 1999); if TEE neg. may only need 2 wks of therapy.
Aortic and/or mitral valve—MRSA	**Staph. aureus, methicillin-resistant**	**Vanco** 1 gm IV q12h **times 4–6 wks**	**Dapto** 6 mg per kg IV q24h	**Quinupristin-dalfopristin** cidal if both components active (both active if S. aureus sensitive to erythro in vitro). Other alternatives less desirable because bacteriostatic, e.g., TMP-SMX, clinda, linezolid. See Table 6.
Tricuspid valve infection (usually IVDUs): **MSSA** (MRSA next page)	**Staph. aureus, methicillin-sensitive**	**Nafcillin** (oxacillin) 2 gm IV q4h PLUS **genta-micin** 1 mg per kg IV q8h **times 2 wks. NOTE: low dose of gent**	If penicillin allergy: Not clear. High failure rate with 2 wks of vanco + gentamicin (CID 33:120, 2001). Can try longer duration rx of **vanco ± RIF** (if sensitive).	**2-week regimen not recommended if metastatic infection (e.g., osteo) or left-sided infection.** 2 reports of success with **4-week oral** regimen: CIP 750 mg bid + RIF 300 mg bid. Less than 10% pts had MRSA (Ln 2:1071, 1989; AJM 101:68, 1996).

¹ Three interesting recent reports: (1) Successful rx of vanco-resistant E. faecium prosthetic valve bacteremia with Synercid without change in MIC (CID 25:163, 1997); (2) resistance to Synercid emerged during therapy of E. faecium bacteremia (CID 24:91, 1997); and (3) super-infection with E. faecalis occurred during Synercid rx of E. faecium (CID 24:91, 1997).
Abbreviations on page 2. NOTE: All dosage recommendations are for adults (unless otherwise indicated) and assume normal renal function.

TABLE 1 (20)

ANATOMIC SITE/DIAGNOSIS/ MODIFYING CIRCUMSTANCES	ETIOLOGIES (usual)	SUGGESTED REGIMENS*		ADJUNCT DIAGNOSTIC OR THERAPEUTIC MEASURES AND COMMENTS
		PRIMARY	ALTERNATIVE§	
HEART, Infective endocarditis—Native valve culture positive/Staphylococcal endocarditis/Tricuspid valve infection (continued)				
Staph. aureus, methicillin-resistant Methicillin resistance (MRSA)	**Staph. aureus, methicillin-resistant**	**Vanco** 15 mg per kg IV q12h (check levels if >2 gm per day) **times 4–6 wks**	Fails/intolerant to vanco, can try **daptomycin, quinu-dalfo,** or **linezolid**[1]	For MRSA, no difference in duration of bacteremia or fever between pts rx with **vanco** or **vanco + RIF** (AnIM 115:674, 1991). **Daptomycin:** Endocarditis studies in progress. **Linezolid:** Bacteriostatic. See Table 6.
Slow-growing fastidious Gm-neg. bacilli	**HACEK group** (see Comments). Change to HABCEK if add Bartonella.	**Ceftriaxone** 2 gm IV q24h **times 4 wks**	**AMP** 12 gm q24h (continuous or div. q4h) **times 4 wks + gentamicin** 1 mg per kg IV/IM q8h **times 4 wks**	**HACEK (acronym for Haemophilus parainfluenzae, H. aphrophilus, Actino-bacillus, Cardiobacterium, Eikenella, Kingella)** H. aphrophilus resistant to vanco, clinda and methicillin. Penicillinase-positive HACEK organisms should be susceptible to AM-SB ± gentamicin. For haemophilus, see CID 24:1087, 1997.
Bartonella species (for bacteremia, see page 43—Urban trench fever) AAC 48:1921, 2004	B. henselae, B. quintana	Optimal rx evolving. Retrospective & open prospective trials support **gentamicin** 3 mg per kg IV once q24h times 14 days + **doxy** 100 mg bid times 4–6 wks		**Dx:** Immunofluorescent antibody titer ≥1:800; blood cultures only occ. positive, or PCR of tissue from surgery. **Surgery:** Over ½ pts require valve surgery; relation to cure unclear. B. quintana transmitted by body lice among homeless; asymptomatic colonization of RBCs described (Ln 360:226, 2002)
Infective endocarditis—"culture negative"	Etiology in 348 cases studied by serology, culture, histopath, & molecular detection: C. burnetii 48%, Bartonella sp. 28%, and rarely (Abiotrophia elegans, Mycoplasma hominis, Legionella pneumophila, Tropheryma whipplei—together 1%), & rest without etiology identified (most on antibiotic).	Fever, valvular disease, and ECHO vegetations ± emboli and neg. cultures. Rev.: Medicine 84:162, 2005		
Infective endocarditis—Prosthetic valve—empiric therapy (cultures pending)				
Early (<2 months post-op)	S. epidermidis, S. aureus. Rarely, Enterobacteriaceae, diphtheroids, fungi	**Vanco** 15 mg per kg IV q12h + **gentamicin** 1 mg per kg IV q8h + **RIF** 600 mg po q24h		Early surgical consultation advised. Watch for evidence of heart failure.
Late (>2 months post-op)	S. epidermidis, viridans strep, enterococci, S. aureus			
Infective endocarditis—Prosthetic valve—positive blood cultures	Staph. epidermidis	**(Vanco** 15 mg per kg IV q12h **times 6 wks + gentamicin** 1 mg IV q8h **times 14 days**	If S. epidermidis is susceptible to nafcillin/oxacillin in vitro (not common), then substitute nafcillin (or oxacillin) for vanco.	
Surgical consultation advised; retrospective analysis shows ↓ mortality of pts with S. aureus during antibiotic rx (CID 26:1302 & 1310, 1996); also, retrospective study showed ↑ risk of death 2° neuro events in assoc. with Coumadin rx (AnIM 159:473, 1999)	Staph. aureus	Methicillin sensitive: **(Nafcillin** 2 gm IV q4h + **RIF** 300 mg po q8h) **times 6 wks + gentamicin** 1 mg per kg IV q8h **times 14 days.** Methicillin resistant: **(Vanco** 1 gm IV q12h + **RIF** 300 mg po q8h) **times 6 wks + gentamicin** 1 mg per kg IV q8h **times 14 days.**		
	Viridans strep, enterococci	See infective endocarditis, native valve, culture positive, pages 21–23		
	Enterobacteriaceae or P. aeruginosa	**Aminoglycoside (tobra** if P. aeruginosa) + **(AP Pen** or **P. Ceph 3 AP** or **P Ceph 4)**	In theory, could substitute CIP for APAG, but no clinical data.	
	Candida, aspergillus	**Ampho B** ± an **azole,** e.g., fluconazole (Table 11, page 77)		High mortality. Valve replacement plus antifungal therapy standard therapy but some success with antifungal therapy alone (CID 22:262, 1996).
Infective endocarditis—Q fever LnID 3:709, 2003	Coxiella burnetii	**Doxy** 100 mg po bid + **hydroxychloroquine** 600 mg per day times 1.5–3 yrs (J Infection 45:127, 2002)		**Dx:** Complement-fix IgG antibody of 1:40 to phase II antigen diagnostic of acute Q fever. IgG C-F antibody of 1:200 to phase I antigen diagnostic of chronic Q fever (LnID 3:709, 2003). Want doxy serum conc. >5 mcg per mL (JID 188:1322, 2003).
Intracardiac-device related infections: Pacemaker/defibrillator, left ventricular assist device	S. aureus, S. epidermidis, rarely others	**Device removal + vanco** 1 gm IV q12h + **RIF** 300 mg po bid	**Device removal + dapto** 6 mg per kg IV q24h[NFDA-1] ± **RIF** (no data) 300 mg po bid	**Duration of rx after device removal:** For "pocket" or subcutaneous infection, 10–14 days; if lead-associated: endocarditis, 4–6 wks depending on organism. Refs.: Circulation 108:2015, 2003; NEJM 350:1422, 2004.

[1] **Daptomycin** 6 mg per kg IV q24h. **Quinupristin/dalfopristin** (Synercid) 7.5 mg per kg IV q24h. **Linezolid** 600 mg IV or po q12h.

Abbreviations on page 2.   NOTE: All dosage recommendations are for adults (unless otherwise indicated) and assume normal renal function.

TABLE 1 (21)

ANATOMIC SITE/DIAGNOSIS/ MODIFYING CIRCUMSTANCES	ETIOLOGIES (usual)	SUGGESTED REGIMENS*		ADJUNCT DIAGNOSTIC OR THERAPEUTIC MEASURES AND COMMENTS
		PRIMARY	ALTERNATIVE§	
HEART (continued)				
Pericarditis, purulent—empiric rx Rev.: Medicine 82:385, 2003	Staph. aureus, Strep. pneumoniae. Group A strep, Enterobacteriaceae	**Vanco + CIP** (Dosage, see footnote†)	**Vanco** or **CFP** (see footnote†)	Drainage required if signs of tamponade. Forced to use empiric vanco due to high prevalence of MRSA.
Rheumatic fever with carditis Ref.: Ln 366:155, 2005 For acute rheumatic fever, see page 44; reactive arthritis, below	Post-infectious sequelae of Group A strep infection (usually pharyngitis)	ASA, and usually prednisone 2 mg per kg po q24h for symptomatic treatment of fever, arthritis, arthralgia. May not influence carditis.		Clinical features: Carditis, polyarthritis, chorea, subcutaneous nodules, erythema marginatum. For Jones criteria: Circulation 87:302, 1993. Prophylaxis: see page 44
JOINT—Also see Lyme Disease, page 42				
Reactive arthritis				
Reiter's syndrome (See Comment for definition)	Occurs wks after infection with C. trachomatis, Campylobacter jejuni, Yersinia enterocolitica, Shigella/Salmonella spp.	Only treatment is non-steroidal anti-inflammatory drugs	Definition: Urethritis, conjunctivitis, arthritis, and sometimes uveitis and rash. Arthritis: asymmetrical oligoarthritis of ankles, knees, feet, sacroiliitis. Rash: palms and soles—keratoderma blennorrhagia; circinate balanitis of glans penis. HLA-B27 positive predisposes to Reiter's.	
Poststreptococcal reactive arthritis (See Rheumatic fever, above)	Immunologic reaction after strep pharyngitis: (1) arthritis onset in <10 days, (2) lasts months, (3) unresponsive to ASA	Treat strep pharyngitis and then NSAIDs (prednisone needed in some pts)	A reactive arthritis after a β-hemolytic strep infection in absence of sufficient Jones criteria for acute rheumatic fever. Ref.: Mayo Clin Proc 75:144, 2000.	
Septic arthritis: Treatment requires prompt and adequate drainage of purulent joint fluid and appropriate antimicrobial therapy				There is no need to inject antimicrobials into joints. Empiric therapy after collection
of blood and joint fluid for culture: review Gram stain of joint fluid. For full arthritis, see Ln 351:197, 1998.				
Infants <3 months (neonate)	Staph. aureus, Enterobacteriaceae, Group B strep, N. gonorrhoeae	**If MRSA no concern:** **(Nafcillin** or **oxacillin)** + **P Ceph 3**	**If MRSA concern: Vanco** + **P Ceph 3**	Blood cultures frequently positive. Adjacent bone involved in 2/3 pts. Group B strep and gonococci most common community-acquired etiologies.
Children (3 months–14 years)	Staph. aureus 27%, S. pyogenes & S. pneumo 14%, H. influenzae 3%, Gm-neg. bacilli 6%, other (GC, N. meningitidis) 14%, unknown 36%	**Vanco + P Ceph 3** until culture results available	(Dosage, see Table 16, page 133) See Table 16 for dosage Steroids ?—see Comment	Marked ↓ in H. influenzae since use of conjugate vaccine. NOTE: Septic arthritis due to salmonella has no association with sickle cell disease, unlike salmonella osteomyelitis. Duration of treatment varies with specific microbial etiology. Short-course steroid: Benefit reported (PIDJ 22:883, 2003).
Adults (review Gram stain): See page 42 for Lyme Disease				
Acute monoarticular At risk for sexually-transmitted disease	**N. gonorrhoeae** (see page 17), S. aureus, streptococci, rarely aerobic Gm-neg. bacilli	**Gram stain negative:** **Ceftriaxone** 1 gm IV q24h or **cefotaxime** 1 gm IV q8h clusters: **vanco** 1 gm or **ceftizoxime** 1 gm IV q8h	If Gram stain shows Gm+ cocci in IV q12h.	For rx comments, see Disseminated GC, page 17
Not at risk for sexually-transmitted disease	S. aureus, streptococci, Gm-neg. bacilli	**All empiric choices guided by Gram stain** **Vanco + P Ceph 3** |**Vanco+ (CIP** or **Levo)** For treatment duration, see Table 3		Differential includes gout and chondrocalcinosis (pseudogout). **Look for crystals in joint fluid.** NOTE: See Table 6 for MRSA treatment.
Chronic monoarticular	Brucella, nocardia, mycobacteria, fungi	See Tables 2, 11, & 12 For dosage, see footnote page 26		
Polyarticular, usually acute	**Gonococci:** B. burgdorferi, acute rheumatic fever; viruses, e.g., hepatitis B, rubella vaccine, parvo B19	Gram stain usually negative for GC. If sexually active, culture urethra, cervix, anal canal, throat, blood, joint fluid, and then: **ceftriaxone** 1 gm IV q24h		If GC, usually associated petechiae and/or pustular skin lesions and tenosynovitis. Consider Lyme disease if exposure areas known to harbor infected ticks. See page 42. Expanded differential includes gout, pseudogout, reactive arthritis (HLA-B27 pos.).

§**APAG** (see Table 10D, page 74), **IMP** 0.5 gm IV q6h, **MER** 1 gm IV q8h, **nafcillin** or **oxacillin** 2 gm IV q4h, **TC-CL** 3.1 gm IV q4h, **PIP-TZ** 3.375 gm IV q6h or 4.5 gm q8h, **AM-SB** 3 gm IV q6h, **P Ceph 1** (**cephalothin** 2 gm IV q4h or **cefazolin** 2 gm IV q8h), **CIP** 750 mg po bid or 400 mg IV bid, **vanco** 1 gm IV q12h, **RIF** 600 mg po q24h, **aztreonam** 2 gm IV q8h, **CFP** 2 gm IV q12h. Abbreviations on page 2.   NOTE: All dosage recommendations are for adults (unless otherwise indicated) and assume normal renal function.

ANATOMIC SITE/DIAGNOSIS/ MODIFYING CIRCUMSTANCES	ETIOLOGIES (usual)	SUGGESTED REGIMENS* PRIMARY	ALTERNATIVE§	ADJUNCT DIAGNOSTIC OR THERAPEUTIC MEASURES AND COMMENTS
JOINT (continued)				
Septic arthritis, post intra-articular injection	MSSE/MRSE 40%, MSSA/ MRSA 20%, P. aeruginosa, Propionibacteria	**NO empiric therapy.** Arthroscopy for culture/sensitivity, crystals, washout		Treat based on culture results x14 days (assumes no foreign body present).
Infected prosthetic joint CID 36:1157, 2003; JAC 53:127, 2004; NEJM 351:1645, 2004 See surgical options in Comments Drug dosages in footnote[1]	See below	**No empiric therapy.** Need culture & sens. results. Surgical options in Comment. Debridement & prosthesis retention; (**Pen G** or **ceftriax**) IV times 4 wks (CID 36:847, 2003) (**Nafcillin/oxacillin** IV + **RIF** po) times 6 wks (**Vanco** IV + **RIF** po) times 6 wks	(**Vanco** IV + **RIF** po) times 6 wks [(**CIP** or **Levo**—if suscepti-ble—po) + (**RIF** po)] **OR** (**linezolid** po) times 6 wks	**Surgical options: 1. 2-stage:** Remove infected prosthesis & leave spacer, anti-microbics, then new prosthesis. Highest cure rate. **2. 1-stage:** Remove infected prosthesis, debride, new prosthesis, then antimicrobics. **3. Extensive debridement & leave prosthesis in place.** Antimicrobic therapy. Other: Remove prosthesis & treat ± bone fusion of joint. Last: Chronic antimicrobic suppression. RIF bactericidal vs surface-adhering, slow-growing, & biofilm-producing bacteria. Never use RIF alone due to rapid development of resistance. Limited linezolid experience favorable (JAC 55:387, 2005). Watch for toxicity, Table 10C, page 70.
	P. aeruginosa	Ceftaz IV + (**CIP** or **Levo** po)		AAC 39:2423, 1995.
Rheumatoid arthritis	TNF inhibitors (adalimumab, etanercept, infliximab) ↑ risk of TBc, fungal infection (CID 38:1261, 2004). Treat latent TBc first (MMWR 53:683, 2004).			
Septic bursitis; Olecranon bursitis; prepatellar bursitis	Staph. aureus >80%, M. tuberculosis (rare), M. marinum (rare)	(**Nafcillin** or **oxacillin** 2 gm IV q4h or **dicloxacillin** 500 mg po qid) if MSSA	(**Vanco** 1 gm IV q12h or **linezolid** 600 mg po bid) if MRSA	**Initially aspirate q24h and treat for a minimum of 2–3 weeks.** If recurrence, surgical excision of bursa—should not be necessary often if treated for at least 3 weeks +. Ref.: Semin Arth & Rheum 24:391, 1995.
		Other doses, see footnote page 26		
KIDNEY, BLADDER AND PROSTATE [For review, see AJM 113(Suppl.1A):1S, 2002 & NEJM 349:259, 2003]				
Acute uncomplicated urinary tract infection (cystitis-urethritis) in females [NOTE: Routine urine culture not necessary; self-rx works (AnIM 135:9, 2001)]. Try to spare FQs (CID 39:75, 2004)				
NOTE: Resistance of E. coli to TMP-SMX approx. 15–20% (CID 36:183, 2003) & correlates with microbiological/ clinical failure (CID 34:1061 & 1165, 2002). **Recent reports of E. coli resistant to CIP & Levo as well**	Enterobacteriaceae (E. coli), Staph. saprophyticus, enterococci	Local E. coli resistant to TMP-SMX <20% & no allergy: **TMP-SMX-DS** bid times 3 days; if sulfa allergy, **NF** times 7 days or **fosfomycin** single dose	Local E. coli resistant ≥20% or TMP-SMX allergy: then 3 days of **CIP** 250 mg bid, **CIP-ER** 500 mg q24h, **Gati** 200 mg q24h, **Levo** 250 mg q24h. **Do not use Moxi or Gemi.**	7-day rx recommended in pregnancy [discontinue or do not use sulfonamides (TMP-SMX) near term (2 weeks before EDC) because of potential ↑ in kernicterus]. If failure on 3-day course, culture and rx 2 weeks. **Fosfomycin** 3 gm po times 1 less effective vs. E. coli than multi-dose TMP-SMX or FQ (Med Lett 39:66, 1997). Fosfo active vs E. faecalis; poor activity vs other coliforms. **Moxifloxacin & gemifloxacin:** Neither approved for UTIs. Do not use; inadequate urine concentration. **Phenazopyridine (Pyridium)**—non-prescription—may relieve dysuria: 200 mg po tid times 2 days. Hemolysis if G6PD deficient.
Risk factors for STD. Dipstick: positive leukocyte esterase or hemoglobin, neg. Gram stain	C. trachomatis	**Doxy** 100 mg po bid times 7 days	**Azithro** 1 gm po single dose	Pelvic exam for vaginitis & herpes simplex, urine LCR/PCR for GC and C. trachomatis.
Recurrent (3 or more episodes/ year) in young women	Any of the above bacteria	Eradicate infection, then TMP-SMX 1 single-strength tab po q24h long term	TMP-SMX 1 single-strength	A cost-effective alternative to continuous prophylaxis is self-administered single dose rx (TMP-SMX DS, 2 tabs, 320/1600 mg) at symptom onset. Another alternative: 1 DS tablet TMP-SMX post-coitus.
Child: ≤5 yrs old and grade 3–4 reflux	Coliforms	**TMP-SMX** (2 mg TMP/10 mg SMX) per kg po q24h		**(TMP-SMX** (2 mg TMP/10 mg SMX) per kg po q24h) or **nitrofurantoin** 2 mg per kg po q24h. **CIP** approved as alternative drug ages 1–17 yrs.
Recurrent UTI in postmenopausal women See CID 30:152, 2000	E. coli & other Enterobacteriaceae, enterococci, S. saprophyticus	Treat as for uncomplicated UTI. Evaluate for potentially correctable urologic factors—see Comment. NF more effective than vaginal cream in decreasing frequency, but Editors worry about pulmonary fibrosis with long-term NF rx (CID 36:1362, 2003).		Definition: ≥3 culture + symptomatic UTIs in 1 year or 2 UTIs in 6 months. Urologic factors: (1) cystocele, (2) incontinence, (3) ↑ residual urine volume (≥50 mL).

[1] **Aqueous Pen G** 2 million units IV q4h, **nafcillin** or **oxacillin** 2 gm IV q4h, **vancomycin** 1 gm IV q12h, **RIF** 300 mg IV/po bid, **CIP** 750 mg IV/po bid, **Levo** 750 mg IV/po q24h, **ceftriaxone** 2 gm IV q24h, **ceftazidime** 2 gm IV q8h
Abbreviations on page 2.   NOTE: All dosage recommendations are for adults (unless otherwise indicated) and assume normal renal function.

TABLE 1 (23)

ANATOMIC SITE/DIAGNOSIS/ MODIFYING CIRCUMSTANCES	ETIOLOGIES (usual)	SUGGESTED REGIMENS* PRIMARY	ALTERNATIVE§	ADJUNCT DIAGNOSTIC OR THERAPEUTIC MEASURES AND COMMENTS
KIDNEY, BLADDER AND PROSTATE *(continued)*				
Acute uncomplicated pyelonephritis (usually women 18–40 yrs, temperature >102°F, definite costovertebral tenderness) [NEJM 335:635, 1996]. **If male, look for obstructive uropathy or other complicating pathology.**				
Moderately ill (outpatient) NOTE: Increasing resistance of E. coli to both TMP-SMX & FQs a concern	Enterobacteriaceae (most likely E. coli), enterococci (Gm stain of **uncentrifuged** urine may allow identification of Gm-neg. bacilli vs Gm + cocci)	An **FQ** po times 7 days: **CIP** 500 mg bid or **CIP-ER** 1000 mg q24h, **Levo** 250 mg q24h, **Oflox** 400 mg bid	**AM-CL,**[1] **O Ceph,** or **TMP-SMX-DS.** Treat for 14 days.	[NOTE: Culture of urine and blood indicated prior to therapy. Report of hemolytic uremic syndrome as result of toxin-producing E. coli UTI (NEJM 335:635, 1996).] In randomized double-blind trial, bacteriologic and **clinical success higher for 7 days of CIP than for 14 days of TMP-SMX;** failures correlated with TMP-SMX in vitro resistance (JAMA 283:1583, 2000). Since CIP worked with 7-day rx, suspect other FQs effective with 7 d. of rx. Do not use Moxi or Gemi due to low urine concentrations.
Hospitalized	E. coli most common, enterococci 2nd in frequency	**FQ (IV)** or **(AMP + genta- micin)** or **P Ceph 3** or **AP Pen.** Treat for 14 days. Do not use cephalosporins for suspect or proven enterococcal infection	**TC-CL** or **AM-SB** or **PIP- TZ** or **ERTA.** Treat for 14 days. Dosages in footnote[1]	Treat IV until pt afebrile 24–48 hrs, then complete 2-wk course with oral drugs (as *Moderately ill, above)*. If no clinical improvement in 3 days, we recommend imaging. On CT if single focal mass-like lesion avg. response requires 6 d., if lesions diffuse avg. response 13 days. (AJM 93:289, 1992). **If pt hypotensive, prompt imaging (Echo or CT) is recommended to ensure absence of obstructive uropathy.** NOTE: **Cephalosporins & ertapenem not active vs enterococci.**
Complicated UTI/catheters Obstruction, reflux, azotemia, transplant, Foley catheter-related	Enterobacteriaceae, P. aeruginosa, enterococci	**(AMP + gent)** or **PIP-TZ** or **TC-CL** or **IMP** or **MER** times 2–3 wks Switch to po **FQ** or **TMP-SMX** when possible For dosages, see footnote[1]	**FQ:** **CIP, Gati, Levo,** **[V FQ:** **CIP, Gati, Levo,** times 2–3 wks	Rule out obstruction. Watch out for enterococci and P. aeruginosa—not all listed drugs have predictable activity. **CIP-ER** oral dose: 1000 mg q24h
Asymptomatic bacteriuria. IDSA Guidelines: CID 40:643, 2005				
Preschool children		Base regimen on C&S, not empirical		Diagnosis requires ≥10^5 CFU per mL urine of same bacterial species in 2 specimens obtained 3–7 days apart.
Pregnancy	Aerobic Gm-neg. bacilli & Staph. hemolyticus	Screen 1st trimester. If positive, rx 3–7 days with **amox, NF, O Ceph, TMP-SMX,** or **TMP** alone	**Vanco** if **MRSA**	Screen monthly for recurrence. Some authorities treat continuously until delivery (stop TMP-SMX 2 wks before EDC). ↑ resistance of E. coli to TMP-SMX.
Before and after invasive urologic intervention, e.g., Foley catheter	Aerobic Gm-neg. bacilli	Obtain urine culture and then rx 3 days with **TMP-SMX** DS, bid		In one study, single dose 2-TMP-SMX DS 80% effective (AnIM 114:713, 1991). Use of silver-alloy Foley catheter may ↓ risk of clinically significant bacteriuria (AJM 105:236, 1998; AnIM 160:3294, 2000).
Neurogenic bladder	No rx in asymptomatic; intermittent catheterization if possible			Ref.: AJM 113(1A):67S, 2002—Bacteriuria in spinal cord injured patient.
Asymptomatic, advanced age, male or female	No rx indicated unless in conjunction with surgery to correct obstructive uropathy; measure residual urine vol. in females; prostate exam/PSA in males.			
Malacoplakia	E. coli	**Bethanechol chloride** + (**CIP** or **TMP-SMX**)		Chronic pyelo with abnormal inflammatory response. See CID 29:444, 1999
Perinephric abscess Associated with staphylococcal bacteremia	Staph. aureus	**Nafcillin/oxacillin** or **P Ceph 1** (Dos- age, see footnote 24) if MSSA	**Vanco** if **MRSA**	Drainage, surgical or image-guided aspiration
Associated with pyelonephritis	Enterobacteriaceae	See pyelonephritis, complicated UTI, above		Drainage, surgical or image-guided aspiration
Prostatitis		See prostatitis, page 20		
Spinal cord injury pts with UTI	E. coli, Klebsiella sp., enterococci	**CIP** 250 mg times 14 days		Suspect assoc. pyelonephritis. In RDBPC* trial microbiologic cure greater after 14 vs 3 days of CIP (CID 39:658 & 665, 2004).

NOTE: bid = twice a day; tid = 3 times a day; qid = 4 times a day.   * RDBPC = Randomized double-blind placebo-controlled

[1] **AM-CL** 875/125 mg po q12h or 500/125 mg po tid or 2000/125 mg po bid. **aztreonam** 2 gm IV q8h. **FQ (IV)** [**CIP** 400 mg bid, **Gati** 400 mg q24h, **Levo** (250 mg po q24h for mild uncomplicated disease, 500 mg IV q24h for hospital pt)], **cefoxitin** 2.0 gm IV q8h, **P Ceph 3** [**cefotaxime** 1 gm IV q8h, **P Ceph 3 AP** [**ceftazidime** 2 gm IV q8h. **P Ceph 4** [**cefepime** 2 gm IV q12h. Enterococci, up to 2 gm IV q4h for life-threatening infections; **ceftriaxone** 1–2 gm IV q24h (use 2 gm under age 65)], **AP Pen** [PIP 3 gm IV q6h], **AM-SB** 3 gm IV q6h, **PIP-TZ** 3.375 gm IV q6h or for nosocomial pneumonia 4.5 gm IV q6h, **gentamicin** (see Table 10D, page 74), **TMP-SMX** 2.0 mg per kg (TMP) IV q6h, **P Ceph 3** 3.1 gm IV q8h), **ERTA** 1 gm IV q24h, **IMP** 0.5 gm IV q6h, **MER** 1 gm IV q8h, **Nafcillin** or **oxacillin** 2 gm IV q4h. For oral cephalosporin dosages, see Table 10C, page 69. **Dicloxacillin** 500 mg po q6h or 15 mg per kg IV q12h (max. 4 gm per day). **Vanco** 1 gm IV q12h, **linezolid** 600 mg IV/po q12h

TABLE 1 (24)

ANATOMIC SITE/DIAGNOSIS/ MODIFYING CIRCUMSTANCES	ETIOLOGIES (usual)	SUGGESTED REGIMENS* PRIMARY	ALTERNATIVE§	ADJUNCT DIAGNOSTIC OR THERAPEUTIC MEASURES AND COMMENTS
LIVER (for spontaneous bacterial peritonitis, see page 34)				
Cholangitis		See Gallbladder, page 13		
Hepatic abscess Pyogenic abscess ref.: CID 39:1654, 2004	Enterobacteriaceae (esp. Klebsiella sp.), bacteroides, enterococci, Entamoeba histolytica, Yersinia entero-colitica (rare) For echinococcus, see Table 13, page 102. For cat-scratch disease (CSD), see pages 33 & 41.	**Metro** + (**P Ceph 3** or **cefoxitin** or **TC-CL** or **PIP-TZ** or **AM-SB** or **FQ**) **AMP + APAG + metro** traditional & effective but AMP-resistant Gm-neg. bacilli increasing.	**Metro** (for amoeba) + either **IMP** or **MER** (Dosage, see footnote page 26)	**Serological tests for amebiasis should be done on all patients;** if neg., surgical drainage or percutaneous aspiration. In pyogenic abscess, ½ have identifiable GI source or underlying biliary tract disease. If amoeba serology positive, treat with metro alone without surgery. Metro included for both E. histolytica & bacteroides. **Hemochromatosis** associated with Yersinia enterocolitica liver abscess (CID 18:938, 1994); regimens listed are effective for yersinia.
Leptospirosis	Leptospirosis, see page 43			
Peliosis hepatis in AIDS pts	Bartonella henselae and B. quintana	See page 41		
Post-transplant biloma (CID 39:517, 2004)	Enterococci (incl. VRE), candi-da, Gm-neg. bacilli (P. aeru-ginosa 8%), anaerobes 5%	**Linezolid** 600 mg IV bid + **CIP** 400 mg IV q12h + **flu-conazole** 400 mg IV q24h	**Dapto** 6 mg per kg per day + **Levo** 750 mg IV q24h + **fluconazole** 400 mg IV q24h	Suspect if fever & abdominal pain post-transplant. Exclude hepatic artery thrombosis. Presence of candida and/or VRE bad prognosticators.
UGI bleeding & cirrhosis		**CIP** 500 mg po bid times 7 days. Cautious support from recent meta-analysis: Cochrane Database 2002 (2): CD002907.		
Viral hepatitis	Hepatitis A, B, C, D, E, G	See Table 14		
LUNG/Bronchi				
Bronchiolitis/wheezy bronchitis (expiratory wheezing)				
Infants/children (≤ age 5) See RSV, Table 14B(3)	Respiratory syncytial virus (RSV) 50%, parainfluenza 25%, other viruses 20%	Antibiotics not useful, mainstay of rx is oxygen. Riba-virin (of no benefit (AJRCCM 160:829, 1999). 2 products available for prevention: **RSV-immune globulin** or a humanized mouse monoclonal antibody, **palivizumab**. See Table 14, page 113		RSV most important. Rapid dx with antigen detection methods. Ribavirin: No data on IV ribavirin but little enthusiasm. Emphasis now on vaccine development and preventive modulation with immunoglobulins. Reviews: PIDJ 19:773, 2000; Red Book of Peds 2003, 26th Ed.
Bronchitis				
Infants/children (≤ age 5)	< Age 2: Adenovirus; age 2–5: parainfluenza 3 virus	Antibiotics indicated only with associated sinusitis or heavy growth on throat culture for S. pneumo., Group A strep, H. influenzae or no improvement in 1 week. Otherwise rx is symptomatic.		
Adolescents and adults with acute tracheobronchitis (Acute bronchitis) Ref.: AnIM 162:256, 2002; AnIM 134:521, 2001	Usually viral. M. pneumoniae 5%; C. pneumoniae 5%. See Persistent cough, below	**Antibiotics not indicated.** Antitussive ± inhaled bronchodilators	Purulent sputum alone not an indication for antibiotic rx. Azithro was no better than low-dose vitamin C in a controlled trial (Ln 359:1648, 2002). Expect cough to last 2 weeks. If fever/rigors, get chest x-ray.	
Persistent cough (>14 d.), afebrile during community outbreak: Pertussis (whooping cough) 10–20% adults with cough > 14 d. have pertussis (CID 32:1691, 2001). Rev.: LnID 2:744, 2002	Bordetella pertussis & occ. Bordetella para-pertussis. Also consi-der asthma, gastro-esophageal reflux, post-nasal drip	**Peds doses: Azithro/ clarithro** (dose in foot-note[1]) OR **erythro esto-late** po 40 mg per kg per day div. q6-12h times14 days OR **erythro base** po 40 mg per kg per d div. q6h times14 days.	**Adult doses: Azithro** po 500 mg day 1, 250 mg q24h days 2–5 OR **erythro esto-late** 500 mg po qid times 14 days OR **TMP-SMX-DS** 1 tab po bid times14 days OR (**clarithro** 500 mg po bid times 7 days) or 1 gm ER q24h times 7 days). **See footnote[1]**	M. pneumoniae & C. pneumoniae ref.: LnID 1:334, 2001. Rare pt with true C. pneumo infection may require 6 wks of clarithro to clear organism (J Med Micro 52:265, 2003) **3 stages of illness:** catarrhal (1–2 wks), paroxysmal coughing (2–4 wks), and convalescence (1–2 wks). Treatment may abort or eliminate pertussis in catarrhal stage, but does not shorten paroxysmal stage. **Diagnosis:** PCR on nasopharyn-geal secretions or ↑ pertussis-toxin antibody. **Azithro** works fastest (PIDJ 22:847, 2003). **Rx at eradication of NP carriage. Azithro** at eradication of NP carriage. Azithro reported in infants under 6 wks of age given erythro (MMWR 48:1117, 1999).
Prophylaxis of household contacts		**Erythromycin—Children: clarithro:** 7.5 mg per kg po q6h times14 days. **Alternative: clarithro** 7.5 mg per kg po q12h times14 days. **Adults:** 500 mg po bid times 14 days. **See footnote[1]**		Recommended by Am. Acad. Ped. Red Book 2003 for all household or close con-tacts; community-wide prophylaxis not recommended.

[1] Peds doses: azithro 10 mg per kg per day on day 1, then 5 mg per kg q24h times 4 days (PIDJ 22:847, 2003) or clarithro 7.5 mg per kg po q12h times 5–7 days.

[2] Compliance with erythro poor due to nausea/vomiting; azithro costs more but compliance should be better.

Abbreviations on page 2. NOTE: All dosage recommendations are for adults (unless otherwise indicated) and assume normal renal function.

TABLE 1 (25)

ANATOMIC SITE/DIAGNOSIS/ MODIFYING CIRCUMSTANCES	ETIOLOGIES (usual)	SUGGESTED REGIMENS*		ADJUNCT DIAGNOSTIC OR THERAPEUTIC MEASURES AND COMMENTS
		PRIMARY	ALTERNATIVE[1]	
LUNG/Bronchi/Bronchitis (continued) **Acute bacterial exacerbation of chronic bronchitis (ABECB), adults (almost always smokers with COPD)** Pertinent refs.: Chest 118: 193, 2000; NEJM 347:465, 2002; CID 39:980 & 987, 2004; AnIM 165:891, 2005	Viruses 20–50%, C. pneumoniae 5%, M. pneumoniae <1%; role of S. pneumo, H. influenzae & M. catarrhalis controversial. Tobacco use, air pollution contribute.	**Severe ABECB** = ↑ dyspnea, ↑ sputum viscosity/purulence, ↑ sputum volume. For severe ABECB: (1) consider chest x-ray, esp. if febrile &/or low O₂ sat.; (2) inhaled anticholinergic bronchodilator; (3) oral corticosteroid; taper over 2 wks; (4) D/C tobacco use; (5) non-invasive positive pressure ventilation. **Role of antimicrobial rx** debated even for severe disease. **For mild or moderate disease, no antimicrobial treatment or maybe** amox, doxy, TMP-SMX, or O Ceph. **For severe disease,** AM-CL, azithro/clarithro, or O Ceph or telithro or FQs with enhanced activity vs drug-resistant S. pneumo (Gati, Gemi, Levo, or Moxi). **Drugs & doses** in footnote[1]. **Duration** varies with drug; range 3–10 d. Limit Gemi to 5 d. Placebo-controlled studies. Pul Pharm & Therap 14:449, 2001; Ln 358:2020, 2001.		
Pneumonia				
Neonatal: Birth to 1 month	**Viruses:** CMV, rubella, H. simplex **Bacteria:** Group B strep, listeria, coliforms, S. aureus, P. aeruginosa **Other:** Chlamydia trachomatis, syphilis	**AMP + gentamicin ± cefotaxime** Add **vanco** if MRSA a concern. For chlamydia rx, **erythro** 12.5 mg per kg po or IV qid times 14 days.		Blood cultures indicated. Consider C. trachomatis if afebrile pneumonia, staccato cough, IgM > 1:8; rx with erythro or sulfisoxazole. If MRSA documented, **vanco. TMP-SMX & linezolid** alternatives. **Linezolid** dosage birth to age 11 yrs is **10 mg per kg q8h.** Ref.: PIDJ 22(Suppl):S158,2003.

CONSIDER TUBERCULOSIS IN ALL PATIENTS; ISOLATE ALL SUSPECT PATIENTS

ANATOMIC SITE/DIAGNOSIS/ MODIFYING CIRCUMSTANCES	ETIOLOGIES (usual)	SUGGESTED REGIMENS*		ADJUNCT DIAGNOSTIC OR THERAPEUTIC MEASURES AND COMMENTS
		PRIMARY	ALTERNATIVE[1]	
Age 1–3 months (Adapted from NEJM 346:429, 2002) Pneumonitis syndrome. Usually afebrile	C. trachomatis, RSV, parainfluenza virus 3, Bordetella, S. pneumoniae, S. aureus (rare)	**Outpatient: po erythro** 10 mg per kg q6h or po **azithro** 10 mg per kg times1 dose, then 5 mg per kg times 4 days.	**Inpatient: If afebrile erythro** 10 mg per kg IV q6h or **azithro** 2.5 mg per kg IV q12h (see Comment). **If febrile,** add **cefotaxime** 200 mg per kg per day div q8h	Pneumonitis syndrome: cough, tachypnea, dyspnea, diffuse infiltrates, afebrile. Usually requires hospital care. Reports of hypertrophic pyloric stenosis after erythro under age 6 wks, not sure about azithro; bid azithro dosing theoretically might ↓ risk of hypertrophic pyloric stenosis. If lobar pneumonia, give AMP 200–300 mg per kg per day for S. pneumoniae. No empiric coverage for S. aureus, as it is rare etiology.
Age 4 months–5 years For RSV, see bronchiolitis, page 27, & Table 14 Refs.: NEJM 346:429, 2002; Ln 364:1141, 2004	RSV, other resp. viruses, S. pneumo, H. flu, mycoplasma, S. aureus (rare), M. tbc	*For RSV see bronchiolitis, page 27* **Outpatient: Amox** 100 mg per kg per day q8h. **Inpatient (not ICU):** No antibiotic if viral or IV **AMP** 200 mg per kg per day div q6h	**Inpatient (ICU): Cefotaxime** 200 mg per kg per day IV div q8h or **ceftriaxone** 50–75 mg per kg per day IV once per day.	Common 'other' viruses: rhinovirus, influenza, parainfluenza, adenovirus (PIDJ 19: 293, 2000). Often of mild to moderate severity. S. pneumo, non-type B H. flu in 4–20%. Treat times 10–14 days. NOTE: High frequency of resistance of DRSP to cefuroxime. See footnote[1], footnote 1 page 27, footnote 2 page 29, and Table 5, page 56, for rx of drug-resistant S. pneumo.
Age 5 years–15 years, Non-hospitalized, immunocompetent NEJM 346:429, 2002; PIDJ 21:592, 2002	Mycoplasma, Chlamydophila pneumoniae, S. pneumoniae, Mycobacterium tuberculosis Respiratory viruses; mixed, e.g., influenza Bacterial/viral infection in 23% (Peds 113:701, 2004)	[(**Amox** 100 mg per kg per day) + (**Clarithro** 500 mg po bid or 1 gm ER q24h; Peds dose: 7.5 mg per kg q12h)] OR (**azithro** 0.5 gm po times 1, then 0.25 gm per day. Peds dose: 10 mg per kg po, then 5 mg per kg per day, max. 250 mg)	[**Amox** 100 mg per kg per day) + [**Doxy** 100 mg po bid (if >8 yrs old) or **erythro** 500 mg po qid. (Peds dose: 10 mg per kg po q6h)]	If otherwise healthy and if not concomitant with (or post-) influenza, S. pneumoniae & S. aureus uncommon in this subset; suspect S. pneumo if sudden onset and large amount of purulent sputum. **Macrolide-resistant S. pneumo** an issue. Higher prevalence of macrolide-resistant S. pneumo in pts <5 yrs old (JAMA 266:1857, 2001). **Mycoplasma** PCR/viral culture usually not done for outpatients. **Mycoplasma requires 2–3 wks of rx,** C. pneumoniae up to 6 wks. (LnID 1:334, 2001; J Med Micro 52:265, 2003). Linezolid approved for peds use for pen-susceptible S. pneumo (including bacteremia) & methicillin-sensitive S. aureus.
		See Comment regarding macrolide resistance		

NOTE: bid = twice q24h; tid = 3 times a day; qid = 4 times a day.

[1] **TMP-SMX** 1 double-strength tab (160 mg TMP) po bid, **doxy** 100 mg po bid, **amox** 500 mg po tid, **AM-CL** 875/125 mg po bid or 500/125 mg po tid or 2000/125 mg po bid, adult dose of **O Ceph** (**cefaclor** 500 mg q8h or 500 mg CD [extended release] po q12h, **cefditoren** 200 mg tabs—2 tabs po bid, **cefpodoxime proxetil** 200 mg po q12h, **cefprozil** 500 mg po q12h, **loracarbef** 400 mg po q12h, **cefuroxime axetil** 250 or 500 mg po q12h, **cefdinir** 300 mg q12h or 600 mg q24h), **azithro** 500 mg po initial dose then 250 mg q24h times 4 or 500 mg po q24h times 3 days, **clarithro** 500 mg po q12h or **clarithro ER** 1000 mg po q24h times 7 days, **dirithromycin** 500 mg po q24h, **Oflox** 400 mg q12h, **Levo** 500 mg po q24h, or **Gati** 400 mg po q24h, **Gemi** 320 mg po q24h times 5 days. **Moxi** 400 mg po q24h times 5 days. **Ketolide: Telithromycin** 800 mg po q24h times 5 days.

NOTE: CIP and ceftibuten have relatively poor in vitro activity vs S. pneumo

NOTE: All dosage recommendations are for adults (unless otherwise indicated) and assume normal renal function.

Abbreviations on page 2.

TABLE 1 (3)

ANATOMIC SITE/DIAGNOSIS/ MODIFYING CIRCUMSTANCES	ETIOLOGIES (usual)	SUGGESTED REGIMENS* PRIMARY	ALTERNATIVE§	ADJUNCT DIAGNOSTIC OR THERAPEUTIC MEASURES AND COMMENTS
LUNG/Pneumonia (continued) **Children, hospitalized, immunocompetent—2–18 yrs**	S. pneumoniae, viruses, mycoplasma; consider S. aureus if abscesses or necrotizing	**Ceftriaxone** 50 mg per kg per day IV (to max 2 gm per day) + **azithro** 10 mg per kg per day up to 500 mg IV div q12h. Add anti-staph drug if evidence of lung necrosis		**Alternatives are a problem in children:** If proven S. pneumo resistant to azithro & ceftriaxone (or severe ceftriaxone allergy): IV vanco, linezolid, or off-label respiratory FQ. No doxy under age 8. Linezolid reported efficacious in children (PIDJ 22:677, 2003). Cefuroxime failures vs drug-resistant S. pneumo (CID 29:462, 1999).
Adults (over age 18)—See IDSA Guidelines (CID 37:1405, 2003; Chest 125:1888 & 1913, 2004; AJM 117(3A):39S, 2004; Thorax 56(Suppl):1, 2001)				
Community-acquired, not hospitalized Guidelines reflect variable approaches: **No co-morbidity** **1.** Focus on S. pneumo, ignore atypicals, & empha-size **high dose amox** or **AM-CL** **2.** If no co-morbidity, focus on atypicals, & emphasize **macrolides** that are still active vs majority of S. pneumo **3.** Focus on both S. pneumo & atypicals by combining (**high dose amox + a macrolide**) OR suggesting a **respiratory FQ** OR **telithromycin**	Varies with clinical setting. **No co-morbidity:** Atypicals—M. pneumoniae, et al., S. pneumo, viral **Co-morbidity:** Alcoholism: S. pneumo, anaerobes, coliforms Bronchiectasis: see Cystic fibrosis, page 32 COPD: H. influenzae, M. catarrhalis, S. pneumo IVDU: Hematogenous S. aureus Post-CVA aspiration: Oral flora, incl. S. pneumo Post-obstruction of bronchi: S. pneumo, anaerobes Post-viral: e.g. influenza	**No co-morbidity:** **Azithro** 0.5 gm po times 1, then 0.25 gm per day or **azithro-ER** 2 gm po times 1 OR **clarithro** 500 mg po bid or **clarithro-ER** 1 gm po q24h OR **doxy** 100 mg po bid **Co-morbidity:** (**amox** or **clarithro**) + (**amox**, high dose **AM-CL**) **Duration of rx:** S. pneumo—Not bacteremic: until afebrile 3 days —Bacteremic: 10–14 days reasonable C. pneumoniae—Unclear. Some reports suggest 21 days. Some bronchitis pts required 5–6 wks of clarithro (J Med Micro 52:265, 2003) Legionella—10–21 days Necrotizing pneumo 2° to coliforms, S. aureus, anaerobes: ≥2 weeks	**Co-morbidity present:** **Respiratory FQ** (see footnote[2]) OR [(**azithro** or **clarithro**) + (high dose **amox**, high dose **AM-CL**, **cefpodoxime** or **cefprozil**)] OR **telithromycin** Doses in footnote[3]	**Azithro/clarithro:** Pro: appropriate spectrum of action; more in vitro resistance than clinical failure [CID 34(Suppl 1):S27, 2002; q24h dosing; better tolerated than erythro Con: Overall S. pneumo resistance in vitro 20–30% [CID 34(Suppl 1):S4, 2002]. If pen G resist. S. pneumo, up to 50%+ resistance. Breakthrough infections reported (NEJM 346:630, 2002; CID 35:556, 2002) **Amoxicillin:** Pro: Active 90–95% S. pneumo at 3–4 gm per day Con: No activity atypicals or β-lactamase + bacteria. Need 3–4 gm per day **AM-CL:** Pro: spectrum includes β-lactamase + H. influenzae, M. catarrhalis, MSSA, & Bacteroides sp. Con: No activity atypicals **Cephalosporins**—po: Cefditoren, cefpodoxime, cefprozil, cefuroxime & others—see footnote[3] Pro: Active 75–85% S. pneumo & H. influenzae. Cefuroxime least active & higher mortality rate when S. pneumo resistant (CID 37:230, 2003) Con: Inactive vs atypical pathogens **Doxycycline:** Pro: Active vs S. pneumo (DMID 49:147, 2004) but resistance may be increasing. Active vs H. influenzae, atypicals, & bioterrorism agents (anthrax, plague, tularemia) Con: Resistance of S. pneumo 18–20% (CID 35:633, 2002). Sparse clinical data (ArIM 159: 266, 1999; CID 37:870, 2003). **FQs—Respiratory FQs:** Pro: In vitro & clinically effective vs pen-sensitive & pen-resistant S. pneumo. **NOTE: dose of Levo is 750 mg q24h.** Q24H dosing. Gemi only available po. Con: Geographic pockets of resistance with clinical failure (NEJM 346:747, 2002). Drug-drug interactions (see Table 22A, page 147). Unique reversible rash in young females given Gemi
Community-acquired, hospitalized—NOT in the ICU Empiric therapy S. pneumo resistance data (TRUST8-2003-2004) %R Penicillin—high level: 18.6 Azithro/Erythro: 26	Etiology by co-morbidity & risk factors as above. Culture sputum & blood. S. pneumo, urine antigen reported helpful (CID 40: 1608, 2005). Legionella urine antigen helpful.	**Ceftriaxone** 2 gm IV q24h (1 gm IV q24h > age 65) + **azithro** 500 mg IV q24h	**Gati** 400 mg IV q24h or **Levo** 750 mg IV q24h or **Moxi** 400 mg IV q24h	**Ceftriaxone/cefotaxime:** Pro: Drugs of choice for pen-sens. S. pneumo, active H. influenzae, M. catarrhalis, & MSSA Con: Not active atypicals or pneumonia due to bioterrorism pathogens. Add macrolide for atypicals. **Telithromycin:** Pro: Virtually no resistant S. pneumo. Active vs atypical pathogens. Con: Only available po. Transient reversible blurry vision due to paralysis of lens accommo-dation; avoid in myasthenia gravis pts.

Footnotes for Ceph dosage: **Cefdinir** 300 mg po q12h, **cefditoren pivoxil** 200 mg, 2 tabs po bid, **cefpodoxime proxetil** 200 mg po q12h, **cefprozil** 500 mg po q12h, **high dose amox** 1 gm po tid; **high dose AM-CL**—use **AM-CL-ER** 1000/62.5 mg, 2 tabs po bid, **telithromycin** 800 mg po q24h times 7–10 days.
Abbreviations on page 2.   NOTE: All dosage recommendations are for adults (unless otherwise indicated) and assume normal renal function.

NOTE: q24h = once q24h; bid = twice q24h; tid = 3 times a day; qid = 4 times a day.

[1] Atypical pathogens: Chlamydophila pneumoniae, C. psittaci, Legionella sp., M. pneumoniae, C. burnetii (Q fever ref.: LnID 3:709, 2003)
[2] Respiratory FQs with enhanced activity vs S. pneumo with HLR to penicillin: **Gati** 400 mg IV/po q24h, **Gemi** 320 mg IV/po q24h, **Levo** 750 mg IV/po q24h, **Moxi** 400 mg IV/po q12h. Ketolide: **telithro** 800 mg po q24h.
[3] High dose amox = 1 gm po tid; high dose AM-CL (see footnote[3])

TABLE 1 (27)

ANATOMIC SITE/DIAGNOSIS/ MODIFYING CIRCUMSTANCES	ETIOLOGIES (usual)	SUGGESTED REGIMENS*		ADJUNCT DIAGNOSTIC OR THERAPEUTIC MEASURES AND COMMENTS
		PRIMARY	ALTERNATIVE§	
LUNG/Pneumonia/Adults (continued)				
Community-acquired, hospitalized—IN ICU Empiric therapy	Severe COPD: S. pneumo, H. influ, M. catarrhalis Legionella Post-influenza S. aureus Coliforms & P. aeruginosa rare unless bronchiectasis (see below)	**Aggressive attempts at micro. diagnosis justified:** Culture sputum, blood, maybe pleural fluid. **Urine antigen tests** for both Legionella & S. pneumoniae. Empiric therapy must be active vs S. pneumo & Legionella. **Gati** 400 mg IV q24h or **Levo** 750 mg IV q24h or **Moxi** 400 mg IV q24h	**Ceftriaxone** 2 gm IV q24h (1 gm IV q24h > age 65) or **azithro** 500 mg IV q24h) or **ERTA** 1 gm IV q24h + **azithro** 500 mg IV q24h (see Comment)	Various studies indicate improved outcome when azithro added to a β-lactam (CID 36:389 & 1239, 2003); AnM 164:1837, 2001 & 159:2562, 1999). Similar results in prospective study of critically ill pts with pneumococcal bacteremia (AJRCCM 170:440, 2004). **Ertapenem** could substitute for ceftriaxone but limited clinical experience. Need azithro for atypical pathogens. Do not use if suspect P. aeruginosa. Not all Legionella species detected by urine antigen; if suspicious culture or PCR on airway secretions.
Hospital-acquired— usually with mechanical ventilation (empiric therapy) Diagnosis confirmed by quantitative cultures (see Comment) Guidelines: AJRCCM 171:388, 2005	Highly variable depending on clinical setting: S. pneumo, S. aureus, Legionella, coliforms, P. aeruginosa, stenotrophomonas, acinetobacter,¹ anaerobes all possible	**(IMP** 0.5 gm IV q6h or **MER** 1 gm IV q8h) plus, if suspect legionella or bioterrorism, **respiratory FQ** (Gati, Levo or Moxi) NOTE: Regimen not active vs **MRSA**—see below	(Cefepime or **high-dose PIP-TZ²**) + tobra. Add resp. **FQ** if suspect legionella or bioterrorism. See Comment regarding diagnosis Dosages: See footnotes pages 19, 26, 28, & 29	**Dx of ventilator-associated pneumonia:** Fever & lung infiltrates often **not** pneumonia (Chest 106:221, 1994). Quantitative cultures helpful: bronchoalveolar lavage (> 10⁴ per ml. pos.) or protect. spec. brush (> 10³ per ml. pos.) Ref.: AJRCCM 165:867, 2002. **Microbial etiology:** No empiric regimen covers all possibilities. Regimens listed active majority of **S. pneumo, legionella, & most coliforms.** Regimens not active vs MRSA, Stenotrophomonas & others; see below: Specific rx when culture results known. **Ventilator-associated pneumonia—Prevention:** If possible, keep head of bed elevated 30° or more. Remove N-G, endotracheal tubes as soon as possible. If available, continuous subglottic suctioning. Limit stress ulcer prophylaxis. Refs.: NEJM 340:627, 1999; CCM 32:1396, 2004.
Hospital- or community-acquired, neutropenic pt (<500 neutrophils per mm³)	Any of organisms listed under community- & hospital-acquired + fungi (aspergillus) See Table 11	See Hospital-acquired, immediately above. Vanco not included in initial rx unless high suspicion of infected IV access or drug-resistant S. pneumo. Ampho not used unless still febrile after 3 days of high clinical likelihood. See Comment		[See consensus document on management of febrile neutropenic pt: CID 34:730, 2002.
Adults—Selected specific rx when culture results (sputum, blood, pleural fluid, etc.) available. Also see Table 2, page 49				
Burkholderia (Pseudomonas) pseudomallei (etiology of melioidosis) Ref.: Ln 361:1775, 2003	Gram-negative	**Initial parenteral rx:** **Ceftazidime** 30-50 mg per kg IV q6h or **IMP** 20 mg per kg IV q8h. Rx minimum 10 days & improving, then po therapy → see Alternative column	**Post-parenteral po rx:** (see Comment for children): **Chloro** 10 mg per kg q6h times 8 wks; **Doxy** 2 mg per kg bid times 20 wks; **TMP-SMX** 5 mg per kg (TMP component) bid times 20 wks	**Children ≤8 yrs old & pregnancy:** For oral regimen, use **AM-CL-ER** 1000/62.5, 2 tabs po bid times 20 wks. Even with compliance, relapse rate is 10%. Max. daily ceftazidime dose: 6 gm.
Haemophilus influenzae	β-lactamase negative	**AMP** IV, **amox** po.	**TMP-SMX, azithro/clarithro, doxy**	
	β-lactamase positive	**AM-CL. O Ceph 2/3. P Ceph 3. FQ, azithro/clarithro,**		
Klebsiella sp.—ESBL pos. & other coliforms⁴	β-lactamase positive	**IMP** or **MER**; if resistant, **polymyxin E (colistin)**		**25–35% strains β-lactamase positive. ↑ resistance to both TMP-SMX and doxy. See Table 10C, page 67 for dosages.** **ESBL⁴** inactivates all cephalosporins, β-lactam/β-lactamase inhibitor drug activ. not predictable; co-resistance to all FQs & often aminoglycosides. Ref.: JAC 51:1119, 2003. Best legionella website: www.legionella.org. Two international observational studies support the superiority of **Levo** over macrolides (CID 40:794 & 800, 2005).
Legionella species	Hospitalized/immunocompromised	**Azithro** IV or **Levo** IV or **Gati** IV or **Moxi** See Table 10C, pages 70 & 71 for dosages. Treat for 7–14 days (CID 39:1734, 2004)		

¹ If Acinetobacter sp., susceptibility to IMP & MER may be discordant (CID 41:758, 2005).

² **PIP-TZ** dose: 4.5 gm IV q6h

³ **Telithro** = telithromycin 800 mg po q24h

⁴ **ESBL** = Extended spectrum beta-lactamase

TABLE 1 (28)

ANATOMIC SITE/DIAGNOSIS/ MODIFYING CIRCUMSTANCES	ETIOLOGIES (usual)	SUGGESTED REGIMENS* PRIMARY	SUGGESTED REGIMENS* ALTERNATIVE§	ADJUNCT DIAGNOSTIC OR THERAPEUTIC MEASURES AND COMMENTS
LUNG/Pneumonia/Adults, when culture results available (continued)				
Moraxella catarrhalis	93% β-lactamase positive	**AM-CL.** O Ceph 2/3, P Ceph 2/3, macrolide,[1] telithro (see footnote 3 page 30). **FQ. TMP-SMX. Doxy** another option. See Table 10C, page 67 for dosages		
Pseudomonas aeruginosa	Often ventilator-associated	**PIP-TZ** 4.5 gm IV q6h + **tobra** 5 mg per kg IV once q24h (see Table 10D, page 74)	**NOTE:** High-dose **PIP-TZ** for P. aeruginosa	
Staphylococcus aureus	Nafcillin/oxacillin susceptible	**Nafcillin/oxacillin** 2 gm IV q4h	**Vanco** 1 gm IV q12h or **linezolid** 600 mg IV q12h	Retrospective analysis of 2 prospective randomized double-blind studies of hospital-acquired MRSA showed enhanced survival with linezolid, p 0.03 (Chest 124:1632, 2003); efficacy perhaps related to superb linezolid lung concentrations. Concern of possible misinterpretation of post hoc subgroup analysis (Chest 126:314, 2004).
	MRSA	**Vanco** 1 gm IV q12h	**Linezolid** 600 mg IV q12h	
Stenotrophomonas maltophilia		**TMP-SMX**	**TC-CL ± aztreonam**	In vitro synergy refs.: AAC 39:2220, 1995; CMR 11:57, 1998
Streptococcus pneumoniae	Penicillin-susceptible	**AMP** 2 gm IV q6h, **amox** 1 gm po tid, **macrolide,**[1] **pen G** IV,[2] **doxy.** O Ceph 2, P Ceph 2/3, **telithro** 800 mg po q24h. See Table 10C, page 67 for other dosages		1. Clinda may block toxin production 2. Rifampin penetrates CSF & intracellular sites. 3. If isolate shown penicillin-susceptible.
	Penicillin-resistant, high level	**FQs** with enhanced activity: **Gati, Gemi, Levo, Moxi** IV—see Table 5, page 56 for more data. If all culture results not possible (e.g., allergy). linezolid active: 600 mg IV or po q12h. **telithro** 800 mg po q24h		a. **Adults: Pen G** 4 million units IV q4h b. **Children: Pen G** <12 y/o: 50,000 units per kg IV q6h; >12 y/o: 4 million units IV q4h c. Constitutive & inducible β-lactamases—do not use pen or amp alone. 4. Do not use cephalosporins or TMP-SMX. 5. Erytho, azithro activity borderline; clarithro active. 6. No person-to-person spread. 7. Antitoxins in development
LUNG—Other				
Anthrax Inhalation (applies to oropharyngeal & gastrointestinal forms): Treatment (Cutaneous: See page 37) Refs.: JAMA 287:2236, 2002 & CID 41:1167, 2005. Clinical experience: JAMA 286:2549, 2001 CIP rationale: CID 39:303, 2004	Bacillus anthracis **To report possible bioterrorism event: 770-488-7100** Plague, tularemia: see Table 1B, page 48 Chest x-ray: mediastinal widening & pleural effusion (AnIM 139:337, 2003; Ln 364:449, 2004)	**Adults (including pregnancy): CIP** 400 mg IV q12h or **Levo** 500 mg IV q24h) **plus (doxy** 100 mg IV q12h) **plus (clindamycin** 900 mg IV q8h and/or **RIF** 300 mg IV q12h) Switch to po when able & lower CIP to 500 mg po q8h; clinda to 450 mg po q8h; & RIF 300 mg po bid Treat times 60 days. Other alternatives: Table 1B, page 48	**Adults (including pregnancy): Doxy 10** mg per kg IV q12h or 15 mg per kg po q12h) or **(Doxy** >8 y/o & > 45 kg: 100 mg IV q12h; >8 y/o & ≤45 kg: 2.2 mg per kg IV q12h; ≤8 y/o: 2.2 mg per kg IV q12h) **plus clindamycin** 7.5 mg per kg IV q6h **and/or RIF** 20 mg per kg (max. 600 mg) IV q24h. Treat times 60 days. See Table 16, page 133 for oral dosage.	1. Clinda may block toxin production 2. Rifampin penetrates CSF & intracellular sites. 3. If isolate shown penicillin-susceptible. a. **Adults: Pen G** 4 million units IV q4h b. **Children: Pen G** <12 y/o: 50,000 units per kg IV q6h; >12 y/o: 4 million units IV q4h c. Constitutive & inducible β-lactamases—do not use pen or amp alone. 4. Do not use cephalosporins or TMP-SMX. 5. Erytho, azithro activity borderline; clarithro active. 6. No person-to-person spread. 7. Antitoxins in development
Post-exposure prophylaxis	Info: www.bt.cdc.gov	**Adults (including pregnancy): CIP** 500 mg IV bid or **Levo** 500 mg po q24h) times 60 days. **Children: CIP** 20–30 mg per kg per day div q12h times 60 days.	**Adults (including pregnancy): Doxy** >8 y/o 100 mg po bid times 60 d. **Children (see Comment): Doxy** >8 y/o & >45 kg: 100 mg po bid; <8 y/o & ≤45 kg; 2.2 mg per kg po bid; ≤8 y/o: 2.2 mg per kg po bid. All for 60 days.	1. Once organism shows suscept. to penicillin, switch to amoxicillin 80 mg per kg per day div. q8h (max. 500 mg q8h); pregnant pt to amoxicillin 500 mg po tid. 2. Do **not** use cephalosporins or TMP-SMX. 3. Other FQs (Gati, Moxi) & clarithro should work but no clinical experience.
Aspiration pneumonia ± lung abscess Refs.: CID 40:015 & 923, 2005	Transthoracic culture in 90 pts—% of total isolates: anaerobes 34%, Gm-pos. cocci 26%, S. milleri 16%, Klebsiella pneumonia 25%, nocardia 3%	**PIP-TZ** 3.375 gm IV q6h (For nocardia, see Table 11, page 82)	**Ceftriaxone** 2 gm IV q24h plus **metro** 500 mg IV q6h or 1 gm IV q12h	Suggested regimens based on retrospective evaluation of 90 pts with cultures obtained by transthoracic aspiration (CID 40:915 & 923, 2005). Surprising frequency of Klebsiella pneumoniae. **Moxi** 400 mg IV/po q24h another option (CID 41:764, 2005).
Chronic pneumonia with fever, night sweats and weight loss	M. tuberculosis, coccidioidomycosis, histoplasmosis	See Tables 11, 12. For risk associated with TNF inhibitors, see CID 41(Suppl 3):S187, 2005.		HIV+, foreign-born, alcoholism, contact with TB, travel into developing countries

[1] **Macrolide** = azithromycin, clarithromycin, dirithromycin, and erythromycin: Dirithromycin serum levels inadequate for bacteremic S. pneumo.

[2] **IV Pen G dosage:** Blood cultures neg., & no meningitis, 2 million units IV q4h; blood cultures pos. & no meningitis, 2 million units IV q4h. Another option is continuous infusion (CI) 3 million units loading dose & then CI of 10–12 million units over 12 hrs (Chest 112:1657, 1997).

Abbreviations on page 2. NOTE: All dosage recommendations are for adults (unless otherwise indicated) and assume normal renal function.

TABLE 1 (29)

ANATOMIC SITE/DIAGNOSIS/ MODIFYING CIRCUMSTANCES	ETIOLOGIES (usual)	SUGGESTED REGIMENS* PRIMARY	ALTERNATIVE§	ADJUNCT DIAGNOSTIC OR THERAPEUTIC MEASURES AND COMMENTS
LUNG/Other *(continued)* **Cystic fibrosis Acute exacerbation of pulmonary symptoms.** Refs.: Ln 361:681, 2003; AJRCCM 168:918, 2003	S. aureus or H. influenzae early in disease; P. aeruginosa later in disease	**For P. aeruginosa: Tobra** 3.3 mg per kg IV q6h or 10 mg per kg IV q24h. Combine tobra with (**PIP or ticarcillin** 100 mg per kg q6h) **or ceftaz** 50 mg per kg IV q8h to max. of 6 gm per day. See footnote	**For S. aureus: (1) MSSA— oxacillin/nafcillin** q4h (Peds dose, Table 16). **(2) MRSA—vanco** 1 gm q12h & check serum levels. See Comment	Other options: **Clarithro** synergistic with **tobra** vs P. aeruginosa (AAC 46: 1105, 2002) + anti-inflammatory properties (Pharmacotherapy 22:227, 2002). **Azithro** modestly improved FEV₁, pts chronically infected with P. aeruginosa (JAMA 290: 1749, 2003). Once-daily aminoglycosides in CF, see JAC 50:553, 2002. For pharmacokinetics of aminoglycosides see footnote. **inhaled phenol-free tobra** 300 mg bid times 28 d., then no rx times 28 d., then repeat cycle (AJRCCM 167:841, 2003)
	Burkholderia (Pseudomonas) cepacia	**TMP-SMX** 5 mg per kg (TMP) IV q6h	**Chloro** 15–20 mg per kg IV/po q6h *For other alternatives, see Table 2*	B. cepacia has become a major pathogen. Patients develop progressive respiratory failure. 62% mortality at 1 year. **Fail to respond to APAG**, piperacillin, & ceftazidime. Patients with B. cepacia should be isolated from other CF patients. **NOTE:** 3- & 4-drug combinations under study in refractory pts (AAC 43:213, 1999)
Empyema. Ref.: CID 22:747, 1996;: Pleural effusion review: NEJM 346:1971, 2002				
Neonatal	Staph. aureus	See Pneumonia, neonatal, page 28		Drainage indicated.
Infants/children (1 month–5 yrs)	Staph. aureus, Strep. pneumoniae, H. influenzae	See Pneumonia, age 1 month–5 years, page 28		Drainage indicated.
Child >5 yrs to ADULT—Diagnostic thoracentesis; chest tube (see Table 10 or footnote page 26)				
Acute, usually parapneumonic *For dosage, see Table 10 or footnote page 26*	Strep. pneumoniae, Group A strep	**Cefotaxime** or **ceftriaxone** (Dosage, see footnote page 26)	**Vanco**	In large multicenter double-blind trial, intrapleural streptokinase did not improve mortality, reduce the need for surgery or the length of hospitalization (NEJM 352:865, 2005).
Subacute/chronic	Staph. aureus.: Check for MRSA H. influenzae	**Nafcillin** or **oxacillin** if MSSA **Ceftriaxone**	**Vanco** if MRSA **TMP-SMX** or **AM-SB**	Usually complication of S. aureus pneumonia &/or bacteremia. Pleomorphic Gm-neg. bacilli. ↑ resistance to TMP-SMX.
	Anaerobic strep, Strep. milleri, Enterobacteriaceae, M. tuberculosis	**Clinda** 450–900 mg IV q8h + **ceftriaxone**	**Cefoxitin** or **IMP** or **TC-CL** or **PIP-TZ** or **AM-SB** (Dosage, see footnote 1 page 26)	Pleomorphic Gm-neg. bacilli. If organisms not seen, treat as subacute. Drainage. If TB suspected, treat as subacute. Pleural biopsy with culture for mycobacteria and histology if TBc suspected (CID 22:747, 1996)
Human immunodeficiency virus infection (HIV+): See SANFORD GUIDE TO HIV/AIDS THERAPY				
CD4 T-lymphocytes <200 per mm³ or clinical AIDS Dry cough, progressive dyspnea, & diffuse infiltrate **Prednisone first if suspect pneumocystis** (see Comment)	Pneumocystis carinii most likely; also M. tbc, fungi, Kaposi's sarcoma, & lymphoma NOTE: AIDS pts may develop pneumonia due to DRSP or other pathogens—see next box below	*Rx listed here is for **severe** pneumocystis; see Table 13, page 98 for po regimens for **mild** disease.* **Prednisone 1st (see Comment), then : TMP-SMX** [IV: 15 mg / kg per day div q8h (TMP component) or po: 2 DS tabs q8h], total of 21 days	**Clinda** 600 mg IV q8h + **primaquine** 30 mg (base) po q24h) **or (pentamidine isethionate** 4 mg per kg per day IV) times 21 days See Comment	Diagnostic procedure of choice is sputum induction; if negative, bronchoscopy. Pts with PCP or <200 CD4 cells per mm³ should be on PCP prophylaxis for life. **Prednisone 40 mg bid po times 5 days then 40 mg q24h po times 5 days then 20 mg q24h po times 11 days is indicated with PCP (pO₂ <70 mmHg), should be given at initiation of anti-PCP rx; don't wait until pt's condition deteriorates** (Table 13, page 98). If PCP studies negative, consider bacterial pneumonia, TBc, cocci, histo, crypto, Kaposi's sarcoma or lymphoma. **Pentamidine not active vs bacterial pathogens.** **NOTE: Pneumocystis resistant to TMP-SMX, albeit rare, does exist.**
CD4 T-lymphocytes normal Acute onset, purulent sputum & pulmonary infiltrates ± pleuritic pain. **Isolate pt until TBc excluded: Adults**	Strep. pneumoniae, H. influenzae, aerobic Gm-neg. bacilli (including P. aeruginosa), Legionella rare, M. tbc	**P Ceph 3** (Dosages in footnotes on page 26) ± **azithro**. Could use **Gati, Levo,** or **Moxi** IV as alternative (see Comment)		If Gram stain of sputum shows Gm-neg. bacilli, options include **P Ceph 3 AP, TC-CL, PIP-TZ, IMP,** or **MER**. FQs: **Levo** 750 mg po/IV q24h; **Gati** 400 mg IV/po q24h; **Moxi** 400 mg po/IV q24h
As above: Children	Same as adult with HIV + lymphoid interstitial pneumonia (LIP)	As for HIV + adults with pneumonia. If diagnosis is LIP, rx with steroids.		In children with AIDS, LIP responsible for 1/3 of pulmonary complications, usually >1 yr of age vs PCP, which is seen at <1 yr of age. Clinically: clubbing, hepatosplenomegaly, salivary glands enlarged (take up gallium), lymphocytosis.

¹ Other options: (Tobra + aztreonam 50 mg per kg IV q8h); (IMP 15-25 mg per kg IV q6h + tobra); **CIP commonly used in children,** e.g., CIP IV/po + ceftaz IV (LnID 3:537, 2003). Abbreviations on page 2. NOTE: All dosage recommendations are for adults (unless otherwise indicated) and assume normal renal function.

TABLE 1 (30)

ANATOMIC SITE/DIAGNOSIS/ MODIFYING CIRCUMSTANCES	ETIOLOGIES (usual)	SUGGESTED REGIMENS* PRIMARY	SUGGESTED REGIMENS* ALTERNATIVE§	ADJUNCT DIAGNOSTIC OR THERAPEUTIC MEASURES AND COMMENTS
LUNG/Other *(continued)* **Viral (interstitial) pneumonia suspected** (See *Table 14, page 106*)	Consider: Adenovirus, coronavirus (SARS), hantavirus, influenza, metapneumovirus, parainfluenza virus, respiratory syncytial virus	**For influenza A or B: oseltamivir** 75 mg po bid times 5 d or **zanamivir** 10 mg inhaled bid times 5 d. Start within 48 hrs of symptom onset.	**For influenza A: rimantadine** 100 mg po q12h or **amantadine** 100 mg po q12h	No known efficacious drugs for adenovirus, coronavirus (SARS), hantavirus, metapneumovirus, parainfluenza or RSV. Need travel (SARS) & exposure (Hanta) history. RSV as serious as influenza in the elderly (*NEJM 352:1749 & 1810, 2005*).
LYMPH NODES (approaches below apply to lymphadenitis without an obvious primary source)				
Lymphadenitis, acute Generalized	Etiologies: EBV, early HIV infection, syphilis, toxoplasma, tularemia, Lyme disease, sarcoid, lymphoma, systemic lupus erythematosus, and **Kikuchi-Fujimoto disease** (*CID 39:138, 2004*). Complete history and physical examination followed by appropriate serological tests. Treat specific agent(s).			
Regional Cervical—**see cat-scratch disease (CSD), below**	CSD (B. henselae), Grp A strep, Staph. aureus, anaerobes, M. TBc (scrofula), M. avium, M. scrofulaceum, M. malmoense, toxo, tularemia.			History & physical exam directs evaluation. If nodes fluctuant, aspirate and base rx on Gram & acid-fast stains. *Review of mycobacterial etiology: CID 20:954, 1995.* **Kikuchi-Fujimoto** disease causes fever and benign self-limited adenopathy; the etiology is unknown (*AJM 171:401, 1996; CID 39:138, 2004*).
Inguinal Sexually transmitted	HSV, chancroid, syphilis, LGV			
Not sexually transmitted	GAS, SA, tularemia, CSD			
Axillary	GAS, SA, CSD, tularemia, Y. pestis, sporotrichosis.			
Extremity, with associated nodular lymphangitis (For full description see *AnIM 118:883, 1993*)	Sporotrichosis, leishmania, Nocardia brasiliensis, Mycobacterium marinum, Mycobacterium chelonae, tularemia			A distinctive form of lymphangitis characterized by subcutaneous swellings along inflamed lymphatic channels. Primary site of skin invasion usually present; regional adenopathy variable.
Cat-scratch disease—immunocompetent patient Axillary/epitrochlear nodes 46%, neck 26%, inguinal 17%	Bartonella henselae Reviews: *AAC 48:1921, 2004; PIDJ 23:1161, 2004*	**Azithro dosage—Adults** (>45.5 kg): 500 mg po times 1, then 250 mg per day times 4 days. **Children** (<45.5 kg): liquid azithro 10 mg per kg times 1, then 5 mg per kg per day times 4 days. Rx is controversial —*see Comment*	No rx: resolves in 2–6 mos. Needle aspiration relieves pain in suppurative nodes. Avoid I&D.	**Clinical:** Approx. 10% nodes suppurate. Atypical presentation in <5% pts, i.e. lung nodules, liver/spleen lesions, Parinaud's oculoglandular syndrome, CNS manifestations in 2% of pts (encephalitis, peripheral neuropathy, retinitis), FUO. **Dx:** Cat exposure. Positive IFA serology. Rarely need biopsy. **Rx:** Only 1 prospective randomized blinded study, used azithro with ↑ rapidity of resolution of enlarged lymph nodes (*PIDJ 17:447, 1998*).
MOUTH Odontogenic infection, including Ludwig's angina Can result in more serious parapharyngeal space infection (*see page 36*)	Oral microflora: infection polymicrobial	**Clinda** 300–450 mg po q6h or 600 mg IV q6-8h	(**AM-CL** 875/125 mg po bid or 500/125 mg tid or 2000/125 mg bid) or **cefotetan** 2 gm IV q12h	Surgical drainage and removal of necrotic tissue essential. β-lactamase producing organisms are ↑ in frequency. Ref.: *Canad Dental Assn J 64.508, 1998* Other parenteral alternatives: AM-SB, PIP-TZ, or TC-CL.
Buccal cellulitis Children <5 yrs	H. influenzae	**Cefuroxime or ceftriaxone** *Dosage: See Table 16, page 133*	**AM-CL or TMP-SMX**	With Hib immunization, invasive H. influenzae infections have ↓ by 95%. Now occurring in infants prior to immunization.
Herpetic stomatitis	Herpes simplex virus 1 & 2	See Table 14		
Aphthous stomatitis, recurrent, HIV-neg.	Etiology unknown	Topical steroids (Kenalog in Orabase) may ↓ pain and swelling; if AIDS, see SANFORD GUIDE to HIV/AIDS THERAPY.		
MUSCLE **"Gas gangrene"** Contaminated traumatic wound Can be spontaneous without trauma (*CID 28:159, 1999*)	Cl. perfringens, other histotoxic Clostridium sp.	(**Clinda** 900 mg IV q8h) + (**pen G** 24 million units per day div. q4–6h IV)	**Ceftriaxone** 2 gm IV q12h or **erythro** 1 gm q6h IV (not by bolus)	Surgical debridement primary rx. Hyperbaric oxygen adjunctive: efficacy debated, consider if debridement not complete or possible (*NEJM 334:1642, 1996*). Clinda decreases toxin production.
Pyomyositis Review: *AJM 117:420, 2004*	Staph. aureus, Group A strep, (rarely Gm-neg. bacilli), variety of anaerobic organisms	**(Nafcillin** or **oxacillin** 2 gm IV q4h) or [**P Ceph 1** (**cefazolin** 2 gm IV q8h)] if MSSA	**Vanco** 1 gm IV q12h if MRSA	Common in tropics; rare, but occurs, in temperate zones (*IDCP 7:265, 1998*). Follows exercise or muscle injury, see *Necrotizing fasciitis*. Now seen in HIV/AIDS. Add **metro** if anaerobes suspected/proven (*IDCP 8:252, 1999*).

Abbreviations on page 2.   *NOTE: All dosage recommendations are for adults (unless otherwise indicated) and assume normal renal function.*

TABLE 1 (31)

ANATOMIC SITE/DIAGNOSIS/ MODIFYING CIRCUMSTANCES	ETIOLOGIES (usual)	SUGGESTED REGIMENS* PRIMARY	ALTERNATIVE§	ADJUNCT DIAGNOSTIC OR THERAPEUTIC MEASURES AND COMMENTS
PANCREAS: Reviews—*Ln 361:1447,* 2003; *JAMA 291:2865,* 2004				
Acute alcoholic (without necrosis) (idiopathic) pancreatitis	Not bacterial	None CT-diagnosed	1–9% become infected but prospective studies show no advantage of prophylactic antimicrobials (*Ln 346:652,* 1995). Observe for pancreatic abscesses or necrosis which require rx.	
Pancreatic abscess, infected pseudocyst, post-necrotizing pancreatitis	Enterobacteriaceae, enterococci, S. aureus, S. epidermidis, anaerobes, candida	Need culture of abscess/infected pseudocyst to direct therapy		Can often get specimen by fine-needle aspiration.
Antimicrobic prophylaxis, necrotizing pancreatitis	As above	Infection of necrotic pancreas occurs in 30–50% of pts leading to multiple clinical trials. An International Consensus Panel reviewed all available data & **conclude that prophylactic antibacterial &/or antifungal agents should not be used** (*CCM 32:2524,* 2004).		
PAROTID GLAND "Hot" tender parotid swelling	S. aureus, oral flora, & aerobic Gm-neg. bacilli (rare), mumps, rarely enteroviruses/ influenza. **Nafcillin** or **oxacillin** 2 gm IV q4h			Predisposing factors: stone(s) in Stensen's duct, dehydration. Rx depends on ID of specific etiologic organism.
"Cold" non-tender parotid swelling	Granulomatous disease (e.g., mycobacteria, fungi, sarcoidosis, Sjögren's syndrome), diabetes, tumors			History/lab results may narrow differential; may need biopsy for dx
PERITONEUM/PERITONITIS: Reference—*CID 31:997,* 2003				
Primary (spontaneous bacterial peritonitis, SBP) Rev. *CID 27:669,* 1998 ESBL ref.: *CID 28:683,* 1999 Microbiology: *CID 33:1513,* 2001	Enterobacteriaceae 63%, S. pneumo 15%, enterococci 6–10%, anaerobes <1%. Extended β-lactamase (ESBL) positive Klebsiella species.	[**Cefotaxime** 2 gm IV q8h (if life-threatening, q4h)] or **TC-CL** or **PIP-TZ** q24h] OR [**ceftriaxone** 2 gm IV q24h] If resistant **E. coli/Klebsiella species (ESBL+), then: (IMP** or **MER)** or **(FQ: CIP, Levo, Gati, Moxi)** *(Dosage in footnote¹)*		One-year **risk of SBP** in pts with ascites and cirrhosis as high as 29% (*Gastro 104:1133,* 1993). 30–40% of pts have neg. cultures of blood and ascitic fluid. % pos. cultures ↑ if 10 mL of pt's ascitic fluid cultured in blood culture bottles. **Duration of rx unclear.** Suggest 2 wks if blood culture pos. One report suggests repeat paracentesis after 48 hrs of cefotaxime. If PMNs <250 per mm³ ascitic fluid sterile, success with 5 days of rx (*AJM 97:169,* 1994). IV albumin (1.5 gm per kg at dx & 1 gm per kg on day 3) may ↓ frequency of renal impairment (p 0.002) & ↓ hospital mortality (p 0.01) (*NEJM 341:403,* 1999)
Prevention of SBP: Cirrhosis & ascites		**TMP-SMX-DS** 1 tab po 5 days per wk or **CIP** 750 mg po q wk	**TMP-SMX** ↓ peritonitis or spontaneous bacteremia from 27% to 3% (*AnIM 122:595,* 1995). Ref. for CIP: *Hpt 22:1171,* 1995	
Secondary (bowel perforation, ruptured appendix, ruptured diverticula) Refs: *NEJM 338:1521,* 1998 & *CID 37:997,* 2003	Enterobacteriaceae, Bacteroides sp., enterococci, P. aeruginosa (3+–15%)	**Mild-moderate disease—parenteral rx:** (e.g., focal periappendiceal, peridiverticular abscess, endometritis) **PIP-TZ** 3.375 gm IV q6h or 4.5 gm IV q8h, **OR AM-SB** 3 gm IV q6h **OR TC-CL** 3.1 gm IV q6h **OR ERTA** 1 gm IV q24h	[(**CIP** 400 mg IV q12h or **Levo** 750 mg IV q24h) + (**metro** 1 gm IV q12h)] or (**CFP** 2 gm q12h + **metro**) or **tigecycline** 100 mg IV times 1 dose, then 50 mg q12h.	Must "cover" both Gm-neg. aerobic & Gm-neg. anaerobic bacteria. **Drugs active only vs anaerobic Gm-neg. bacilli:** clinda, metro. **Drugs active only vs aerobic Gm-neg. bacilli:** APAG, P Ceph 2/3/4, aztreonam, AP Pen, CIP, Levo. **Drugs active vs both aerobic/anaerobic Gm-neg. bacteria:** cefoxitin, cefotetan, TC-CL, PIP-TZ, AM-SB, IMP, MER, Gati, Moxi.
		Severe life-threatening disease—ICU patient: **IMP** 500 mg IV q6h or **MER** 1 gm IV q8h	[**AMP** + metro + (**CIP** 400 mg IV q12h or **Levo** 750 mg IV q24h)] **OR** [**AMP** 2 gm IV q4h + **metro** 500 mg IV q6h + **APAG** (see Table 10D, page 74)]	Increasing resistance (R) of Bacteroides species:

	Cefoxitin	Cefotetan	Clindamycin
% R	4–25	17–87	16–44

Essentially no resistance: **metro**, **PIP-TZ** (*CID 35(Suppl.1):S126,* 2000). Case reports of metro resistance: *CID 40:e67,* 2005; *JCM 42:4127,* 2004. Mechanisms of resistance: *CID 33:92,* 2004.
Ertapenem not active vs P. aeruginosa/Acinetobacter species. Based on in vitro activity, could sub **Gati/Moxi** for **CIP/Levo**, but insufficient clinical data.
If absence of ongoing fecal contamination, aerobic/anaerobic culture of peritoneal exudate/abscess of help in guiding specific therapy.
Less need for aminoglycosides. **With severe pen allergy,** can "cover" Gm-neg. aerobes with CIP or aztreonam. **Remember IMP/MER are β-lactams.**

Concomitant surgical management important.

¹ Parenteral **IV therapy** for peritonitis: **TC-CL** 3.1 gm q6h, **PIP-TZ** 3.375 gm q6h or 4.5 gm q8h, **AM-SB** 3 gm q6h, **IMP** 0.5 gm q6h, **MER** 1 gm q8h, **FQ** (**CIP** 400 mg q12h, **Oflox** 400 mg q12h, **Levo** 750 mg q24h, **Gati** 400 mg q24h, **Moxi** 400 mg q24h), **AP Pen** 1 gm q6h, **Moxi** (see Table 10D, page 74), **cefotetan** 2 gm q12h, **cefoxitin** 2 gm q6h, **cefotaxime** 2 gm q4–8h, **ceftriaxone** 1–2 gm q12h, **ceftizoxime** 2 gm q8–12h, **P Ceph 4** (**CFP** 2 gm q12h), **cefpirome**AUS 2 gm q12h), **clinda** 450–900 mg q8h, **metro** 1 gm loading then 0.5 gm q6h or 1 gm q12h, **aztreonam** 2 gm q8h.
PIP 4 gm q6h, **aztreonam** 2 gm q8h.
NOTE: All dosage recommendations are for adults (unless otherwise indicated) and assume normal renal function.
Abbreviations on page 2.

TABLE 1 (32)

ANATOMIC SITE/DIAGNOSIS/ MODIFYING CIRCUMSTANCES	ETIOLOGIES (usual)	SUGGESTED REGIMENS*		ADJUNCT DIAGNOSTIC OR THERAPEUTIC MEASURES AND COMMENTS
		PRIMARY	ALTERNATIVE§	
PERITONEUM/PERITONITIS (continued) **Associated with chronic ambulatory peritoneal dialysis** (defined as >100 WBC per mcL, >50% PMNs)	Staph. aureus (most common), Staph. epidermidis, P. aeruginosa 7%, Gm-neg. bacilli 11%, sterile 20%, M. fortuitum (rare)	If of moderate severity, can rx by adding drug to dialysis fluid—see Table 17 for dosage. Reasonable empiric combinations: (**vanco + ceftazidime**) or (**vanco + APAG**) If severely ill, rx with same drugs IV (adjust dose for renal failure, Table 17) & via addition to dialysis fluid. Excellent ref.: Perit Dialysis Int 13:14, 1993		For diagnosis: concentrate several hundred mL of removed dialysis fluid by centrifugation. Gram stain concentrate and then inject into aerobic/anaerobic blood culture bottles. A positive Gram stain will guide initial therapy. If culture shows Staph. epidermidis, good chance of "saving" dialysis catheter; if multiple Gm-neg. bacilli cultured, consider bowel perforation and catheter removal.
PHARYNX **Pharyngitis/Tonsillitis**—Reviews: NEJM 344:205, 2001; AnIM 139:113, 2003. Guideline for Group A strep: CID 35:113, 2002				
Exudative or diffuse erythema For relationship to acute rheumatic fever, see footnote[1] Rheumatic fever ref.: Ln 366:155, 2005	Group A,C,G strep, "viral," infectious mononucleosis (NEJM 329:156, 1993), C. diphtheriae, A. haemolyticum, Mycoplasma pneumoniae In adults, only 10% pharyngitis due to Group A strep	**Pen V** po times 10 days or (if compliance unlikely) **benzathine pen** IM times 1 dose. Up to 35% of isolates resistant to erythro, azithro, clarithro, clinda (AAC 48:473, 2004) See footnote[2] for adult and pediatric dosages Acetaminophen effective for pain relief (Br J Gen Prac 50:817, 2000). If macrolide-resistant & pen-allergy: Clinda—Linezolid should work; Adults—FQ or telithro	**O Ceph 2** times 10 days (CID 38:1526 & 1535, 2004) or **clinda** or **azithro** times 5 days or **clarithro** times 10 days or **dirithro** times10 days or **erythro** times 10 days, azithro	**Dx:** In children & adults—Rapid strep test or culture. (Some debate: JAMA 291:1587, 2004, & 292:767, 2004) **Pen allergy & macrolide resistance:** No penicillin or cephalosporin-resistant S. pyogenes, but now **macrolide-resist. S. pyogenes** (7% 2000–2003). Culture & susceptibility testing if clinical failure with azithro/clarithro (CID 41:599, 2005). **S. pyogenes Groups C & G cause pharyngitis but not a risk for post-strep rheumatic fever.** To prevent rheumatic fever, eradicate Group A strep. Requires 10 days of pen V po; 4–6 days of po O Ceph 2; 5 days of po azithro; 10 days of clarithro. In controlled trial, better eradication rate with 10 days clarithro (91%) than 5 days azithro (82%)(CID 32: 1798,2001)
	Gonococci	**Ceftriaxone** 125 mg IM times 1 dose + (**azithro** times 1 or **doxy**) (see Comment)	(**CIP** 500 mg po times 1) or (**Levo** 250 mg po times 1) (see Comment)	(**Gati** 400 mg po times 1) Because of risk of concomitant genital C. trachomatis, add either (azithro 1 gm po times 1) or (doxy 100 mg po q12h times 7 days). See page 17 for more options.
Asymptomatic post-rx carrier Multiple repeated culture-positive episodes (CID 25:574, 1997)	Group A strep	No rx required	Clinda or AM-CL po	Parenteral **benzathine pen G ± RIF** (see Comment) Routine post-rx throat culture not advised. Small % of pts have recurrent culture-pos. Group A strep with symptomatic tonsillo-pharyngitis. Hard to tell if true Group A Strep infection or active viral infection in carrier of Group A Strep. Addition of RIF may help: 20 mg per kg per day times 4 days to max. of 300 mg (J Ped 106:481 & 876, 1995). Dosages in footnote[2]
Whitish plaques; HIV+ (thrush) **Vesicular, ulcerative**	Candida albicans (see Table 11, page 78); Coxsackie A9, B1-5, ECHO (multiple types); Enterovirus 71; Herpes simplex 1,2	Antibacterial agents not indicated, but for HSV-1,2: **acyclovir** 400 mg tid po times 10 days.		
Membranous—Diphtheria or Vincent's angina	C. diphtheriae	[**Antitoxin + erythro** 20–25 mg per kg IV q12h times 7–14 days (JAC 35:717, 1995)] or [**benzyl pen G** 50,000 units per kg per day times 5 days, then po **pen VK** 50 mg per kg per day times 5 days]		Diphtheria occurs in immunized individuals. Antibiotics may ↓ toxin production, ↓ spread of organisms. Penicillin superior to erythro in randomized trial (CID 27:845, 1998).
	Vincent's angina (anaerobes/spirochetes)	**Pen G** 4 million units IV q4h	**Clinda** 600 mg IV q8h	May be complicated by F. necrophorum bacteremia, see jugular vein phlebitis (Lemierre's), page 36.

[1] Primary rationale for rx is eradication of Group A strep (GAS) and prevention of acute rheumatic fever (ARF). Subsequent studies have been based on cultures, not actual prevention of ARF. Benzathine penicillin G has been shown in clinical trials to ↓ rate of ARF from 2.8 to 0.2%. This was associated with clearance of GAS on pharyngeal cultures (CID 19:1110, 1994). Treatment decreases duration of symptoms.

[2] Treatment of Group A strep: **All po unless otherwise indicated. PEDIATRIC DOSAGE: Benzathine penicillin** 25,000 units per kg IM to max. 1.2 million units; **Pen V** 25–50 mg per kg per day div. q6h times10 days; **AM-CL** 45 mg per kg per day div. q12h times 10 days; **erythro estolate** 20 mg per kg per day div. bid times 10 days; **succinate** 40 mg per kg per day div. bid times 10 days; **cefadroxil** 20 mg per kg per day div. bid or 4–10 days (PIDJ 14:295, 1995); **cefpodoxime proxetil** 10 mg per kg per day div. bid times 5–10 days or 14 mg per kg q24h times 10 days; **cefdinir** 7 mg per kg q12h times 5–10 days; **cefprozil** 15 mg per kg per day div. bid times 10 days; **clarithro** 15 mg per kg per day div. bid times 10 days; **azithro** 12 mg per kg per day q24h times 5 days; **clinda** 20–30 mg per kg per day q8h times 10 days **ADULT DOSAGE: Benzathine penicillin** 1.2 million units IM times 1; **Pen V** 500 mg bid or 250 mg qid times 10 days; **erythro**, dosage varies—with erythro base 500 mg qid times 10 days; **cefadroxil** 1 gm q24h; **cefpodoxime proxetil** 100 mg bid times 4 days; **cefdinir** 300 mg q12h times 5–10 days or 600 mg q24h times 10 days; **cefditoren** 200 mg bid times 10 days; **cefprozil** 500 mg q24h times 10 days; **cefuroxime axetil** 250 mg bid times 4 days; **cefpodoxime proxetil** 100 mg q24h times 10 days; **NOTE:** All O Ceph 2 drugs approved for 10-day rx of strep. pharyngitis; increasing number of studies show efficacy of 4–6 days; **clarithro** 250 mg bid times 10 days; **azithro** 500 mg times 1 and then 250 mg times 4 days or 500 mg q24h times 3 days; **dirithro** 500 mg q24h times 10 days.

Abbreviations on page 2. NOTE: All dosage recommendations are for adults (unless otherwise indicated) and assume normal renal function.

TABLE 1 (33)

ANATOMIC SITE/DIAGNOSIS/ MODIFYING CIRCUMSTANCES	ETIOLOGIES (usual)	SUGGESTED REGIMENS*		ADJUNCT DIAGNOSTIC OR THERAPEUTIC MEASURES AND COMMENTS
		PRIMARY	ALTERNATIVE§	
PHARYNX (continued)				
Epiglottitis Children	H. influenzae (rare), S. pyogenes, S. pneumoniae, S. aureus	**Peds dosage: Cefotaxime** 50 mg per kg IV q8h or **ceftriaxone** 50 mg per kg IV q24h	**Peds dosage: AM-SB** 100–200 mg per kg per day div q6h or **TMP-SMX** 8–12 mg TMP component per kg per day q12h (rare) **Adult dosage:** See footnote¹	Have tracheostomy set "at bedside." Chloro is effective, but potentially less toxic alternative agents available. Review (adults): JAMA 272:1358, 1994)
Adults	Group A strep, H. influenzae			
Parapharyngeal space infection Poor dental hygiene, dental extractions, foreign bodies (e.g., toothpicks, fish bones)	[Spaces include: sublingual, submaxillary, submandibular (Ludwig's angina, used loosely for these), lateral pharyngeal, retropharyngeal, pretracheal] Polymicrobic: Strep sp., anaerobes, Eikenella corrodens	**Clinda** 600–900 mg IV q8h) or (**pen G** 24 million units by cont. infusion or div. q4–6h IV) + **metro** 1 gm IV load and then 0.5 gm IV q6h)	**Cefoxitin** 2 gm IV q8h or **clinda** or **TC-CL** or **PIP-TZ** or **AM-SB** (Dosage, see footnote 1)	Close observation of airway; 1/3 require intubation, MRI or CT to identify abscess; If present, surgical drainage. **Metro** may be given 1 gm IV q12h.
Jugular vein septic phlebitis (Lemierre's disease) (PID 22:921, 2003; CID 31:524, 2000)	Fusobacterium necrophorum in vast majority	**Pen G** 24 million units q24h by cont. infusion or div. q4–6h	**Clinda** 600–900 mg IV q8h	Usual rx includes external drainage of lateral pharyngeal space. Emboli, pulmonary and systemic common. Erosion into carotid artery can occur.
Laryngitis (hoarseness)/tracheitis	Viral (90%)	Not indicated		
SINUSES, PARANASAL **Sinusitis, acute; current terminology: acute rhinosinusitis Obstruction of sinus ostia, viral infection, allergens** Refs.: Otolaryn-Head & Neck Surgery 130/S1, 2004; AnIM 134:495 & 498, 2001. For rhinovirus infections (common cold), see Table 14, page 113 Pediatric Guidelines: Peds 108:798, 2001	Strep. pneumoniae 31%, H. influenzae 21%, M. catarrhalis 2%, Group A strep 2%, anaerobes 6%, viruses 15%, Staph. aureus 4% By CT scans, sinus mucosa inflamed in 87% of viral URIs; only 2% develop bacterial rhinosinusitis	Reserve antibiotic rx for pts given decongestants/ analgesics for 7 days who have (1) maxillary/facial pain & (2) purulent nasal discharge; if severe illness (pain, fever), treat sooner—usually treat spontaneous resolution. **For mild/mod. disease: Ask if antibiotics in prior month** **NO:** **Amox-HD** or **AM-CL-ER** or **cefdinir** or **cefpodoxime** or **cefprozil** or **telithro** _In general, treat times 10 days; exceptions in adult and pediatric doses, footnote² and footnote 2 page 2_	**YES:** **AM-CL-ER** (adults) or resp. **FQ** (adults). For pen. allergy, see Comments. Use **AM-CL** susp. in peds.	**Rx goals:** (1) Resolve infection, (2) prevent complications, e.g., meningitis, brain abscess, (3) avoid chronic sinus disease, (4) avoid unnecessary antibiotic rx. High rate of spontaneous resolution. **For pts with pen/cephalosporin allergy, esp. severe IgE-mediated allergy, e.g., hives, anaphylaxis, treatment options: telithro, clarithro, azithro, TMP-SMX, doxy or FQs. Telithro listed 1st because of activity vs S. pneumo, resistant to clarithro/azithro. Avoid FQs if under age 18. Dosages in footnote 2 page 35.** If allergy just skin rash, po cephalosporin OK. **Usual rx 10 days.** In 1 study, results of 3 & 10 d. of TMP-SMX the same (JAMA 273:1015, 1995). Telithro approved for 5 days. Watch for pts with fever & fascial erythema, ↑ risk of S. aureus infection, requires IV **nafcillin/oxacillin (antistaphylococcal penicillin, penicillinase-resistant for MSSA or vanco for MRSA).** Pts aged 1–18 yrs with clinical diagnosis of sinusitis randomized to placebo, amox, or AM-CL for 14 d. **No difference** in multiple measures of efficacy (Peds 107:619, 2001). Similar study in adults: AnIM 163:1793, 2003. Hence, without bacteriologic endpoints, data are hard to interpret. AM-CL-ER ref.: AJM 117(Suppl.3A):23S, 2004
Clinical failure after 3 days	As above; consider diagnostic tap/aspirate	**Mild/Mod. Disease: AM-CL-ER** (**cefpodoxime, cefprozil,** or **cefdinir**) or **telithro**	**Severe Disease: Gati, Gemi, Levo,** or **Moxi**	See footnote 2 & Comment _Treat 10 days. Adult doses in footnote 2 & Comment_

¹ **Ceftriaxone** 2 gm IV q24h; **cefotaxime** 2 gm IV q4–8h; **AM-SB** 3 gm IV q6h; **PIP-TZ** 3.375 gm IV q6h; **TC-CL** 3.1 gm IV q4–6h; **TMP-SMX** 8–10 mg per kg per day (based on TMP component) div q6h, q8h, or q12h.

² **Pediatric doses for sinusitis (all oral): Amoxicillin** high dose 90 mg per kg per day div. q8h or q12h. **AM-CL-ES** (extra strength) pediatric susp.: 90 mg amox component per kg per day div. q12h, **azithro** 10 mg per kg times 1, then 5 mg per kg per day times 3 days, **clarithro** 15 mg per kg per day div. q12h, **cefpodoxime** 10 mg per kg per day (max. 400 mg). div. q12–24h, **cefuroxime axetil** 30 mg per kg per day div. q12h, **cefdinir** 14 mg per kg per day once q24h or div q12h, **TMP-SMX** 8–12 mg TMP/40–60 mg SMX per kg per day div. q12h.
Adult doses for sinusitis (all oral): AM-CL-ER (Augmentin XR) 2000/125 mg bid, **amox high-dose (HD)** 1 gm tid, **clarithro** 500 mg bid or **clarithro ext. release** 1 gm q24h, **doxy** 100 mg bid, **respiratory FQs** (**Gati** 400 mg q24h, **Gemi** 320 mg q24h (not FDA indication but should work), **Levo** 750 mg q24h, **Moxi** 400 mg q24h), **O Ceph** (**cefdinir** 300 mg q12h or 600 mg q24h, **cefpodoxime** 200 mg bid, **cefprozil** 250–500 mg bid, **cefuroxime** 250 mg bid), **TMP-SMX** 1 double-strength (160 mg/800 mg) q12h, **telithro** 800 mg q24h

NOTE: All dosage recommendations are for adults (unless otherwise indicated) and assume normal renal function.
Abbreviations on page 2.

TABLE 1 (34)

ANATOMIC SITE/DIAGNOSIS/ MODIFYING CIRCUMSTANCES	ETIOLOGIES (usual)	SUGGESTED REGIMENS* PRIMARY	ALTERNATIVE§	ADJUNCT DIAGNOSTIC OR THERAPEUTIC MEASURES AND COMMENTS
SINUSES, PARANASAL/Sinusitis, Acute *(continued)*				
Diabetes mellitus with acute ketoacidosis; neutropenia; deferoxamine rx.	Rhizopus sp., (mucor), aspergillus	*See Table 11, pages 75 & 82.* Ref.: *NEJM 337:254, 1997*		
Hospitalized + nasotracheal or nasogastric intubation	Gm-neg. bacilli 47% (pseudomonas, acinetobacter, E. coli common), Gm+ (S. aureus 35%, yeasts 18%. Polymicrobial in 80%	Remove nasotracheal tube and if fever persists, recommend sinus aspiration for C/S prior to empiric rx. **IMP** 0.5 gm IV q6h or **MER** 1 gm IV q8h. Add vanco for MRSA if Gram stain suggestive.	(**Ceftaz** 2 gm IV q8h + **vanco**) or (**CFP** 2 gm IV q12h + **vanco**). Vanco if possible MRSA.	After 7 d. of nasotracheal or gastric tubes, 95% have x-ray "sinusitis" (fluid in sinuses), but on transnasal puncture only 38% culture + (*AJRCCM 150:776, 1994*). For pts requiring mechanical ventilation for ≥1 wk, bacterial sinusitis occurs in <10% (*CID 27:851, 1998*). May need fluconazole if yeast on Gram stain of aspirate. Review: *CID 25:1441, 1997.* Epidemiology study *CID 27:463, 1998.*
Sinusitis, chronic Adults	Prevotella, anaerobic strep, & fusobacterium—common anaerobes. Strep sp., haemophilus, P. aeruginosa, S. aureus, & moraxella-aerobes. (*CID 35:428, 2002*)	Antibiotics usually not effective	Otolaryngology consultation. If acute exacerbation, rx as acute	Pathogenesis unclear and may be polyfactorial: damage to ostiomeatal complex during acute bacterial disease, allergy ± polyps, occult immunodeficiency, and/or odontogenic disease (periodontitis in maxillary teeth).
SKIN				
Acne vulgaris (*JAMA 292:726, 2004; NEJM 352:1463, 2005; Ln 364:2188, 2004; Cochrane Database Syst Rev 2000, 2:CD002086*)				
Comedonal acne. "blackheads," "whiteheads," earliest form, no inflammation	Excessive sebum production & gland obstruction. No Propionibacterium acnes	All once-q24h: Topical **tretinoin** (cream 0.025 or 0.05%) or (gel 0.01 or 0.025%)	Topical **adapalene** 0.1% gel OR **azelaic acid** 20% cream or **tazarotene** 0.1% cream.	Goal is prevention, ↓ number of new comedones and create an environment unfavorable to P. acnes. Adapalene causes less irritation than tretinoin. Azelaic acid less potent but less irritating than retinoids. Expect 40–70% ↓ in comedones in 12 weeks.
Mild inflammatory acne: small papules or pustules	Proliferation of P. acnes + abnormal desquamation of follicular cells	Topical **erythro** 3% + **benzoyl peroxide** 5%, bid	Can substitute **clinda** 1% gel for erythro	In random. controlled trial, topical benzoyl peroxide + erythro of equal efficacy to oral minocycline and tetracycline and not affected by antibiotic resistance of propionibacteria (*Ln 364:2188, 2004*).
Inflammatory acne: comedones, papules & pustules. Less common: deep nodules (cysts)	Progression of above events	(Topical **erythro** 3% + **benzoyl peroxide** 5% bid) ± oral antibiotic. *See Comment for mild acne.*	Oral drugs: (**doxy** 100 mg bid) or (**minocycline** 50 mg bid). Others: **tetracycline, erythro, TMP-SMX, clinda**	Systemic **isotretinoin** reserved for pts with severe widespread nodular cystic lesions that fail oral antibiotic rx: 4–5 mo. course of 0.1–1 mg per kg per day. Aggressive/violent behavior reported. Tetracyclines stain developing teeth. Doxy can cause photosensitivity. Minocycline side-effects: urticaria, vertigo, pigment deposition in skin or oral mucosa.
Acne rosacea *NEJM 352:793, 2005*	? skin mite: Demadex folliculorum	**Azelaic acid gel** bid, topical	**Metro** topical cream bid	More pt satisfaction with azelaic acid (*J Am Acad Derm 40(6, Pt.1):961, 1999*). More options listed in *NEJM 352:793, 2005.*
Anthrax, cutaneous, inhalation (pulmonary, mediastinal) **To report bioterrorism event:** 770-488-7100; **For info: www.bt.cdc.gov** Refs.: *JAMA 281:1735, 1999, & MMWR 50:909, 2001*	B. anthracis *See Lung, page 31, and Table 1B, page 48*	**Adults (including pregnancy):** CIP 500 mg po bid or Levo 500 mg IV/po q24h) times 60 days **Children:** CIP 20–30 mg per kg per day div q12h po (to max. 1 gm per day) times 60 days	**Adults (including pregnancy): Doxy** 100 mg po bid times 60 days. **Children: Doxy** >8 y/o & >45 kg: 100 mg po bid; >8 y/o & ≤45 kg: 2.2 mg per kg po bid; ≤8 y/o: 2.2 mg per kg po bid All for 60 days.	1. If penicillin susceptible, then: **Adults: Amox** 500 mg po q8h times 60 days. **Children: Amox** 80 mg per kg per day div. q8h (max. 500 mg q8h) 2. Usual treatment of cutaneous anthrax is 7–10 days; 60 days in setting of bioterrorism with presumed aerosol exposure 3. Other **FQs** (Gati, Levo, Moxi) should work based on in vitro susceptibility data
Bacillary angiomatosis: For other Bartonella infections, see *Cat-scratch disease lymphadenitis, page 33, and Bartonella, page 41* In immunocompromised (HIV-1, bone marrow transplant) patients *Also see SANFORD GUIDE TO HIV/AIDS THERAPY*	Bartonella henselae and quintana	**Adults:** CIP 500 mg po bid or ext. release 1 gm po q24h or **azithro** 250 mg po q24h or **CIP** 500–750 mg po bid (see Comment)	**Clarithro** 500 mg po bid or **Erythro** 500 mg po qid or **doxy** 100 mg po bid	In immunocompromised pts with severe disease, doxy 100 mg po/IV bid + RIF 300 mg po bid reported effective (*IDC No. Amer 12:37, 1998; Adv PID 11:1, 1996*).

Abbreviations on page 2.   *NOTE: All dosage recommendations are for adults (unless otherwise indicated) and assume normal renal function.*

TABLE 1 (35)

ANATOMIC SITE/DIAGNOSIS/ MODIFYING CIRCUMSTANCES	ETIOLOGIES (usual)	SUGGESTED REGIMENS*		ADJUNCT DIAGNOSTIC OR THERAPEUTIC MEASURES AND COMMENTS
		PRIMARY	ALTERNATIVE§	
SKIN (continued)				
Bite: Remember tetanus prophylaxis—see Table 20. See Table 20C for rabies prophylaxis				
Bat, raccoon, skunk	Strep & staph from skin; rabies	AM-CL 875/125 mg po bid or 500/125 mg po tid	Doxy 100 mg po bid	In Americas, **antirabies rx indicated**, rabies immune globulin + vaccine. (See *Table 20D, pages 144–145*)
Cat (Ref.: *NEJM 340:85 & 138, 1999*) Cat-scratch disease: *page 33*	**Pasteurella multocida**, Staph. aureus	AM-CL 875/125 mg po bid or 500/125 mg po tid	**Cefuroxime axetil** 0.5 gm po q12h or **doxy** 100 mg po bid. **Do not use cephalexin.** Sens. to FQs in vitro.	80% cat bites become infected. **P. multocida resistant to dicloxacillin, cephalexin, clinda; many strains resistant to erythro** (most sensitive to azithro but no clinical data). P. multocida infection develops within 24 hrs. Observe for osteomyelitis. If culture + for only P. multocida, can switch to pen G IV or pen VK po.
Catfish sting	Toxins	See Comments		Presents as immediate pain, erythema and edema. Resembles strep cellulitis. May become secondarily infected; AM-CL is reasonable choice for prophylaxis
Dog (Ref.: *NEJM 340:85 & 138, 1999*)	**P. multocida**, S. aureus, Bacteroides sp., Fusobacterium sp., EF-4, Capnocytophaga	AM-CL 875/125 mg po bid or 500/125 mg po tid	Clinda 300 mg po qid + FQ (adults) or clinda + TMP-SMX (children)	Only 5% dog bites become infected. Prophylaxis may be worthwhile (*AnEM 23:535, 1994*). Consider antirabies rx; rabies immune globulin + vaccine (*Table 20C*). Capnocytophaga in splenectomized pts may cause local eschar, sepsis with DIC. **P. multocida resistant to diclox, cephalexin, clinda and erythro; sensitive to FQs in vitro** (*AAC 43:1475, 1999*).
Human For bacteriology, see *CID 37:1481, 2003*	Viridans strep 100%, Staph epidermidis 53%, corynebacterium 41%, **Staph. aureus 29%, eikenella 15%**, bacteroides 82%, peptostrep 26%	**Early** (not yet infected): AM-CL 875/125 mg po bid times 5 days. **Later**: Signs of infection (usually in 3–24 hrs): **(AM-SB** 1.5 gm IV q6h or **cefoxitin** 2 gm IV q8h or **TC-CL** 3.1 gm IV q6h) or **(PIP-TZ** 3.375 gm IV q6h or 4.5 gm q8h)	AM-CL 875/125 mg po qid + either CIP or TMP-SMX	Cleaning, irrigation and debridement most important. X-rays should be obtained. Bites inflicted by hospitalized pts. consider aerobic Gm-neg. bacilli. **Eikenella resistant to clinda, nafcillin/oxacillin, metro, P Ceph 1, and erythro; susceptible to FQs and TMP-SMX.**
		Pen allergy: **Clinda** + (either CIP or TMP-SMX)		
Pig (swine)	Polymicrobic: Gm+ cocci, Gm-neg. bacilli, anaerobes, Pasteurella sp.	AM-CL 875/125 mg po bid	P Ceph 3 or TC-CL or AM-SB or IMP	Information limited but infection is common and serious (*Ln 348:888, 1996*).
Prairie dog	Monkeypox	See Table 14A, page 112.	No rx recommended	
Primate, non-human	Microbiology?	Acyclovir: See Table 14B, page 114		*CID 20:421, 1995*
Rat	Spirillum minus & Streptobacillus moniliformis	AM-CL 875/125 mg po bid	Doxy	Antirabies rx is not indicated.
Seal	Marine mycoplasma	Tetracycline times 4 wks.		
Snake: pit viper (Ref.: *NEJM 347:347, 2002*)	Pseudomonas sp., Enterobacteriaceae, Staph. epidermidis, Clostridium sp.			Can take weeks to appear after bite (*Ln 364:549, 2004*) or MRSA infection. Primary therapy is antivenom. Penicillin generally used but would not be effective vs organisms isolated. Tetanus prophylaxis indicated.
Spider bite: Most necrotic ulcers attributed to spiders are probably due to another cause, e.g., cutaneous anthrax (*Ln 364:549, 2004*) or MRSA infection				
Widow (Latrodectus)	Not infectious	None		May be confused with "acute abdomen." Diazepam or calcium gluconate helpful to control pain, muscle spasm. Tetanus prophylaxis.
Brown recluse (Loxosceles) *NEJM 352:700, 2005*	Not infectious "Overdiagnosed! Spider distribution limited to South Central & desert SW of USA.	Bite usually self-limited & self-healing. No therapy of proven efficacy.	Dapsone 50 mg po q24h often used despite marginal supportive data	Dapsone causes hemolysis (check for G6PD deficiency). Can cause hepatitis; baseline & weekly liver panels suggested.
Boils—Furunculosis—Subcutaneous abscesses in drug addicts ("skin poppers"). Carbuncles = multiple connecting furuncles				
Active lesions See *Table 6, page 57*	Staph. aureus, both MSSA & MRSA concern for community-acquired MRSA	**If afebrile & abscess <5 cm in diameter:** I&D, culture, hot packs. No drugs. **If ≥5 cm in diameter: TMP-SMX-DS** 2 tabs po bid times 5–10 days. **Doxy/mino** alternatives.	**Febrile, large &/or multiple abscesses; outpatient care:** I&D, culture abscess & maybe blood, hot packs. (**TMP-SMX-DS** 2 tabs po bid times 10 days **or RIF** 300 mg po bid + **RIF** 300 mg po bid) times 10 days	Epidemic of **community-acquired MRSA**: currently susceptible to TMP-SMX, clinda, minocycline, & linezolid. If erythro-resistant, probably clinda-resistant. **Alternatives for febrile pt, multiple abscesses: Linezolid** 600 mg po bid times 10 days or **dalbavancin** 1000 mg IV times 1 dose.

Abbreviations on page 2. NOTE: All dosage recommendations are for adults (unless otherwise indicated) and assume normal renal function.

ANATOMIC SITE/DIAGNOSIS/ MODIFYING CIRCUMSTANCES	ETIOLOGIES (usual)	SUGGESTED REGIMENS* PRIMARY	ALTERNATIVE§	ADJUNCT DIAGNOSTIC OR THERAPEUTIC MEASURES AND COMMENTS
SKIN/Boils/Furunculosis—Subcutaneous abscesses in drug addicts (continued)				
To lessen number of recurrences	MSSA & MRSA	Guided by in vitro susceptibilities: (**Diclox 500 mg po qid** or **TMP-SMX-DS** 2 tabs po bid) + **RIF** 600 mg po q24h, all times 10 days	**Plus:** Nasal & under finger-nail treatment with **mupirocin ointment bid**	**Plus:** Shower with Hibiclens q24h times 3 days & then 3 times per week. Others have tried 5% povidone-iodine cream intranasal qid. times 5 days. Reports of S. aureus resistant to mupirocin. Not sure about bacitracin ointment; no contemporary in vitro susceptibility studies vs MRSA. Mupirocin prophylaxis of non-surgical hosp. pts had no effect on S. aureus infection in placebo-controlled study (AnIM 140:419 & 484, 2004).
Hidradenitis suppurativa	Lesions secondarily infected: S. aureus, Enterobacteriaceae, pseudomonas, anaerobes	Aspirate, base rx on culture	Many pts ultimately require surgical excision.	Caused by keratinous plugging of apocrine glands of axillary and/or inguinal areas.
Burns. For overall management: NEJM 350:810, 2004—step-by-step case outlined & explained				
Initial burn wound care (CID 37:543, 2003)	Not infected	Early excision & wound closure; shower hydrotherapy. Role of topical antimicrobics unclear.	**Silver sulfadiazine** cream, 1%, apply 1–2 times per day or 0.5% **silver nitrate** solution or **mafenide** acetate cream. Apply bid.	Marrow-induced neutropenia can occur during 1st wk of sulfadiazine but resolves even if use is continued. Silver nitrate leaches electrolytes from wounds & stains everything. Mafenide inhibits carbonic anhydrase and can cause metabolic acidosis.
Burn wound sepsis Variety of skin grafts and skin substitutes; see JAMA 283:717, 2000	Strep. pyogenes, Enterobacter sp. S. aureus, S. epidermidis, E. faecalis, E. coli, P. aeruginosa. Fungi rare. Herpesvirus rare.	(**Vanco** 1 gm IV q12h) + (**amikacin** 10 mg per kg loading dose then 7.5 mg per kg IV q12h) + **PIP** 4 gm IV q4h (give ½ q24h dose of **piperacillin** into subeschar tissues with surgical eschar removal within 12 hours). Can use PIP-TZ if PIP not available.		Monitor serum levels, ½ of most antibiotics ↓. Staph. aureus tend to remain localized to burn wound; if toxic, consider toxic shock syndrome. Candida sp. colonize but seldom invade. Pneumonia is the major infectious complication, often staph. Complications include septic thrombophlebitis. Dapto (4 mg per kg IV q24h) alternative for vanco.
Cellulitis, erysipelas: Be wary of macrolide (erythro)-resistant S. pyogenes. Review: NEJM 350:904, 2004. **NOTE:** Consider diseases that masquerade as cellulitis (AnIM 142:47, 2005)				
Extremities, not associated with venous catheter (see Comments); non-diabetic For diabetes, see below	Group A strep, occ. Group B, C, G; Staph. aureus (uncommon but difficult to exclude)	**Pen G** 1–2 million units IV q6h or (**Nafcillin** or **oxacillin** 2 gm IV q4h). If not severe, **dicloxacillin** 500 mg po q6h or **cefazolin** 1 gm IV q8h. See Comment	**Erythro** 1 or **P Ceph 1** or **AM-CL** or **azithro** or **clarithro** or **dirithro** or **tigecycline**. (Dosage, see footnote page 28 or Table 10C)	**"Spontaneous" erysipelas of leg in non-diabetic is usually due to strep. Gps A,B,C or G.** Hence OK to **start with IV pen G 1–2 million units q6h** & observe for localized S. aureus infection. Look for tinea pedis with fissures, a common portal of entry; can often culture strep from between toes (CID 23:1162, 1996). For rx of pts with lymphedema & recurrent erysipelas, see prophylaxis, Table 15. Other alternatives: **clinda, Gati, Levo, Moxi**
Facial, adult (erysipelas)	Group A strep, Staph. aureus	**Vanco** 1 gm IV q12h	**Dapto** 4 mg per kg per day	**Choice of empiric therapy must have activity vs S. aureus.** S. aureus erysipelas of face can mimic S. pyogenes erysipelas of an extremity. Forced to treat empirically for MRSA until in vitro susceptibilities available.
Diabetes mellitus and erysipelas (See Foot, "Diabetic", page 12)	Group A strep, Staph. aureus, Enterobacteriaceae; clostridia (rare)	**Early mild: TMP-SMX-DS** 2 tabs po bid + **RIF** 300 mg po. **For severe disease: IMP** or **MER** or **ERTA** IV + (**linezolid** 600 mg IV/po bid or **vanco** (IV) Dosage, see page 12, Diabetic foot	See Comment	Prompt surgical debridement indicated to rule out necrotizing fasciitis and to obtain cultures. If septic, consider x-ray of extremity to demonstrate gas. **Prognosis dependent on blood supply: assess arteries.** See diabetic foot, page 12.
Erysipelas 2° to lymphedema (congenital = Milroy's disease); post-breast surgery with lymph node dissection	S. pyogenes, Groups A, C, G	**Benzathine pen G** 1.2 million units IM q4 wks [of minimal benefit in reducing recurrences under underlying predisposing conditions (CID 25:685, 1997)]		Indicated only if pt is having frequent episodes of cellulitis. Pen V 250 mg po bid should be effective but not aware of clinical trials. In pen-allergic pts: erythro 500 mg po q24h, azithro 250 mg po q24h, or clarithro 500 mg po q24h.
Dandruff (seborrheic dermatitis)	Malassezia species	**Ketoconazole shampoo** 2% or **selenium sulfide** 2.5%	(see page 8, chronic external otitis)	
Decubitus or venous stasis or arterial insufficiency ulcers: with sepsis	Polymicrobic: S. pyogenes (Gps A,C,G), enterococci, anaerobic strep, Enterobacteriaceae, Pseudomonas sp., Bacteroides sp., Staph. aureus	**IMP** or **MER** or **TC-CL** or **PIP-TZ** or **ERTA**	(**CIP Gati, Levo,** or **Moxi**) + (**clinda** or **metro**) Dosages, see footnotes pages 12, 19, 24, 45	Without sepsis or extensive cellulitis local care may be adequate. Debride as needed. Topical mafenide or silver sulfadiazine adjunctive. R/O underlying osteomyelitis. May need wound coverage with skin graft or skin substitute (JAMA 283:716, 2000).
Erythema multiforme	H. simplex type 1, mycoplasma, Strep. pyogenes, drugs (sulfonamides, phenytoin, penicillins)			**Rx: Acyclovir** if due to H. simplex

Abbreviations on page 2.   NOTE: All dosage recommendations are for adults (unless otherwise indicated) and assume normal renal function.

TABLE 1 (37)

ANATOMIC SITE/DIAGNOSIS/ MODIFYING CIRCUMSTANCES	ETIOLOGIES (usual)	SUGGESTED REGIMENS* PRIMARY	ALTERNATIVE§	ADJUNCT DIAGNOSTIC OR THERAPEUTIC MEASURES AND COMMENTS
SKIN (continued)				
Erythema nodosum	Sarcoidosis, inflammatory bowel disease, M. tbc, coccidioidomycosis, yersinia, sulfonamides			**Rx: NSAIDs; glucocorticoids** if refractory.
Erythrasma	Corynebacterium minutissimum	**Erythro** 250 mg po q6h times 14 days		Coral red fluorescence with Wood's lamp. Alt: 2% aqueous clinda topically.
Folliculitis	Many etiologies: S. aureus, candida, P. aeruginosa, malassezia, demadex.	See individual entities. See Whirlpool folliculitis, page 41.		
Furunculosis	Staph. aureus	See Boils, pages 38-39		
Hemorrhagic bullous lesions				
Hx of sea water-contaminated abrasion or eating raw seafood, shock	Vibrio vulnificus, V. damsela (CID 37:272, 2003)	**Ceftazidime** 2 gm IV q8h + **doxy** 100 mg IV/po bid	Either **cefotaxime** 2 gm IV q8h or (**CIP** 750 mg po bid or 400 mg IV bid)	¾ pts have chronic liver disease with mortality in 50% (NEJM 312:343, 1985). In Taiwan, where a number of cases are seen, the impression exists that ceftazidime is superior to tetracyclines (CID 15:271, 1992) hence both.
Herpes zoster (shingles) See Table 14				
Impetigo, ecthyma—usually children				
"Honey-crust" lesions (non-bullous)	**Group A strep impetigo**; crusted lesions can be Staph. aureus + strepto-cocci	Mupirocin ointment 2% tid or fusidic acid cream^NUS 2% times 3–5 days	**Azithro** or **clarithro** or **erythro** or **O Ceph 2**	In meta-analysis that combined strep & staph impetigo, mupirocin had higher cure rates than placebo. Mupirocin superior to oral erythro. Penicillin inferior to erythro. Few placebo-controlled trials. Ref: Cochrane Database Systemic Reviews, 2004 (2): CD003261.
		For dosages, see Table 10C for adults and Table 16, page 133 for children.		
Bullous (if ruptured; thin "varnish-like" crust)	**Staph. aureus impetigo** MSSA & MRSA	For MSSA: po therapy with **dicloxacillin, oxacillin, cephalexin, AM-CL, azithro, clarithro,** or **mupirocin** ointment	**For MRSA: Mupirocin** ointment, **TMP-SMX-DS, minocycline**	
		For dosages, see Table 10C		
Infected wound, extremity—Post-trauma (for bites, see page 38; for post-operative, see below)**—Gram stain indicated.**				**Culture & sensitivity, check Gram stain. Tetanus toxoid if indicated.**
Mild to moderate; uncomplicated	Polymicrobic: Staph. aureus (MSSA & MRSA), Group A & anaerobic strep, Enterobacteriaceae, Cl. tetani; if water exposure, Aeromonas sp.	**TMP-SMX-DS** 2 tabs po bid or **clinda** 300–450 mg po tid (see Comment)	**Minocycline** 100 mg po bid or **linezolid** 600 mg po bid (see Comment)	**Mild infection:** Suggested drugs focus on S. aureus & Strep species. If suspect Gm-neg. bacilli, add **AM-CL-ER** 1000/62.5 two tabs po bid. If MRSA is erythroresistant, may have inducible resistance to clinda.
Febrile with sepsis—hospitalized		**AM-SB** or **TC-CL** or **PIP-TZ** or **IMP** or **MER** or **ERTA** (Dosage, page 19)	**Vanco** 1 gm IV q12h (see Comment) + (**CIP** or **Levo** IV—dose in Comment)	**Fever—sepsis:** Alternative to vanco is **linezolid** 600 mg IV/po q12h. If Gm-neg. bacilli & severe pen allergy, **CIP** 400 mg IV q12h or **Levo** 750 mg IV q24h.
		+ **vanco** 1 gm IV q12h		
		For dosages, see Table 10C		
Infected wound, post-operative—Gram stain negative				
Surgery not involving GI or female genital tract				
Without sepsis (mild)	Staph. aureus, Group A, B, C or G step	**TMP-SMX-DS** 2 tabs po bid **Vanco** 1 gm IV q12h	**Clinda** 300–450 mg po bid **Dapto** 6 mg per kg IV q24h	Check Gram stain of exudate. If (Gm-neg. bacilli, **add** β-lactam/β-lactamase inhibitor: **AM-CL-ER** po or (**ERTA** or **PIP-TZ** or **TC-CL**) V. Dosage on page 19.
With sepsis (severe)				
Surgery involving GI tract (includes oropharynx, esophagus) or female genital tract—fever, neutrophilia	MSSA/MRSA, coliforms, bacteroides & other anaerobes	[**PIP-TZ** or (**P Ceph 3** + **metro**) or **ERTA** or **IMP** or **MER**] + **vanco** 1 gm IV q12h **if severely ill.** **Mild infection: AM-CL-ER** 2 tabs po bid Add **TMP-SMX-DS** 2 tabs po bid if Gm+ cocci on Gram stain.		For all treatment options, see Peritonitis, page 34. Most important: Drain wound & get cultures. Can sub linezolid for vanco. Can sub CIP or Levo for β-lactams.
Meleney's synergistic gangrene	See Necrotizing fasciitis, page 41			
Infected wound, febrile patient—Gram stain: Gram-positive cocci in clusters	S. aureus, possibly MRSA	**Oral: TMP-SMX-DS** 2 tabs po bid or **clinda** 300–450 mg po tid (see Comment)	**Do culture & sensitivity** **IV: Vanco** 1 gm IV q12h or **daptomycin** 4 mg per kg IV q24h or 6 mg per kg IV q24h if septic	↑ in community-acquired MRSA (CA-MRSA). Need culture & sensitivity to verify. Other po options for CA-MRSA include minocycline 100 mg po q12h (inexpensive) & linezolid 600 mg po q12h (expensive). If MRSA clinda-sensitive but erythro-resistant, watch out for inducible clinda resistance. IV alternative: **tigecycline** 100 mg times 1 dose, then 50 mg per day

ANATOMIC SITE/DIAGNOSIS/ MODIFYING CIRCUMSTANCES	ETIOLOGIES (usual)	SUGGESTED REGIMENS* PRIMARY	ALTERNATIVE§	ADJUNCT DIAGNOSTIC OR THERAPEUTIC MEASURES AND COMMENTS
SKIN (continued) **Necrotizing fasciitis ("flesh-eating bacteria")** Post-surgery, trauma, strepto- coccal skin infections See Gas gangrene, page 33, & Toxic shock, page 46	**4 types:** (1) Streptococci, Grp A, C, G; (2) Clostridia sp.; (3) polymicrobic: aerob- ic + anaerobic (if S. aureus + anaerobic strep = Mele- ney's synergistic gangrene); (4) Community-acquired MRSA	For treatment of clostridia, see Muscle, gas gangrene, page 33. The terminology of **polymicrobic** wound infections is not precise: Meleney's synergistic gangrene, Fournier's gangrene, necrotizing fasciitis have a common pathophysiology. **All require prompt surgical debridement** as well as antibiotics. Dx of necrotizing fasciitis requires incision and probing. If no resistance to probing subcutaneously (fascial plane), dx = necrotizing fasciitis. **Need Gram stain/culture** to determine if etiology is strep, clostridia, polymicrobial, or S. aureus. **Treatment: Pen G** if strep or clostridia; **IMP** or **MER** if polymicrobial, add **vanco** if MRSA suspected. **NOTE:** If strep necrotizing fasciitis, reasonable to treat with penicillin & clinda (SMJ 96:968, 2003); if clostridia ± gas gangrene, add clinda to penicillin (see page 33). MRSA ref: NEJM 352:1445, 2005		
Puncture wound—nail	Through tennis shoe: P. aeruginosa	Local debridement to remove foreign body & tetanus prophylaxis		Osteomyelitis evolves in only 1–2% of plantar puncture wounds.
Staphylococcal scalded skin syndrome Ref.: PIDJ 19.819, 2000	Toxin-producing S. aureus	**Nafcillin** or **oxacillin** 2 gm IV q4h (children: 150 mg per kg per day div. q6h) times 5–7 days for MSSA; **vanco** 1 gm IV q12h (children 40–60 mg per kg per day div q6h).		Toxin causes **intraepidermal split** and positive Nikolsky sign. Drugs cause epiderm/dermal split. **called toxic epidermal necrolysis**—more serious (Ln 351:1417, 1998). Biopsy differentiates.
Ulcerated skin lesions	Consider: anthrax, tularemia, plague, blastomycosis, ecthyma gangrenosum), P. aeruginosa (ecthyma gangrenosum), plague, blastomycosis, mucormycosis, mycobacteria, leishmania, arterial insuffi- ciency, venous stasis, and others			
Whirlpool (Hot Tub) folliculitis See Folliculitis, page 40	Pseudomonas aeruginosa	Usually self-limited, treatment not indicated		Decontaminate hot tub: drain and chlorinate. Also associated with exfoliative beauty aids (loofah sponges) (J Clin Micro 31:480, 1993).
SPLEEN. For post-splenectomy prophylaxis, see Table 15B, page 125				
Splenic abscess Endocarditis, bacteremia Contiguous from intra-abdominal site Immunocompromised	Staph. aureus, streptococci Polymicrobic Candida sp.	**Nafcillin** or **oxacillin** 2 gm IV q4h if MSSA Treat as Peritonitis, secondary, page 34 **Amphotericin B** (Dosage, see Table 11, page 76)	**Vanco** 1 gm IV q12h if MRSA **Fluconazole, caspofungin**	Burkholderia (Pseudomonas) pseudomallei is common cause of splenic abscess in SE Asia.
SYSTEMIC FEBRILE SYNDROMES Spread by infected **TICK, FLEA, or LICE** (CID 29:888, 1999): Epidemiologic history crucial. **Babesiosis, Lyme disease, & granulocytic Ehrlichiosis** have same reservoir & tick vector. **Babesiosis:** see NEJM 343: 1454, 2000 Do not treat if asymptomatic, young, has spleen, and immunocompetent	Etiol: B. microti et al. Vector: Usually Ixodes ticks Host: White-footed mouse & others	**(Atovaquone** 750 mg po q12h) + (**azithro** 500 mg po day 1, then 250 mg po per day) times 7 days] OR [**clinda** 1.2 gm IV bid or 600 mg po tid times 7 days + **quinine** 650 mg po tid times 7 days. **Ped. dosage: Clinda** 20–40 mg per kg per day and **quinine** 25 mg per kg per day] plus **exchange transfusion**		Exposure endemic areas May to Sept. Can result from blood transfusion (JAMA 281: 927, 1999). Usually subclinical. Illness likely in asplenic pts, pts with concomitant Lyme disease, older pts, pts with HIV. Dx: Giemsa-stained blood smear; antibody test available. PCR under study. **Rx: Exchange transfusions successful adjunct, used early, in severe disease.**
Bartonella infections: CID 35:684, 2002 Asymptomatic bacteremia	B. quintana	**Doxy** 100 mg po/IV times 15 days		Can lead to endocarditis &/or trench fever; found in homeless, esp. if lice/leg pain.
Cat-scratch disease	B. henselae	**Azithro** (or symptomatic only—see page 33, usually lymphadenitis, can involve CNS, liver in immunocompetent pts)		
Bacillary angiomatosis; Peliosis hepatis—pts with AIDS	B. henselae, B. quintana	(**Claritho** 500 mg bid or **claritho** ER 1 gm po q24h or **azithro** 250 mg po q24h or **CIP** 500–750 mg po bid) times 8 wks	(**Erythro** 500 mg po qid or **doxy** 100 mg po bid) times 8 wks or if severe, combina- tion of **doxy** 100 mg po/IV bid + **RIF** 300 mg po bid	**Manifestations of Bartonella infections: Immunocompetent Patient:** Bacteremia/endocarditis/FUO/ encephalitis Cat scratch disease Vertebral osteo Trench fever Parinaud's oculoglandular syndrome **HIV/AIDS Patient:** Bacillary angiomatosis Bacillary peliosis Bacteremia/endocarditis/FUO
Endocarditis (see page 23) (AAC 47:2204, 2003)	B. henselae, B. quintana	**Gentamicin** 3 mg per kg IV once q24h times minimum 14 days + **doxy** 200 mg po once q24h times 4–6 wks		Hard to detect with automated blood culture systems. Need lysis-centrifugation and/or blind subculture onto chocolate agar at 7 & 14 days. Diagnosis often by antibody titer ≥1:800.
Trench fever (FUO)	B. quintana	**Doxy** 100 mg po bid (doxy alone if **no** endocarditis)		Same as Urban Trench Fever (page 43)

Abbreviations on page 2.   NOTE: All dosage recommendations are for adults (unless otherwise indicated) and assume normal renal function.

TABLE 1 (39)

ANATOMIC SITE/DIAGNOSIS/ MODIFYING CIRCUMSTANCES	ETIOLOGIES (usual)	SUGGESTED REGIMENS*		ADJUNCT DIAGNOSTIC OR THERAPEUTIC MEASURES AND COMMENTS
		PRIMARY	ALTERNATIVE§	
SYSTEMIC FEBRILE SYNDROMES. Spread by infected **TICK, FLEA or LICE** (continued)				
Ehrlichiosis*. CDC def. is one of: (1) 4x ↑ IFA antibody, (2) detection of Ehrlichia DNA in blood or CSF by PCR, (3) visible morulae in WBC and IFA ≥1:64 [MMWR 46(RR-10):1–55, 1997]				
Human monocytic ehrlichiosis (HEM) (JAMA 292:2263, 2004)	Ehrlichia chaffeensis (Lone Star tick is vector)	**Doxy** 100 mg po/IV bid times 7–14 days	**Tetracycline** 500 mg po qid times 7–14 days. No current recommendation for children or pregnancy.	30 states: mostly SE of line from NJ to Ill. to Missouri to Oklahoma to Texas. History of outdoor activity and tick exposure. April-Sept. Fever, rash (36%), leukopenia and thrombocytopenia. Blood smears no help. PCR for early dx.
Human granulocytic ehrlichiosis (HGE) (JAMA 292:2263, 2004)	Anaplasma (Ehrlichia) phagocytophilum (Ixodes sp. ticks are vector). Dog variant is Ehrlichia ewingii (NEJM 341:148 & 195, 1999)	**Doxy** 100 mg bid po or IV times 7–14 days	**Tetracycline** 500 mg po qid times 7–14 days. Not in children or pregnancy. See Comment	Upper Midwest, NE, West Coast & Europe. H/O tick exposure. April-Sept. Febrile flu-like illness after outdoor activity. No rash. Leukopenia/thrombocytopenia common. **Dx:** Up to 80% have positive blood smear. Antibody test for confirmation. **Rx:** RIF successful in pregnancy (CID 27:213, 1998) but worry about resistance developing. Based on in vitro studies, no clear alternative rx—Levo activity marginal (AAC 47:413, 2003).
Lyme Disease Tick bite; possible Ixodes acquired in endemic area	NOTE: Think about concomitant tick-borne disease—babesiosis (JAMA 275:1657, 1996) or ehrlichiosis. Reviews: LnID 3:489 & 761, 2003; Ln 362:1639, 2003. www.cdc.gov			
	Borrelia burgdorferi Urine antigen test reported unreliable (AJM 110:217 & 236, 2001).	**If endemic area,** if nymphal partially engorged deer tick: **doxy** 200 mg po times 1 dose with food.	**If not endemic area.** not engorged deer tick: No treatment	Prophylaxis study in endemic area: erythema migrans developed in 3% of the control group and 0.4% doxy group (NEJM 345:79 & 133, 2001).
Early (erythema migrans) See Comment	Terminology ref.: AnIM 136:413, 2002 **Lyme Disease National Surveillance Case Definition** available at either NEJM 345:115, 2001 or JAMA 288:1002, 2002	**Doxy** 100 mg po bid, or **amoxicillin** 500 mg po tid or **cefuroxime axetil** 500 mg po bid or **erythro** 250 mg po qid. All regimens for 14–21 days. (10 days as good as 20: AnIM 138:697, 2003) See Comment for peds doses		High rate of clinical failure with azithro & erythro (Drugs 57:157, 1999). **Peds** (all po for 14–21 days): **Amox** 50 mg per kg per day in 3 div. doses or **cefuroxime axetil** 30 mg per kg per day in 2 div. doses or **erythro** 30 mg per kg per day in 3 div. doses. Lesions usually homogeneous—not target-like (AnIM 136:423, 2002).
Carditis See Comment		**Ceftriaxone** 2 gm IV q24h) or **(cefotaxime** 2 gm IV q4h) or **(pen G** 24 million units IV q24h) times 14–21 days	**Doxy** (see Comments) 100 mg po bid times 14–21 days or **amoxicillin** 250–500 mg po bid times 14–21 days.	First degree AV block: Oral regimen. High degree AV block (PR >0.3 sec.): IV therapy—permanent pacemaker not necessary.
Facial nerve paralysis (isolated finding, early)		**(Doxy** 100 mg po bid) or **amoxicillin** 500 mg po) tid times 14–21 days	**Ceftriaxone** 2 gm IV q24h times 14–21 days	LP suggested to exclude neurologic disease. If LP neg., oral regimen OK. If abnormal or not done, suggest parenteral regimen.
Meningitis, encephalitis For encephalopathy, see Comment		**Ceftriaxone** 2 gm IV q24h times 14–28 days	**(Pen G** 20 million units IV q24h in div. dose) or **(cefotaxime** 2 gm IV q8h) times 14–28 days	Encephalopathy: memory difficulty, depression, somnolence, or headache. CSF abnormalities. 89% had objective CSF abnormalities. 18/18 pts improved with ceftriaxone 2 gm per day times 30 days (JID 180:377, 1999).
Arthritis		**(Doxy** 100 mg po bid) or **amoxicillin** 500 mg po qid), both times 30–60 days	**(Ceftriaxone** 2 gm IV q24h) or **(pen G** 20–24 million units per day IV) times 14–28 days	
Pregnant women		Choice should **not** include doxy: **amoxicillin** 500 mg po tid times 21 days.	**If pen. allergic: (azithro** 500 mg po q24h times 7–10 days) or **(erythro** 500 mg po qid times 14–21 days)	
Asymptomatic seropositivity and symptoms post-rx		None indicated		No benefit from rx (NEJM 345:85, 2001).
Plague **As biological weapon:** JAMA 283:2281, 2000, and Table 1B, page 48	Yersinia pestis Reservoir: rat Vector: rat flea	**Gentamicin** 2 mg per kg IV loading dose then 1.7 mg per kg IV q8h or **streptomycin** 1 gm IM/IV q12h	**(Doxy** 100 mg IV/po bid or **(chloro** 500 mg IV/po qid)	Reference IV streptomycin: CID 19:1150, 1994. Septicemic form can occur without buboes. **CIP** effective in vitro + in animal models (JAC 41:301, 1998); CIP success in 1 pt (CID 36:521, 2003).
Relapsing fever Can be tick-borne or louse-borne (MMWR 52:809, 2003)	Borrelia recurrentis, B. hermsii, & other borrelia sp.	**Doxy** 100 mg bid	**Erythro** 500 mg po qid	Jarisch-Herxheimer (fever, ↑ pulse, ↑ resp., ↓ blood pressure) in most patients (occurs in ~2 hrs). Not prevented by prior steroids. **Dx: Examine peripheral blood smear during fever for spirochetes.** Can relapse up to 10 times.

[1] In endemic area (New York), high % of both adult ticks and nymphs are jointly infected with both HGE and B. burgdorferi (NEJM 337:49, 1997).

ANATOMIC SITE/DIAGNOSIS/ MODIFYING CIRCUMSTANCES	ETIOLOGIES (usual)	SUGGESTED REGIMENS* PRIMARY	SUGGESTED REGIMENS* ALTERNATIVE§	ADJUNCT DIAGNOSTIC OR THERAPEUTIC MEASURES AND COMMENTS
SYSTEMIC FEBRILE SYNDROMES. Spread by infected **TICK, FLEA or LICE** (*continued*)				
Rickettsial diseases. Review—Disease in travelers (*CID 39:1493, 2004*)				
Spotted fevers (NOTE: Rickettsial pox not included)				
Rocky Mountain spotted fever (RMSF) (*AJTMH 63:21, 2000; ArIM 163:769, 2003*)	R. rickettsii (Dermacentor ticks)	**Doxy** 100 mg po/IV bid times 7 days or for 2 days after temp. normal	**Chloro** use found as risk factor for fatal RMSF (*JID 184:1437, 2001*)	Fever, rash (95%), petechiae 40–50%. **Rash spreads from distal extremities to trunk.** Dx: Immunohistology on skin biopsy; confirmation with antibody titers. Highest incidence in Mid-Atlantic states; also seen in Oklahoma, S. Dakota, Montana. **NOTE: Only 3–18% of pts present with fever, rash, and hx of tick exposure; esp. in children many early deaths & empiric doxy reasonable** (*MMWR 49: 888, 2000*).
NOTE: Can mimic ehrlichiosis. Pattern of rash important—*see Comment*				
Other spotted fevers, e.g., Boutonneuse fever. *LnID 3:557, 2003*	6 species: R. conorii et al. (multiple ticks). In sub-Saharan Africa, R. africae	**Doxy** 100 mg po bid times 5 days	**Chloro** 500 mg po/IV bid times 5 days Children <8 y.o.: **azithro** or **clarithro** (*see Comment*)	Clarithro 7.5 mg per kg q12h & azithro 10 mg per kg per day times 1 or 3 days equally efficacious in children with Mediterranean spotted fever (*CID 34:154, 2002*). R. africae review: *CID 36:1411, 2003.* R. parkeri in U.S.: *CID 38:805, 2004.*
Typhus group—Consider in returning travelers with fever				
Louse-borne	R. prowazekii (body louse)	**Doxy** 100 mg IV/po bid times 7 days	**Chloro** 500 mg IV/po qid times 7 days	**Brill-Zinsser disease** (*Ln 357:1198, 2001*) is a relapse of remote past infection, e.g., WW II. Truncal rash spreads centrifugally—opposite of RMSF. A winter disease.
Murine typhus (cat flea typhus similar)	R. typhi (rat reservoir and flea vector)	**Doxy** 100 mg IV/po bid times 7 days	**Chloro** 500 mg IV/po qid times 7 days	Most U.S. cases south Texas and southern Calif. Flu-like illness. Rash in <50%. Dx based on suspicion, confirmed serologically.
Scrub typhus	O. tsutsugamushi [rodent reservoir; vector is larval stage of mites (chiggers)]	**Doxy** 100 mg IV/po bid times 7 days. NOTE: Reports of doxy and chloro resistance from northern Thailand (*Ln 348:86, 1996*). In pregnancy, single 500 mg dose of **azithro** as effective as **doxy** (*CID 39:1329, 2004*)		Limited to Far East (Asia, India). Cases imported into U.S. Evidence of chigger bite: flu-like illness. Rash like louse-borne typhus. **RIF** alone 450 mg bid po times 7 days reported effective (*Ln 356:1057, 2000*). Worry about RIF resistance.
Tularemia, typhoidal type Ref. **bioterrorism**, *see Table 1B, page 48, & JAMA 285:2763, 2001*	Francisella tularensis. (Vector depends on geography; ticks, biting flies, mosquitoes identified)	**Gentamicin** or **tobra** 5 mg per kg per day div. q8h IV times 7–14 days	Add **chloro** if evidence of meningitis. **CIP** reported effective in 12 children (*PIDJ 19:449, 2000*).	Typhoidal form in 5–30% pts. No lymphadenopathy. Diarrhea, pneumonia common. Dx: blood cultures. Antibody confirmation. Rx: Jarisch-Herxheimer reaction may occur. Clinical failures with rx with P Ceph 3 (*CID 17:976, 1993*).
Urban trench fever (endocarditis) (*AAC 47:2204, 2003*)	Bartonella quintana Vector: Body louse	**Gentamicin** 3 mg per kg IV once q24h times min. of 14 days + **doxy** 200 mg po single q24h dose times 28 days		One of many Bartonella syndromes; *see pages 23 & 41*
Other Zoonotic Systemic Bacterial Febrile Illnesses: Obtain careful epidemiologic history				
Brucellosis Review: *NEJM 352:2325, 2005*	Brucella sp. B. abortus—cattle B. suis—pigs B. melitensis—goats B. canis—dogs	Adult or child >8 years: [**Doxy** 100 mg po bid times 6 wks + **gentamicin** times 2–3 wks (*see Table 10D, page 74*)] or [**doxy** times 6 wks + **streptomycin** 1 gm IM q24h times 2–3 wks] *See Comment*	[**Doxy** + **RIF** 600–900 mg po q24h, both times 6 wks] or [**TMP-SMX** 1 DS tab (160 mg TMP) po q12h times 6 wks + **gentamicin** times 2 wks]	**Clinical disease:** Protean. Fever in 91%. **Malodorous perspiration almost pathognomonic.** Osteoarticular disease in approx. 20%, epididymitis/orchitis 6%. **Lab:** Mild hepatitis. Leukopenia & relative lymphocytosis. **Diagnosis:** Serology, bone marrow culture, real-time PCR if available. **Treatment:** Drugs must penetrate macrophages & act in acidic milieu. **Pregnancy:** TMP-SMX-DS + RIF reasonable.
Child <8 years		**TMP-SMX** 5 mg per kg TMP po q12h times 6 wks + **gentamicin** q24h times 2 wks		
Leptospirosis (*CID 36:1507 & 1514, 2003; LnID 3:757, 2003*)	Leptospira—in urine of domestic livestock, dogs, small rodents	**Pen G** 1.5 million units IV q6h or **ceftriaxone** 1 gm q24h. Duration: 7 days	**Doxy** 100 mg IV/po q12h or **AMP** 0.5–1 gm IV q6h	**Severity varies.** Two-stage mild anicteric illness to severe icteric disease (Weil's disease) with renal failure and myocarditis. **Rx:** Penicillin, doxy, & cefotaxime of equal efficacy in severe lepto (*CID 39:1417, 2004*).

Abbreviations on page 2.   NOTE: All dosage recommendations are for adults (unless otherwise indicated) and assume normal renal function.

TABLE 1 (41)

ANATOMIC SITE/DIAGNOSIS/ MODIFYING CIRCUMSTANCES	ETIOLOGIES (usual)	SUGGESTED REGIMENS* PRIMARY	ALTERNATIVE§	ADJUNCT DIAGNOSTIC OR THERAPEUTIC MEASURES AND COMMENTS
SYSTEMIC FEBRILE SYNDROMES/Other Zoonotic Systemic Bacterial Febrile Illnesses *(continued)*				
Salmonella bacteremia (enteric fever most often caused by S. typhi)	Salmonella enteritidis—a variety of serotypes	CIP 400 mg IV q12h times 14 days (switch to po 750 mg bid when clinically possible)	Ceftriaxone 2 gm IV q12h times 14 days (switch to po CIP when possible)	Usual exposure is contaminated poultry and eggs. Many others. Myriad of complications to consider, e.g., mycotic aneurysm (10% of adults over age 50, *AJM 110:60, 2001*), septic arthritis, osteomyelitis, septic shock. Sporadic reports of resistance to CIP. Ref.: *LnID 5:341, 2005*
Miscellaneous Systemic Febrile Syndromes				
Kawasaki syndrome Acute, 3 mos to 12 yrs of age, peak at 1 yr of age; 85% below age 5 (*Ln 364:533, 2004*)	Acute self-limited vasculitis with ↑ temp., rash, conjunctivitis, stomatitis, cervical adenitis, red hands/feet & coronary artery aneurysms (25% if untreated)	**IVIG** 2 gm per kg over 12 hrs + **ASA** 20-25 mg per kg qid **THEN** **ASA** 3–5 mg per kg per day po q24h times 6–8 wks	If still febrile after 1st dose of IVIG, some give 2nd dose (*PIDJ 17:1144, 1998*)	IV gamma globulin (2 gm per kg over 10 hrs) in pts rx before 10th day of illness ↓ coronary artery lesions (*Ln 347:1128, 1996*). See *Table 14B, page 116* for IVIG adverse effects and expense.
Rheumatic Fever, acute Ref.: *Ln 366:155, 2005*	Post–Group A strep pharyngitis (not Group B, C, or G).	(1) Symptom relief: **ASA** 80–100 mg per kg per day in children; 4–8 gm per day in adults. **Pen** times 10 days. (2) Eradicate Group A strep: (See *Pharyngitis, page 35*). (3) Start prophylaxis: *see below*		
Prophylaxis Primary prophylaxis		**Benzathine pen G** 1.2 million units IM (see *Pharyngitis, p. 32*)		**Penicillin** for 10 days, prevents rheumatic fever even when started 7–9 days after onset of illness.
Secondary prophylaxis (previous documented rheumatic fever)		**Benzathine pen G** 1.2 million units IM q3–4 wks		Alternative: **Penicillin V** 250 mg po bid or **sulfadiazine (sulfisoxazole)** 1 gm po q24h or **erythro** 250 mg po bid. Duration of 2° prophylaxis varies: with carditis continue 10 yrs or until age 25; without carditis continue 5 yrs or until age 18 (*AnIM 118:401, 1993*).
Typhoidal syndrome (typhoid fever, enteric fever) (*Ln 366:749, 2005; LnID 5:623, 2005*)	Salmonella typhi, S. paratyphi NOTE: In vitro resistance to nalidixic acid often predicts clinical failure of CIP (FQs) (*Ln 366:749, 2005*)	(**CIP** 500 mg po bid times 10 days) or (**ceftriaxone** 2 gm IV q24h times 14 days). If associated shock, give **dexamethasone** a few minutes before antibiotic (See *Comment*). In children, CIP superior to ceftriaxone (*LnID 3:537, 2003*)	**Azithro** 1 gm po day 1, then 500 mg po times 6 days (*AAC 43:1441, 1999*) or 1 gm po q24h times 5 days (*AAC 44:1855, 2000*) (See *Comment*)	**Dexamethasone dose:** 3 mg per kg then 1 mg per kg q6h times 8 doses ↓ mortality (*NEJM 310:82, 1984*). **Complications:** perforation of terminal ileum &/or cecum, osteo, septic arthritis, **mycotic aneurysm** (approx. 10% over age 50, *AJM 110:62, 2001*), meningitis. **Other rx options:** Controlled trial of CIP vs chloro. Efficacy equivalent. After 5 days, blood culture positive: CIP 18%, chloro 36% (*AAC 47:1727, 2003*). **Children & adolescents: Ceftriaxone** (75 mg per kg per day) and **azithro** (20 mg per kg per day to 1 gm max.) equal efficacy. More relapses with ceftriaxone (*CID 38:951, 2004*).
Sepsis: Following suggested **empiric** therapy assumes pt is bacteremic; mimicked by viral, fungal, rickettsial infections and pancreatitis				
Neonatal—early onset <1 week old	Group B strep, E. coli, klebsiella, enterobacter, Staph. aureus (uncommon), listeria (rare in U.S.)	**AMP** 25 mg per kg IV q8h + **cefotaxime** 50 mg per kg q12h	(**AMP** + **APAG** 2.5 mg per kg IV/IM q12h) or (**AMP** + **ceftriaxone** 50 mg per kg IV/IM q24h)	Blood cultures are key but only 5–10% +. Discontinue antibiotics after 72 hrs if cultures and course do not support diagnosis. In Spain, listeria predominates; in S. America, salmonella.
Neonatal—late onset 1–4 weeks old	As above + H. influenzae & S. epidermidis	(**AMP** 25 mg per kg IV q6h + **cefotaxime** 50 mg per kg q8h) or (**AMP** + **ceftriaxone** 75 mg per kg IV q24h)	(**AMP** + **APAG** 2.5 mg per kg IV or IM	If MSSA/MRSA a concern, add **vanco.**
Child; not neutropenic	Strep. pneumoniae, meningococci, Staph. aureus (MSSA & MRSA), H. influenzae now rare	(**Cefotaxime** 50 mg per kg IV q8h or **ceftriaxone** 100 mg per kg IV q24h) + **vanco** 15 mg per kg IV q6h	**Aztreonam** 7.5 mg per kg IV q6h + **linezolid** (see *Table 16, page 133* for dose)	Major concerns are S. pneumoniae & community-acquired MRSA. Coverage for Gm-neg. bacilli included but H. influenzae infection now rare. Meningococcemia mortality remains high (*Ln 356:961, 2000*).

TABLE 1 (42)

ANATOMIC SITE/DIAGNOSIS/ MODIFYING CIRCUMSTANCES	ETIOLOGIES (usual)	SUGGESTED REGIMENS*		ADJUNCT DIAGNOSTIC OR THERAPEUTIC MEASURES AND COMMENTS
		PRIMARY	ALTERNATIVE§	
SYSTEMIC FEBRILE SYNDROMES/Sepsis *(continued)*				
Adult; not neutropenic; NO HYPOTENSION but LIFE-THREATENING. Source unclear—consider intra-abdominal or skin source. **Life-threatening.**	Aerobic Gm-neg. bacilli; S. aureus; streptococci; others	**(For Septic Shock, see page 46** (IMP or MER or ERTA) + vanco	(Dapto 6 mg per kg IV q24h) + (P Ceph 3/4 or PIP-TZ or TC-CL) Could substitute linezolid for vanco or dapto; however, linezolid bacteriostatic vs S. aureus. *Dosages in footnote[1]*	Systemic inflammatory response syndrome (SIRS): 2 or more of the following: 1. Temperature >38°C or <36°C 2. Heart rate >90 beats per min. 3. Respiratory rate >20 breaths per min. 4. WBC >12,000 per mcL or >10% bands Sepsis: SIRS + a documented infection (+ culture) Severe sepsis: Sepsis + organ dysfunction: hypotension or hypoperfusion abnormalities (lactic acidosis, oliguria, ↓ mental status) **Septic shock:** Sepsis-induced hypotension (systolic BP <90 mmHg) not responsive to 500 mL IV fluid challenge + peripheral hypoperfusion.
if suspect biliary source *(see p.10)*	Enterococci + aerobic Gm-neg. bacilli	AM-SB, PIP-TZ, or TC-CL	P Ceph 3 + metro; (CIP or Levo) + metro. Dosages—footnote[1]	
if illicit use IV drugs	S. aureus	Vanco if high prevalence of MRSA. Some empirically use vanco + oxacillin pending susceptibility results. Dosages—footnote[1]		
if suspect intra-abdominal source	Mixture aerobic & anaerobic Gm-neg. bacilli	*[See secondary peritonitis, page 34]*		
if petechial rash	Meningococcemia	Ceftriaxone 2 gm IV q12h (until sure no meningitis); consider Rocky Mountain spotted fever—*see page 43*		
if suspect urinary source	Aerobic Gm-neg. bacilli & enterococci	*[See pyelonephritis, page 26]*		
Neutropenia: Child or Adult (absolute PMN count <500 per mm³). Guideline: CID 34:730, 2002				
Prophylaxis—afebrile Post-chemotherapy—impending neutropenia	Aerobic Gm-neg. bacilli, pneumocystis (PCP)	Meta-analysis demonstrates substantive reduction in mortality with **CIP** 500 mg po bid *(AnIM 142:979, 2005)*. Similar results in observational study using **Levo** 500 mg po q24h *(CID 40:1087 & 1094, 2005)*. Also *NEJM 353:977, 988 & 1052, 2005*.		
Post-chemotherapy in ↑ risk patient	↑ risk pneumocystis (PCP)	**TMP-SMX-DS** po bid—adults; 10 mg per kg per day div bid po—children		Need TMP-SMX to prevent PCP. Hard to predict which leukemia/lymphoma/solid tumor pt at ↑ risk of PCP.
AIDS patient		**TMP-SMX** as above + (either **acyclovir** or **ganciclovir**) + **fluconazole**		Combined regimen justified by combined effect of neutropenia and immunosuppression.
Allogeneic hematopoietic stem-cell transplant	↑ risk pneumocystis, herpes viruses, candida			
Empiric therapy—febrile neutropenia (≥38.3°C x1 or ≥38°C for ≥1 hr)				
Low-risk adults Peds data pending *(Def. low risk in Comment)*	As above	**CIP** 750 mg po bid + AM-CL 875 mg po bid	**Treat as outpatients with 24/7 access to inpatient care if: no focal findings, no hypotension, no COPD, no fungal infection, age <60 & >16.** Neutropenic children with neg. blood cultures, safely switched to po cefixime 4 mg per kg q12h *(CID 32:36, 2001)*.	
High-risk adults and children	Aerobic Gm-neg. bacilli; ceph-resistant viridans strep, MRSA	**Monotherapy:** CFP or ceftaz or IMP or MER	**Combination therapy:** (Gent or tobra) + (TC-CL or PIP-TZ) *Dosages: Footnote[1] and Table 10* Include empiric vanco if: suspect IV access infected; colonized with drug-resistant S. pneumo or MRSA; blood culture pos. for Gm-pos. cocci; pt hypotensive	Increasing resistance of viridans streptococci to penicillins, cephalosporins & FQs *(CID 34:1469 & 1524, 2002; CID 31:1726, 2000; JAC 47:87, 2001)*. **What if severe IgE-mediated β-lactam allergy?** No formal trials, but [APAG (or CIP) + aztreonam] ± vanco should work.
Persistent fever and neutropenia after 5 days of empiric antibacterial therapy—see CID 34:730, 2002—General guidelines				
	Candida species, aspergillus	Add either **caspofungin** 70 mg IV day 1, then 50 mg IV q24h **OR voriconazole** 6 mg per kg IV q12h times 2 doses, then 3 mg per kg IV q12h		Conventional ampho B more fever & nephrotoxicity & lower efficacy than liposomal ampho B *(NEJM 340:764, 1999)*; both caspofungin & voriconazole better tolerated & perhaps more efficacious than liposomal ampho B *(NEJM 346:225, 2002 & 351:1391 & 1445, 2005)*.

---

[1] **P Ceph 3 (cefotaxime** 2 gm IV q8h, use q4h if life-threatening; **ceftizoxime** 2 gm IV q8h; **ceftriaxone** 2 gm IV q4h; **ceftazidime** 2 gm IV q8h). **AP Pen (piperacillin** 3 gm IV q12h), **AP Pen (piperacillin** 3 gm IV q12h), **TC-CL** 3.1 gm IV q4h, **ticarcillin** 3 gm IV q4h, **PIP-TZ** 3.375 gm IV q4h, **AM-SB** 3 gm IV q6h, **APAG** (see *Table 10D, page 74*), **AMP** 30 mg per kg IV q4h, **clinda** 900 mg IV q8h, **MER** 1 gm IV q8h, **Nafcillin** or **oxacillin** 2 gm IV q4h, **aztreonam** 2 gm IV q8h, **metro** 1 gm loading dose then 0.5 gm q6h or 1 gm IV q12h, **vanco** 1 gm IV q12h, **linezolid** 600 mg IV q12h. **P Ceph 3 AP (ceftazidime** 2 gm IV q8h), **P Ceph 4 |CFP** 2 gm IV q12h (q8h if neutropenic), **cefpirome[NUS]**, **cefepime**) **CIP** 400 mg IV q12h, **levo** 750 mg IV q24h, **linezolid** 600 mg IV q12h.
NOTE: All dosage recommendations are for adults (unless otherwise indicated) and assume normal renal function.
Abbreviations on page 2.

TABLE 1 (43)

ANATOMIC SITE/DIAGNOSIS/ MODIFYING CIRCUMSTANCES	ETIOLOGIES (usual)	SUGGESTED REGIMENS*		ADJUNCT DIAGNOSTIC OR THERAPEUTIC MEASURES AND COMMENTS
		PRIMARY	ALTERNATIVE§	
SYSTEMIC FEBRILE SYNDROMES (continued)				
Shock syndromes				
Septic shock: Fever & hypotension Bacteremic shock, endotoxin shock Overall review: Ln 365:63, 2005 Antimicrobial therapy: CCM 32(Suppl.):S495, 2004 Management consensus: CCM 32:858, 2004	Bacteremia with aerobic Gm-neg. bacteria or Gm+ cocci	**Proven therapy: (1) Replete intravascular volume, (2) correct, if possible, disease that allowed bloodstream infection, (3) appropriate empiric antimicrobial rx**, see suggestions under life-threatening sepsis, page 45. **(4)** Decreased indication for recombinant **activated Protein C** (drotrecogin alfa), see Comment. **(5) Low-dose steroids** if document adrenal insufficiency (see Comment for criteria). [Hydrocortisone 50 mg IV q6h + fludrocortisone (Florinef) 50 mcg via NG once q24h] times 7 days. **(6)** Low-dose **vasopressin** reported effective for catecholamine-resistant septic shock (Sem Resp Crit Care Med 25:705, 2004). **(6) Blood glucose control:** 80–110 mg per dL.		**Activ. Protein C: Drotrecogin (Xigris):** In a prospective randomized double-blind study (NEJM 344:699, 2001), 28-d. mortality ↓ from 31 to 25% in sickest pts. Study in less ill pts (APACHE II score <25) showed no benefit. Xigris not indicated in pts with single organ dysfunction & surgery within last 30 days due to evidence of increased mortality (NEJM 353:1332 & 1398, 2005). **Hemorrhage** (3.5% drotrecogin, 2% placebo) in initial NEJM trial. Stop 2 hrs before & restart 12 hrs after surgery. Approx. **cost** of drug for 4-day course: $8000. **Low-dose steroids:** In controlled random double-blind trial, rx if low baseline cortisol & ≤9 mcg per dL response to 250 mg IV cosyntropin. 28-day mortality 63% placebo & 53% steroid group (JAMA 288:862 & 886, 2002). Results in question because "total" & not "free" plasma cortisol was measured (NEJM 350:1601 & 1629, 2004). Confirm. trial in process. **Low-dose vasopressin:** Dose should not exceed 0.04 units per min. **Targeted glucose levels:** Tight plasma glucose control appears to reduce mortality (AnM 164:2005, 2004).
Septic shock: post-splenectomy (asplenia)	S. pneumoniae, N. meningitidis, H. influenzae, Capnocytophaga (DF-2)	**Ceftriaxone** 2 gm IV q24h (↑ to 2 gm q12h if meningitis)	**Gati** 400 mg or **Levo** 750 mg q24h or **Moxi** 400 mg) all once IV q24h	Howell-Jolly bodies in peripheral blood smear confirm absence of functional spleen. Often results in **symmetrical peripheral gangrene of digits** due to severe DIC. For prophylaxis, see Table 15A, page 124.
Toxic shock syndrome, Clostridium sordelli [CID 35:1441, 2002; www.fda.gov/cder/drug/advisory/mifeprex.htm]				
Post-partum, post-abortion, post-mifepristone MMWR 54:724, 2005	Clostridium sordelli	Other management as per Septic shock, above	Several deaths reported after use to abortifacient regimen of mifepristone (RU486) & misoprostol. Clinically: often afebrile, rapid progression, hypotension, hemoconcentration (high Hct), neutrophilia.	
Toxic shock syndrome, staphylococcal. Superantigen review: LnID 2:156, 2002				
Colonization by toxin-producing Staph. aureus of vagina (tampon-assoc.), surgical/traumatic wounds, endometrium, nares.	Staph. aureus (toxic shock toxin-mediated)	(**Nafcillin** or **oxacillin** 2 gm IV q4h) or (if MRSA, **vanco** 1 gm IV q12h) + IVIG	(**Cefazolin** 1–2 gm IV q8h) or (if MRSA, **vanco** 1 gm IV q12h) + **IVIG**	Nafcillin/oxacillin/cefazolin have no effect on initial syndrome, but ↓ recurrences. Seek occult abscess. TSS may occur with "clean" colonized post-op wounds. Case fatality 5–15% **IVIG reasonable** (see Streptococcal TSS)— dose 1 gm per kg day 1, then 0.5 gm per kg days 2 & 3.
Toxic shock syndrome, streptococcal [Ref.: JID 179(Suppl 2):S366–374, 1999]. NOTE: For necrotizing fasciitis without toxic shock, see page 41				
Associated with invasive disease, i.e., erysipelas, necrotizing fasciitis; secondary strep infection of varicella. Secondary cases TSS reported (NEJM 335:547 & 590, 1996; CID 27:150, 1998).	Group A, B, C, & G Strep. pyogenes	(**Pen G** 24 million units per day IV in div. doses) + **clinda** 900 mg IV q8h) **IVIG** associated with ↓ in sepsis-related organ failure	**Ceftriaxone** 2 gm IV q24h + **clinda** 900 mg q8h	Definition: Isolation of Group A strep, hypotension and ≥2 of: renal impairment, coagulopathy, liver involvement, ARDS, generalized rash, soft tissue necrosis (JAMA 269:390, 1993). Associated with invasive disease. **Surgery usually required.** Mortality with fasciitis 30–50%, myositis 80% even with early rx (CID 14:2, 1992). Clinda ↓ toxin production. Use of NSAID may predispose to TSS. For discussion of possible reasons pen G may fail in fulminant S. pyogenes infections, see JID 167:1401, 1993).
		(IVIG dose: 1 gm per kg day 1, then 0.5 gm per kg days 2 & 3.		
Other Toxin-Mediated Syndromes—no fever unless complicated				
Botulism (CID 41:1167, 2005. As **biologic weapon**: JAMA 285:1059, 2001; Table 1B, page 48; www.bt.cdc.gov)				
	C. botulinum	For all types: Follow vital capacity, other supportive care. If no ileus, purge GI tract	Trivalent (types A, B, E) equine serum antitoxin— State Health Dept. or CDC (see Comment)	**Equine antitoxin:** Obtain from State Health Depts. or CDC (404-639-2206 M-F OR 404-639-2888 evenings/weekends). Skin test first & desensitize if necessary. One vial IV and one vial IM.
Food-borne Dyspnea at presentation bad sign (CID 39:357 & 363, 2004)				**Antimicrobials:** May make infant botulism worse. Untested in wound botulism. When used, pen G 10–20 million units per day usual dose. If complications (pneumonia, UTI) occur, avoid antimicrobials with assoc. neuromuscular blockade, i.e., aminoglycosides, tetracycline.
Infant		Human botulinum immunoglobulin (BIG) IV, single dose. Call 510-540-2646. Do not use equine antitoxin.	No antibiotics; may lyse C. botulinum in gut and ↑ load of toxin	**Differential dx:** Guillain-Barré, myasthenia gravis, tick paralysis, organophosphate toxicity, West Nile virus

Abbreviations on page 2   NOTE: All dosage recommendations are for adults (unless otherwise indicated) and assume normal renal function.

TABLE 1 (44)

ANATOMIC SITE/DIAGNOSIS/ MODIFYING CIRCUMSTANCES	ETIOLOGIES (usual)	SUGGESTED REGIMENS* PRIMARY	ALTERNATIVE§	ADJUNCT DIAGNOSTIC OR THERAPEUTIC MEASURES AND COMMENTS
SYSTEMIC FEBRILE SYNDROMES/Other Toxin-Mediated Syndromes/Botulism *(continued)*				
Wound		Debridement & anaerobic cultures. No proven value of local antitoxin. Role of antibiotics untested.	Trivalent equine antitoxin (see Comment)	Can result from spore contamination of tar heroin.
Tetanus	C. tetani	**Pen G** 24 million units per day in div. dose or **doxy** 100 mg IV q12h times 7–10 days	**Metro** 500 mg po q6h or 1 gm IV q12h times 7–10 days (See Comment)	Multifaceted treatment: Wound debridement, tetanus immunoglobulin (250–500 units IM), antimicrobics, & tetanus toxoid (tetanus does not confer immunity). Options for control of muscle spasms: continuous infusion of midazolam, IV propofol, and/or intrathecal baclofen (CID 38:321, 2004).
VASCULAR				
Cavernous sinus thrombosis	Staph. aureus, Group A strep, H. influenzae, aspergillus/mucor/rhizopus	**Vanco** 1 gm IV q12h + **ceftriaxone** 2 gm IV q24x	**(Dapto** 6 mg per kg IV q24x[NFDA-approved] or **linezolid** 600 mg IV q12h) + **ceftriaxone** 2 gm IV q24h	CT or MRI scan for diagnosis. Heparin indicated (Ln 338:597, 1991). If patient diabetic with ketoacidosis or post-desferrioxamine rx or neutropenic, consider fungal etiology: aspergillus, mucor, rhizopus, see Table 11A, pages 75 & 82.
IV line infection (see IDSA Guidelines: CID 32:1249, 2001); **Treatment:** (For Prevention, see below)	Staph. epidermidis, Staph. aureus (MSSA/MRSA)	**Vanco** 1 gm IV q12h. **Linezolid alternative—see Comment.** Other rx and duration: (1) If S. aureus, remove catheter. Can use TEE result to determine if 2 or 4 wks of rx. (2) If S. epidermidis, can try to "save" catheter. 80% cure after 7–10 days of rx. **Catheter-hub/lumen: Infections may respond to "antibiotic lock" rx & allow salvage of catheter.** Drug (**vanco, gent, CIP**) at 1–5 mg per mL mixed with 50–100 units heparin (or saline) in 2–5 mL volume; fill catheter when not in use. Continue 2 wks. **For S. aureus, need full course of parenteral therapy** (JAC 48:597, 2001 & 55:90, 2005). If fungal, see Hyperalimentation below and Table 11A, pages 76–77.		If no response to, or intolerant of, **vanco**: switch to **daptomycin** 6 mg per kg IV q24h. If definitely no endocarditis or osteomyelitis, could use **linezolid** 600 mg IV po q12h. **Dalbavancin** an option (if vanco cross-allergenicity is not an issue): 1000 mg IV, 500 mg IV 8 days later if needed. See Table 6, page 57. Culture removed catheter. With "roll" method, >15 colonies (NEJM 312:1142, 1985) suggests infection. Lines do not require "routine" changing when not infected. When infected, do not insert new catheter over a wire. Antimicrobial-impregnated catheters may ↓ infection risk; the debate is lively (CID 37:65, 2003 & 38:1287, 2004 & 39:1829, 2004). **If S. epidermidis & catheter left in, vanco can cure 80%** of infections limited to exit site but only 25% cure if infection in subcutaneous tunnel between skin and subclavian vein. **If S. aureus & catheter left in, vanco cure rate 10% at exit site & 0% with tunnel infection** (AJM 89:137, 1990). Similar statistics for infected "ports" (CID 29: 102, 1999). Infected hemodialysis access catheters should be removed (AnIM 127: 275, 1997).
Heparin lock, midline catheter, non-tunneled central venous catheter (subclavian, internal jugular), peripherally inserted central catheter (PICC) Avoid femoral vein if possible. ↑ risk of infection and/or thrombosis (JAMA 286:700, 2001)				
Tunnel type indwelling venous catheters and ports (Broviac, Hickman, Groshong, Quinton), dual lumen hemodialysis catheters (Perma-cath)	Staph. epidermidis, Staph. aureus, (Candida sp.). Rarely: leuconostoc or lactobacillus—both resistant to vanco (see Table 2)			
Impaired host (burn, neutropenic)	As above + Pseudomonas sp. Enterobacteriaceae, Corynebacterium jeikeium, aspergillus, rhizopus	(**Vanco + P Ceph 3 AP**) or (**vanco + AP Pen** or **IMP** or (**P Ceph 4 + APAG**) (Dosage, see page 45)		Usually have associated septic thrombophlebitis. Biopsy of vein to rule out fungi. If fungal, surgical excision + amphotericin B. Surgical drainage, ligation or removal often indicated.
Hyperalimentation	As with tunnel + Candida sp. common (see Table 11, resistant Candida species)	If candida, **voriconazole** 3 mg per kg bid IV or **caspofungin** 70 mg IV day 1, then 50 mg IV q24h		Remove venous catheter and discontinue antimicrobial agents if possible. Ophthalmologic consultation recommended. **Rx all patients with + blood cultures.** See Table 11A, Candidiasis.
Intravenous lipid emulsion	Staph. epidermidis Malassezia furfur	**Vanco** 1 gm IV q12h	**Amphotericin B**	Discontinue intralipid AJM 90:129, 1991
IV line infection: Prevention (CID 35:1281, 2002; NEJM 348:1123, 2003) To minimize risk of infection: 1. Maximal sterile barrier precautions during catheter insertion 2. Use 2% chlorhexidine for skin antisepsis 3. If infection rate high despite # 1 & 2, use either chlorhexidine/silver sulfadiazine or minocycline/rifampin-impregnated catheters. 4. If possible, use subclavian vein			Tunneled hemodialysis catheters: Small study, ↓ infection rate when catheter locked with gentamicin (5 mg per mL) + heparin 5000 units per mL), p < 0.02 (Kidney Intl 66:801, 2004)	
Septic pelvic vein thrombophlebitis (with or without septic pulmonary emboli) Postpartum or postabortion or postpelvic surgery	Streptococci, bacteroides, Enterobacteriaceae	**Metro + P Ceph 3 cefoxitin †C-CL, PIP-TZ, AM-SB**	**IMP** or **MER** or **ERTA** or **clinda + (aztreonam** or **APAG)** Dosages: Table 10B	Use heparin during antibiotic regimen. Continued oral anticoagulation not recommended. Cefotetan less active than cefoxitin vs non-fragilis bacteroides. Cefotetan has methyltetrazole side-chain which is associated with hypoprothrombinemia (prevent with vitamin K).

Abbreviations on page 2.   NOTE: *All dosage recommendations are for adults (unless otherwise indicated) and assume normal renal/renal function.*

TABLE 1B: PROPHYLAXIS AND TREATMENT OF ORGANISMS OF POTENTIAL USE AS BIOLOGICAL WEAPONS (See page 2 for abbreviations)

DISEASE	ETIOLOGY	SUGGESTED EMPIRIC TREATMENT REGIMENS		SPECIFIC THERAPY AND COMMENTS
		PRIMARY	**ALTERNATIVE**	
Anthrax **Cutaneous, inhalational, gastrointestinal** Refs: *Ln 364:393 & 449, 2004; MMWR 50:909, 2001; NEJM 345:1607 & 1621, 2001; CID 35:851, 2002* or www.bt.cdc.gov *Also see Table 1, pages 31 & 37* To report bioterrorism event: 770-488-7100 Rationale for CIP: *CID 39:303, 2004*	Bacillus anthracis Post-exposure **prophylaxis**	**Adults (including pregnancy): Doxy** (CIP) 500 mg po bid or **Levo** 500 mg IV/po q24h) times 60 days **Children: CIP** 20–30 mg per kg per day div q12h times 60 days	**Adults (including pregnancy): Doxy** 100 mg po bid times 60 days. **Children** *(see Comment)*: **Doxy** >8 y/o & >45 kg: 100 mg po bid; >8 y/o & ≤45 kg: 2.2 mg per kg po bid; ≤8 y/o: 2.2 mg per kg po bid. All for 60 days.	1. Once organism shows susceptibility to penicillin, switch children to amoxicillin 80 mg per kg per day div. q8h (max. 500 mg q8h); switch pregnant pt to **amoxicillin** 500 mg po tid. 2. Do **not** use cephalosporins or TMP-SMX. 3. Other **FQs** (Gati, Moxi) & clarithro should work but no clinical experience.
	Treatment—**Cutaneous** anthrax *NEJM 345:1611, 2001*	**Adults (including pregnancy): Doxy** (CIP) 500 mg po bid or **Levo** 500 mg IV/po q24h) times 60 days **Children: CIP** 20–30 mg per kg per day div q12h po (to max. 1 gm per day) times 60 days	**Adults (including pregnancy): Doxy** 100 mg po bid times 60 days. **Children: Doxy** >8 y/o & >45 kg: 100 mg po bid; >8 y/o & ≤45 kg: 2.2 mg per kg po bid ≤8 y/o: 2.2 mg per kg po bid All for 60 days.	1. If penicillin susceptible, then: **Adults: Amox** 500 mg po q8h times 60 days **Children: Amox** 80 mg per kg per day div. q8h (max. 500 mg q8h) 2. Usual treatment of cutaneous anthrax is 7–10 days; 60 days in setting of bioterrorism with presumed aerosol exposure 3. Other **FQs** (Gati, Levo, Moxi) should work based on in vitro susceptibility data

	Treatment—**Inhalational,** gastrointestinal, or oropharyngeal
	
	Characteristic signs & symptoms—**Present:** Dyspnea, N/V; **Absent:** Rhinorrhea, sore throat
	(AnIM 139:337, 2003)
		Adults (including pregnancy): CIP 400 mg IV q12h) or (**Levo** 500 mg IV q24h) or (**doxy** 100 mg IV q12h) **+ clinda** 900 mg IV q8h **+ RIF** 300 mg IV q12h. Switch to po when able & ↓ **CIP** to 500 mg po bid; **clinda** to 450 mg po q8h; & **RIF** 300 mg po bid.
		Treat times 60 days. *See Table 2, page 49 for other alternatives.*
			Children: CIP 10 mg per kg IV q12h or 15 mg per kg po q12h) or (**Doxy** >8 y/o & >45 kg: 100 mg IV q12h; >8 y/o & ≤45 kg: 2.2 mg per kg IV q12h; ≤8 y/o: 2.2 mg per kg IV q12h) **plus clindamycin** 7.5 mg per kg IV q6h **plus RIF** 20 mg per kg IV qd.
			Treat times 60 days. *See Table 16, page 133 for oral dosage.*
				1. Clinda may block toxin production.
				2. Rifampin penetrates CSF & intracellular sites.
				3. If isolate shown penicillin-susceptible:
				  a. **Adult: Pen G** 4 million units IV q4h
				  b. **Child: Pen G** <12 y/o: 50,000 units per kg IV q6h; >12 y/o: 4 million units IV q4h
				  c. Constitutive & inducible β-lactamases—do not use pen or AMP alone.
				4. Do not use cephalosporins or TMP-SMX.
				5. Erythro, azithro activity borderline; clarithro active.
				6. No person-to-person spread.

Botulism: *CID 41:1167, 2005; JAMA 285:1059, 2001* **Food-borne** *See Table 1, page 46*	Clostridium botulinum	Purge GI tract if no ileus. **Trivalent antitoxin** (types A, B, & E): single 10 ml vial per pt. diluted in saline IV (slowly)	Antibiotics have no effect on toxin	Supportive care for all types. Follow vital capacity. Submit suspect food for toxin testing. Ref.: *CID 39:357 & 363, 2004*
Hemorrhagic fever viruses Ebola, Lassa, Hanta, yellow fever, & others	Ebola, Lassa, Hanta, yellow fever, & others	Fluid/electrolyte balance. Optimize circulatory volume.	For Lassa & Hanta: **Ribavirin** dose same as Adults. Pregnancy, Children: LD 30 mg per kg (max. 2 gm) IV times 1, then 16 mg per kg IV (max. 1 gm per dose) q6h times 4 days, then 8 mg per kg IV (max. 500 mg) q8h times 6 days	Ribavirin active in vitro; not FDA-approved for this indication. NOTE: Ribavirin contraindicated in pregnancy. However, in this setting, the benefits outweigh the risks.
Plague Ref.: *JAMA 283:2281, 2000* **Inhalation pneumonic plague** *See Table 1, page 42*	Yersinia pestis **Treatment**	**Gentamicin** 5 mg per kg IV q24h or **streptomycin** 15 mg per kg IV bid. Tobramycin should work.	**(Doxy** 200 mg IV times 1, & then 100 mg po or IV bid) or (**CIP** 500 mg po bid or 400 mg IV q12h) or **gentamicin plus doxy**. Ref.: *CID 38:663, 2004*	1. **Chloro** also active: 25 mg per kg IV qid. 2. In mass casualty situation, may have to treat po 3. Pediatric doses: *see Table 16, page 133*. 4. Pregnancy: *as for non-pregnant adults*
	Post-exposure prophylaxis	**Doxy** 100 mg po bid times 7 days	**CIP** 500 mg po bid times 7 days	5. Isolate during first 48 hrs of treatment For community with pneumonic plague epidemic. Pediatric doses: *see Table 16, page 133*. Pregnancy: *As for non-pregnant adults*
Smallpox Ref.: *NEJM, 346:1300, 2002* *See Table 14, page 113*	Variola virus	Smallpox vaccine up to 4 days after exposure; isolation; gloves, gown; NAS respirator	**Cidofovir** protected mice against aerosol cowpox *(JID 181:10, 2000)*	**Immediately notify State Health Dept.** & State notifies CDC (770-488-7100). Vaccinia immune globulin of no benefit. For vaccination complications, see *JAMA 288:1901, 2002.*
Tularemia **Inhalational tularemia** Ref.: *JAMA 285:2763, 2001* *See Table 1, page 43*	Francisella tularemia **Treatment**	(**Streptomycin** 15 mg per kg IV bid) or (**gentamicin** 5 mg per kg IV qd) times 10 days	**Doxy** 100 mg IV or po bid times 14–21 days or **CIP** 400 mg IV (or 750 mg po) bid times 14–21 days	For pediatric doses, *see Table 16, page 133*. Pregnancy. *As for non-pregnant adults.* **Tobramycin** should work.
	Post-exposure prophylaxis	**Doxy** 100 mg po bid times 14 days	**CIP** 500 mg po bid times 14 days	For pediatric doses, *see Table 16, page 133*. Pregnancy. *As for non-pregnant adults*

TABLE 2: RECOMMENDED ANTIMICROBIAL AGENTS AGAINST SELECTED BACTERIA

BACTERIAL SPECIES	ANTIMICROBIAL AGENT *(See page 2 for abbreviations)*		
	RECOMMENDED	ALTERNATIVE	ALSO EFFECTIVE[1] (COMMENTS)
Alcaligenes xylosoxidans (Achromobacter xylosoxidans)	IMP, MER, AP Pen	TMP-SMX. Some strains susc. to ceftaz *(AAC 32: 276, 1988)*	Resistant to APAG; P Ceph 1, 2, 3, 4; aztreonam; FQ *(AAC 40:772, 1996)*
Acinetobacter calcoaceticus–baumannii complex	IMP or MER or [FQ + (amikacin or ceftaz)]	AM-SB *(CID 24:932, 1997; CID 34:1425, 2002).* Sulbactam[NUS] also effective *(JAC 42:793, 1998)*;colistin *(CID 36:1111, 2003)*	Up to 10% isolates resistant to IMP; resistance to FQs, amikacin increasing. Doxy + amikacin effective in animal model *(JAC 45: 493, 2000). (See Table 5, page 56)*
Actinomyces israelii	AMP or Pen G	Doxy, ceftriaxone	Clindamycin, erythro
Aeromonas hydrophila	FQ	TMP-SMX or (P Ceph 3, 4)	APAG; ERTA; IMP; MER; tetracycline (some resistant to carbapenems)
Arcanobacterium (C.) haemolyticum	Erythro	Benzathine Pen G	Sensitive to most drugs, resistant to TMP-SMX *(AAC 38:142, 1994)*
Bacillus anthracis (anthrax): inhalation *[See Table 1B, page 48*			
Bacillus cereus, B. subtilis	Vancomycin, clindamycin	FQ, IMP	
Bacteroides fragilis (ssp. fragilis)	Metronidazole	Clindamycin	Cefoxitin, ERTA, IMP, MER, TC-CL, PIP-TZ, AM-SB, cefotetan, AM-CL
"DOT" group of bacteroides			(not cefotetan)
Bartonella (Rochalimaea) henselae, quintana *See Table 1, pages 33, 37, 41*	Azithro or clarithro or CIP (bacillary angiomatosis) or azithro (cat-scratch) *(PIDJ 17:447, 1998; AAC 48:1921, 2004)*	Erythro or doxy	Other drugs: TMP-SMX *(IDC No. Amer 12:137, 1998).* Consider doxy + RIF for severe bacillary angiomatosis *(IDC No. Amer 12:137, 1998)*; doxy + gentamicin optimal for endocarditis *(AAC 47:2204, 2003)*
Bordetella pertussis	Erythro	TMP-SMX	An erythro-resistant strain reported in Arizona *(MMWR 43:807, 1994)*
Borrelia burgdorferi, B. afzelii, B. garinii	Ceftriaxone, cefuroxime axetil, doxy, amox *(See Comments)*	Penicillin G (HD), cefotaxime	Clarithro. Choice depends on stage of disease, *Table 1, page 42*
Borrelia sp.	Doxy	Erythro	Penicillin G
Brucella sp.	Doxy + either gentamicin or streptomycin *(IDCP 7, 2004)*	(Doxy + RIF) or (TMP-SMX + gentamicin)	FQ + RIF *(AAC 41:80, 1997; EID 3:213, 1997; CID 21:283, 1995).* Minocycline + RIF *(J Chemother 15:248, 2003).*
Burkholderia (Pseudomonas) cepacia	TMP-SMX or MER or CIP	Minocycline or chloramphenicol	(Usually resistant to APAG, AG, polymyxins) *(AAC 37: 123, 1993 & 43:213, 1999; Inf Medicine 18:49, 2001)* (Some resistant to carbapenems). Combination rx may be necessary *(AJRCCM 161:1206, 2000).*
Burkholderia (Pseudomonas) pseudomallei *See Table 1, page 30, & Ln 361:1715, 2003*	Initially, IV ceftaz or IMP *(CID 29:381, 1999)*	Then, combination of po chloro, doxy, & TMP-SMX	(In Thailand, 12–80% strains resistant to TMP-SMX). FQ active in vitro. Combination of chloro, TMP-SMX, doxy more effective than doxy alone for maintenance rx *(CID 29:375, 1999).* MER also effective *(AAC 48: 1763,2004)*
Campylobacter jejuni	Erythro	FQ (↑ resistance, *NEJM 340: 1525,1999)*	Clindamycin, doxy, azithro, clarithro *(see Table 5, page 57)*
Campylobacter fetus	IMP	Gentamicin	AMP, chloramphenicol, erythro
Capnocytophaga ochracea (DF-1) and	Clindamycin or AM-CL	CIP, Pen G	P Ceph 3, IMP, cefoxitin, FQ, (resistant to APAG, TMP-SMX). C. haemolytica & C. granulosa are often resistant to β-lactams & aminoglycosides [CID 35 (Suppl.1):S17, 2002].
canimorsus (DF-2)	AM-CL		
Chlamydophila pneumoniae	Doxy	Erythro, FQ	Azithro, clarithro, telithro
Chlamydia trachomatis	Doxy or azithro	Erythro or oflox	Levofloxacin
Chryseobacterium (Flavobacterium) meningosepticum	Vancomycin ± RIF *(CID 26:1169, 1998)*	CIP, levofloxacin	In vitro susceptibilities may not correlate with clinical efficacy *(AAC 41:1301, 1997; CID 26:1169, 1998)*
Citrobacter diversus (koseri), C. freundii	CARB	FQ	APAG
Clostridium difficile	Metronidazole (po)	Vancomycin (po)	Bacitracin (po)
Clostridium perfringens	Pen G ± clindamycin	Doxy	Erythro, chloramphenicol, cefazolin, cefoxitin, AP Pen, CARB
Clostridium tetani	Metronidazole or Pen G	Doxy	CARB
Corynebacterium jeikeium	Vancomycin	Pen G + APAG	
C. diphtheriae	Erythro	Clindamycin	RIF. Penicillin reported effective *(CID 27:845, 1998)*
Coxiella burnetii (Q fever) acute disease	Doxy *(see Table 1, page 23)*	Erythro	In meningitis consider FQ *(CID 20:489, 1995).* Endocarditis: doxy + hydroxy-chloroquine *(JID 188:1322, 2003; LnID 3:709, 2003).*
chronic disease	(CIP or doxy) + RIF	FQ + doxy x3 yrs *(CID 20:489, 1995)*	Chloroquine + doxy *(AAC 37:1773, 1993).* ? gamma interferon *(Ln 20:546, 2001)*
Ehrlichia chaffeensis, Ehrlichia ewubguum Anaplasma (Ehrlichia) phagocytophilium	Doxy	Tetracycline, RIF *(CID 27:213, 1998)*	CIP, oflox, chloramphenicol also active in vitro. Resistant to clinda, TMP-SMX, IMP, AMP, erythro, & azithro *(AAC 41:76, 1997).*

TABLE 2 (2)

BACTERIAL SPECIES	ANTIMICROBIAL AGENT *(See page 2 for abbreviations)*		
	RECOMMENDED	ALTERNATIVE	ALSO EFFECTIVE[1] (COMMENTS)
Eikenella corrodens	Penicillin G or AMP or AM-CL	TMP-SMX, FQ	Doxy, cefoxitin, cefotaxime, IMP (Resistant to clindamycin, cephalexin, erythromycin, and metronidazole)
Enterobacter species	Recommended agents vary with clinical setting. *See Tables 1 & 4*		
Enterococcus faecalis	*See Table 5, page 56*		
Enterococcus faecium, β-lactamase +, high-level aminoglycoside resist., vancomycin resist.: *See Table 5, page 56*			
Erysipelothrix rhusiopathiae	Penicillin G or AMP	P Ceph 3, FQ	IMP, AP Pen (vancomycin, APAG, TMP-SMX resistant)
Escherichia coli	Recommended agents vary with clinical setting. *See Tables 1 & 4*		
Francisella tularensis (tularemia) *See Table 1B, page 48*	Gentamicin, tobramycin, or streptomycin	Doxy or CIP	Chloramphenicol, RIF. Doxy/chloro bacteriostatic → relapses
Gardnerella vaginalis (bacterial vaginosis)	Metronidazole	Clindamycin	*See Table 1, page 20 for dosage*
Hafnia alvei	*Same as Enterobacter spp.*		
Helicobacter pylori	*See Table 1, page 16*		Drugs effective in vitro often fail in vivo.
Hemophilus aphrophilus	[(Penicillin or AMP) ± gentamicin] or [AM-SB ± gentamicin]	P Ceph 2, 3 ± gentamicin	(Resistant to vancomycin, clindamycin, methicillin)
Hemophilus ducreyi (chancroid)	Azithro or ceftriaxone	Erythro, CIP	Most strains resistant to tetracycline, amox, TMP-SMX
Hemophilus influenzae Meningitis, epiglottitis & other life-threatening illness	Cefotaxime, ceftriaxone	TMP-SMX, CARB, FQs (AMP if β-lactamase negative) (U.S. 25–30% AMP resistance, Japan 35%)	Chloramphenicol (downgraded from 1st choice because of hematotoxicity). 9% of U.S. strains resistant to TMP-SMX *(AAC 41:292, 1997)*
non-life threatening illness	AM-CL, O Ceph 2/3, TMP-SMX, AM-SB		Azithro, clarithro, telithro
Klebsiella ozaenae/rhinoscleromatis	FQ	RIF + TMP-SMX	*(Ln 342:122, 1993)*
Klebsiella species	Recommended agents vary with clinical setting. *See Tables 1 & 4*		
Lactobacillus species	(Pen G or AMP) ± gentamicin	Clindamycin, erythro	**May be resistant to vancomycin**
Legionella sp. *(42 species & 60 serotypes recognized) (Sem Resp Inf 13:90, 1998)*	FQ, or azithro, or (erythro ± RIF)	Clarithro	TMP-SMX, doxy. Most active FQs in vitro: Gemi, Gati, Levo, Moxi. *See AnIM 129: 328, 1998.* Telithro active in vitro.
Leptospira interrogans	Penicillin G	Doxy	Ceftriaxone *(CID 36:1507, 2003)*, cefotaxime *(CID 39:1417, 2004)*
Leuconostoc	Pen G or AMP	Clindamycin, erythro, minocycline	APAG **NOTE: Resistant to vancomycin**
Listeria monocytogenes	AMP	TMP-SMX	Erythro, penicillin G (high dose), APAG may be synergistic with β-lactams. **Cephalosporin-resistant!**
Moraxella (Branhamella) catarrhalis	AM-CL or O Ceph 2/3, TMP-SMX	Azithro, clarithro, dirithromycin, telithro	Erythro, doxy, FQs
Morganella species	Recommended agents vary with clinical setting. *See Tables 1 & 4*		
Mycoplasma pneumoniae	Erythro, azithro, clarithro, dirithro, telithro,or FQ	Doxy	(Clindamycin and β lactams NOT effective)
Neisseria gonorrhoeae (gonococcus)	Ceftriaxone, cefixime, cefpodoxime	Ofloxacin & other FQs *(Table 1, pages 17–18),* spectinomycin	Kanamycin (used in Asia). FQ resistance in Asia; rare in U.S., but ↑ *(MMWR 47:405, 1998)*
Neisseria meningitidis (meningococcus)	Penicillin G	Ceftriaxone, cefuroxime, cefotaxime	Sulfonamide (some strains), chloramphenicol. Chloro-resistant strains found in SE Asia *(NEJM 339:868, 1998)* (Prophylaxis: *page 8*)
Nocardia asteroides	TMP-SMX, sulfonamides (high dose),	Minocycline	Amikacin + (IMP or ceftriaxone or cefuroxime) for brain abscess
Nocardia brasiliensis	TMP-SMX, sulfonamides (high dose)	AM-CL	Amikacin + ceftriaxone
Pasteurella multocida	Pen G, AMP, amox	Doxy, AM-CL, P Ceph 2, TMP-SMX	Ceftriaxone, cefpodoxime, FQ (active in vitro), azithro (active in vitro) *(DMID 30:99, 1998; AAC 43:1475, 1999)*
Plesiomonas shigelloides	CIP	TMP-SMX	AM-CL, P Ceph 1,2,3,4, IMP, MER, tetracycline, aztreonam
Proteus mirabilis (indole–)	AMP	TMP-SMX	Most agents except nafcillin/oxacillin. β-lactamase (including ESBL) production now being described in P. mirabilis *(J Clin Micro 40:1549, 2002)*
vulgaris (indole +)	P Ceph 3 or FQ	APAG	CARB, aztreonam, BL/BLI
Providencia sp.	Amikacin or P Ceph 3 or FQ	TMP-SMX	AP Pen + amikacin, IMP
Pseudomonas aeruginosa	AP Pen, AP Ceph 3, IMP, MER, tobramycin, CIP, aztreonam. For serious inf., use AP β-lactam + tobramycin or CIP *(LnID 4:519, 2004)*	For UTI, single drugs usually effective: AP Pen, AP Ceph 3, cefepime, IMP, MER, APAG, CIP, aztreonam	Resistance to β-lactams (IMP, ceftaz) may emerge during rx. β-lactam inhibitor adds nothing to activity of TC or PIP against P. aeruginosa. Clavulanic acid has been shown to antagonize TC in vitro *(AAC 43:882, 1999)*. (See also Table 5A). Editors recommend combination therapy for serious infections, but value of combinations remains controversial *(LnID 5:192, 2005)*.

TABLE 2 (3)

BACTERIAL SPECIES	ANTIMICROBIAL AGENT *(See page 2 for abbreviations)*		
	RECOMMENDED	ALTERNATIVE	ALSO EFFECTIVE[1] (COMMENTS)
Rhodococcus (C. equi)	IMP, APAG, erythro, vancomycin, or RIF (consider 2 agents)	CIP (variable) [resistant strains SE Asia *(CID 27: 370, 1998)*], TMP-SMX, tetracycline, or clindamycin	Vancomycin active in vitro but intracellular location of R. equi may impair efficacy *(Sem Resp Inf 12:57, 1997; CID 34:1379, 2002)*
Rickettsiae species	Doxy	Chloramphenicol	FQ; clari, azithro effective for Mediterranean spotted fever in children *(CID 34:154, 2002)*.
Salmonella typhi	FQ, ceftriaxone	Chloramphenicol, amox, TMP-SMX, azithro (for uncomplicated disease: *AAC 43:1441, 1999)*	Multi drug resistant strains (chloramphenicol, AMP, TMP-SMX) common in many developing countries, seen in immigrants. FQ resistance now being reported *(AJTMH 61:163, 1999)*.
Serratia marcescens	P Ceph 3, ERTA, IMP, MER, FQ	Aztreonam, gentamicin	TC-CL, PIP-TZ
Shigella sp.	FQ or azithro	TMP-SMX and AMP (resistance common in Middle East, Latin America). Azithro ref.: *AnIM 126:697, 1997*	
Staph. aureus, methicillin-susceptible	Oxacillin/nafcillin	P Ceph 1, vancomycin, teicoplanin[NUS], clindamycin, dalbavancin	ERTA, IMP, MER, BL/BLI, FQ, erythro, clarithro, dirithromycin, azithro, telithro, quinu-dalfo, linezolid, dapto
Staph. aureus, methicillin-resistant (health-care associated)	Vancomycin	Teicoplanin[NUS], TMP-SMX (some strains resistant), quinu-dalfo, linezolid, daptomycin, dalbavancin	Fusidic acid[NUS]. >60% CIP-resistant in U.S. (Fosfomycin + RIF), novobiocin. Partially vancomycin-resistant strains (GISA, VISA) & highly resistant strains now described—*see Table 6, page 57.*
Staph. aureus, methicillin-resistant [community-acquired (CA-MRSA)]			CA-MRSA usually not multiply-resistant *(Ln 359: 1819, 2002; JAMA 286: 1201, 2001)*. Often resist. to erythro & variably to FQ. Vanco, teico[NUS], daptomycin or dalbavancin can be used in pts requiring hospitalization *(see Table 6, page 57)*.
Mild-moderate infection	(TMP-SMX or doxy or mino) ± RIF *(CID 40: 1429, 2005)*	Clinda (if susceptible to erythro & clinda)	
Severe infection	Vanco or teico[NUS]	Linezolid or daptomycin or dalbavancin	
Staph. epidermidis	Vancomycin ± RIF	RIF + (TMP-SMX or FQ), dalbavancin, daptomycin	Cephalothin or nafcillin/oxacillin if sensitive to nafcillin/oxacillin but 75% are resistant. FQs. *(See Table 5)*
Staph. haemolyticus	TMP-SMX, FQ, nitrofurantoin	Oral cephalosporin	Recommendations apply to UTI only.
Staph. lugdunensis	Oxacillin/nafcillin or penicillin G (if β-lactamase neg.) *(Inf Dis Alert 22:193, 2003)*	P Ceph 1 or vancomycin or teico[NUS]	Approx. 75% are penicillin-susceptible. Usually susceptible to gentamicin, RIF *(AAC 32:2434, 1990)*.
Staph. saprophyticus (UTI)	Oral cephalosporin or AM-CL	FQ	Susceptible to most agents used for UTI; occ. failure of sulfonamides, nitrofurantoin reported *(JID 155:170, 1987)*. Resistant to fosfomycin.
Stenotrophomonas (Xanthomonas, Pseudomonas) maltophilia	TMP-SMX	TC-CL or (aztreonam + TC-CL) *(AAC 41:2612, 1997)*	Minocycline, doxy, ceftaz. [In vitro synergy (TC-CL + TMP-SMX) and (TC-CL + CIP), *AAC 39:2220, 1995; CMR 11:57, 1998]*
Streptobacillus moniliformis	Penicillin G or doxy	Erythro, clindamycin	
Streptococcus, anaerobic (Peptostreptococcus)	Penicillin G	Clindamycin	Erythro, doxy, vancomycin
Streptococcus pneumoniae penicillin-susceptible	Penicillin G	Multiple agents effective, e.g., amox	*See footnote 2 page 9*
penicillin-resistant (MIC ≥2.0)	(Vancomycin ± RIF) or (Gati, Levo, or Moxi) *See footnote 1 page 6 and Table 5, page 56)*		For non-meningeal infections: P Ceph 3/4, CARB, quinu-dalfo, linezolid, telithro
Streptococcus pyogenes, Groups A, B, C, G, F, **Strep. milleri** (constellatus, intermedius, anginosus)	Penicillin G or V (some add gentamicin for serious Group B strep infections & some add clinda for serious invasive Group A strep infections) *(SMJ 96:968, 2003)*	All β lactams, erythro, azithro, dirithromycin, clarithro, telithro	Macrolide resistance increasing.
Vibrio cholerae	Doxy, FQ	TMP-SMX	Strain 0139 is resistant to TMP-SMX
Vibrio parahemolyticus	Antibiotic rx does not ↓ course		Sensitive in vitro to FQ, doxy
Vibrio vulnificus, alginolyticus, damsela	Doxy + ceftaz	Cefotaxime, FQ (e.g., levo, *AAC 46:3580, 2002)*	APAG often used in combination with ceftaz
Yersinia enterocolitica	TMP-SMX or FQ	P Ceph 3 or APAG	*CID 19:655, 1994*
Yersinia pestis (plague)	*See Table 1B, page 48*		

[1] These agents are more variable in effectiveness than the "Recommended" or "Alternative". Selection of "Alternative" or "Also Effective" agents is based on in vitro susceptibility testing, pharmacokinetics, host factors such as auditory, renal, hepatic function, and cost.

52

TABLE 3: SUGGESTED DURATION OF ANTIBIOTIC THERAPY IN IMMUNOCOMPETENT PATIENTS[1,2]

SITE	CLINICAL DIAGNOSIS	DURATION OF THERAPY (Days)
Bacteremia	Bacteremia with removable focus (no endocarditis)	10–14 *(CID 14:75, 1992) (See Table 1)*
Bone	Osteomyelitis, adult; acute	42
	adult; chronic	Until ESR normal (often > 3 months)
	child; acute; staph. and enterobacteriaceae[3]	21
	child; acute; strep., meningococci, hemophilus[3]	14
Ear	Otitis media with effusion	<2 yrs: 10 (or 1 dose ceftriaxone) ; ≥2 yrs: 5–7
	Recent meta-analysis suggests 3 days of azithro *(JAC 52:469, 2003)* or 5 days of "short-acting" antibiotics effective for uncomplicated otitis media *(JAMA 279:1736, 1998)*, but may be inadequate for severe disease *(NEJM 347:1169, 2002)*.	
Endocardium	Infective endocarditis, native valve	
	Viridans strep	14 or 28 *(See Table 1, pages 21–22)*
	Enterococci	28 or 42 *(See Table 1, page 22)*
	Staph. aureus	14 (R-sided only) or 28 *(See Table 1, pages 22–23)*
Gastrointestinal *Also see Table 1*	Bacillary dysentery (shigellosis)/traveler's diarrhea	3
	Typhoid fever (S. typhi): Azithro	5 (children/adolescents)
	Ceftriaxone	14*
	FQ	5–7
	Chloramphenicol	14
		*[Short courses less effective *(AAC 44:450, 2000)*]
	Helicobacter pylori	10–14
	Pseudomembranous enterocolitis (C. difficile)	10
Genital	Non-gonococcal urethritis or mucopurulent cervicitis	7 days doxy or single dose azithro
	Pelvic inflammatory disease	14
Heart	Pericarditis (purulent)	28
Joint	Septic arthritis (non-gonococcal) Adult	14–28 *(Ln 351:197, 1998)*
	Infant/child	Rx as osteomyelitis above
	Gonococcal arthritis/disseminated GC infection	7 *(See Table 1, page 17)*
Kidney	Cystitis (bladder bacteriuria)	3
	Pyelonephritis	14 (7 days if CIP used)
	Recurrent (failure after 14 days rx)	42
Lung	Pneumonia, pneumococcal	Until afebrile 3–5 days (minimum 5 days)
	Pneumonia, enterobacteriaceae or pseudomonal	21, often up to 42
	Pneumonia, staphylococcal	21–28
	Pneumocystis carinii, in AIDS;	21
	other immunocompromised	14
	Legionella, mycoplasma, chlamydia	7–14
	Lung abscess	Usually 28–42[4]
Meninges[5] *(CID 39:1267, 2004)*	N. meningitidis	7
	H. influenzae	7
	S. pneumoniae	10–14
	Listeria meningoencephalitis, gp B strep, coliforms	21 (longer in immunocompromised)
Multiple systems	Brucellosis *(See Table 1, page 43)*	42 (add SM or gent for 1st 7–14 days)
	Tularemia *(See Table 1, pages 33, 43)*	7–14
Muscle	Gas gangrene (clostridial)	10
Pharynx *Also see Pharyngitis, Table 1, page 35*	Group A strep pharyngitis	10 O Ceph 2/3, azithromycin effective at 5 days *(JAC 45, Topic TI 23, 2000)*. 3 days less effective *(Inf Med 18:515, 2001)*
	Diphtheria (membranous)	7–14
	Carrier	7
Prostate	Chronic prostatitis (TMP/SMX)	30–90
	(FQ)	28–42
Sinuses	Acute sinusitis	10–14[6]
Skin	Cellulitis	Until 3 days after acute inflammation disappears
Systemic	Lyme disease	See Table 1, page 42
	Rocky Mountain spotted fever *(See Table 1, page 43)*	Until afebrile 2 days

[1] It has been shown that early change from parenteral to oral regimens (about 72 hours) is cost-effective with many infections, i.e., intra-abdominal *(AJM 91:462, 1991)*
[2] The recommended duration is a minimum or average time and should not be construed as absolute
[3] These times are with proviso: sx & signs resolve within 7 days and ESR is normalized *(J.D. Nelson, APID 6:59, 1991)*
[4] After patient afebrile 4-5 days, change to oral therapy
[5] In children relapses seldom occur until 3 days or more after termination of rx. Practice of observing in hospital for 1 or 2 days after rx is expensive and non-productive. For meningitis in children, *see Table 1, page 6.*
[6] If pt not sx-free at 10 days, sinus puncture and/or rx for 7 more days *(NEJM 326:319, 1992)*. One study reports 3 days of TMP-SMX effective *(JAMA 273:1015, 1995)*. Therapy with azithro for 3 & 6 days as effective as 10 days of AM/CL *(AAC 47:2770, 2003)*.

53

TABLE 4
COMPARISON OF ANTIMICROBIAL SPECTRA*
(These are generalizations; there are major differences between countries, areas and hospitals depending upon antibiotic usage patterns—verify for individual location. See Table 5 for resistant bacteria)

Organisms	Penicillin G	Penicillin V	Methicillin	Nafcillin/Oxacillin	Cloxacillin[NUS]/Diclox.	AMP/Amox	Amox/Clav	AMP-Sulb	Ticarcillin	Ticar-Clav	Pip-Tazo	Piperacillin	Ertapenem	Imipenem	Meropenem	Aztreonam	Ciprofloxacin	Ofloxacin	Lomefloxacin	Pefloxacin[NUS]	Levofloxacin	Moxifloxacin	Gemifloxacin	Gatifloxacin
GRAM-POSITIVE:																								
Strep, Group A,B,C,G	+	+	+	+	+	+	+	+	+	+	+	+	+	+	+	0	±	±	0	0	+	+	+	+
Strep. pneumoniae	+	+	+	+	+	+	+	+	+	+	+	+	+	+	+	0	±	±	0	0	+	+	+	+
Viridans strep	±	±	±	±	±	±	±	±	±	±	±	±	+	+	+	0	0	0			+	+	+	+
Strep. milleri	+	+	+	+	+	+	+	+	+	+	+	+	+	+	+	0	0	0			+	+	+	+
Enterococcus faecalis	+	+	0	0	0	+	+	+	±	±	+	+	±	±	±	0	**	**			0	+	+	+
Enterococcus faecium	±	±	0	0	0	+	+	+	±	±	±	±	0	±	0	0	0	0			0	0	±	±
Staph. aureus (MSSA)	0	0	+	+	+	0	+	+	0	+	+	0	+	+	+	0	+	+	+	+	+	+	+	+
Staph. aureus (MRSA)	0	0	0	0	0	0	0	0	0	0	0	0	0	0	0	0	0	0	0	0	0	±	±	±
Staph. epidermidis	0	0	+	+	+	+	+	+	±	±	+	0	+	+	+	0	+	+	+	+	+	+	+	+
C. jeikeium	0	0	0	0	0	0	0	0	0	0	0	0	0	0	0	0	0	0						
L. monocytogenes	+	0	0	0	0	+		+	+			+	±	+	+	0	+	0	0	0	+	+	+	+
GRAM-NEGATIVE:																								
N. gonorrhoeae	0	0	0	0	0	0	+	+	+	+	+	+	+	+	+	+								+
N. meningitidis	+	0	0	0	0	+	+	+	+	+	+	+	+	+	+	+	+	+			+	+		+
M. catarrhalis	0	0	0	0	0	0	+	+	0	+	±	+	+	+	+	+	+	+	+	+	+	+	+	+
H. influenzae	0	0	0	0	0	±	+	+	±	+	+	+	+	+	+	+	+	+	+	+	+	+	+	+
E. coli	0	0	0	0	0	±	+	+	±	+	+	+	+	+	+	+	+	+	+	+	+	+	+	+
Klebsiella sp.	0	0	0	0	0	0	+	+	0	+	+	+	+	+	+	+	+	+	+	+	+	+	+	+
Enterobacter sp.	0	0	0	0	0	0	0	0	+	+	+	+	+	+	+	+	+	+	+	+	+	+	+	+
Serratia sp.	0	0	0	0	0	0	0	0	+	+	+	0	+	+	+	+	+	+			+	+	+	+
Salmonella sp.	0	0	0	0	0	±	+	+	±	+	+	+	+	+	+	+	+	+			+	+	+	+
Shigella sp.	0	0	0	0	0	±	+	+	+	+	+	+	+	+	+	+	+	+			+	+	+	+
Proteus mirabilis	0	0	0	0	0	+	+	+	+	+	+	+	+	+	+	+	+	+	+	+	+	+	+	+
Proteus vulgaris	0	0	0	0	0	0	+	+	+	+	+	+	+	+	+	+	+	+	+	+	+	+	+	+
Providencia sp.	0	0	0	0	0	0	+	+	+	+	+	+	+	+	+	+	+	+	+		+	+		+
Morganella sp.	0	0	0	0	0	0	±	+	+	+	+	+	+	+	+	+	+	+	+		+	+		+
Citrobacter sp.	0	0	0	0	0	0	0	0	+	+	+	+	+	+	+	+	+	+	+		+	+		+
Aeromonas sp.	0	0	0	0	0	0	+	+	+	+	+	+	+	+	+	+	+	+			+	+		+
Acinetobacter sp.	0	0	0	0	0	0	0	0	+	0	+	0	±	±		±	±				±	±	±	±
Ps. aeruginosa	0	0	0	0	0	0	0	0	+	+	+	+	0	+	+	+	±	±	±		±	±		±
B. (Ps.) cepacia§	0	0	0	0	0	0	0	0	0		0	0		0	+	0	0	0			0		0	0
S. (X.) maltophilia§	0	0	0	0	0	0	0	0	0	±	±	±		0	0	0	0	0	0	0	±	+		
Y. enterocolitica	0	0	0	0	0	0	±	±	±	+		+		+		+	+	+	+		+	+		+
Legionella sp.	0	0	0	0	0	0	0	0	0	0	0	0	0	0	0	0	+	+			+	+	+	+
P. multocida	+	+				+	+	+		+	+		+	+	+	+	+	+			+	+		+
H. ducreyi	+					0	+	+																
MISC.:																								
Chlamydia sp.	0	0	0	0	0	0	0	0	0	0	0	0	0	0	0	0	+	+	+	+	+	+	+	+
M. pneumoniae	0	0	0	0	0	0	0	0	0	0	0	0	0	0	0	0	+	+	+	+	+	+	+	+
ANAEROBES:																								
Actinomyces	+	±	0	0	0	+	+	+				+	+	+		0	0	±					+	+
Bacteroides fragilis	0	±	0	0	0	0	+	+	0	+	+	0	+	+	+	0	0	0	0	0	0	0	+	±
P. melaninogenica§	+	0	0	0	0	+	+	+	+	+	+		+	+	+	0	0	±	0		+	+		±
Clostridium difficile	+[1]					+[1]					+[1]	+[1]	+[1]	+[1]	0	0	0			0		0	0	0
Clostridium *(not difficile)*	+	+				+	+	+	+	+	+	+	+	+	+	0	±	±	0		+	+		+
Peptostreptococcus sp.	+	+	+	+	+	+	+	+	+	+	+	+	+	+	+	0	±	±	0		+	+		+

+ =usually effective clinically or >60% susceptible; ± = clinical trials lacking or 30–60% susceptible; 0 = not effective clinically or <30% susceptible; blank = data not available

§ B. melaninogenicus → Prevotella melaninogenica, Pseudomonas cepacia → Burkholderia cepacia, Xanthomonas → Stenotrophomonas

** Most strains ±, can be used in UTI, not in systemic infection

[1] No clinical evidence that penicillins or fluoroquinolones are effective for C. difficile enterocolitis (but they may cover this organism in mixed intra-abdominal and pelvic infections)

TABLE 4 (2)

Organisms	Cefazolin	Cefotetan	Cefoxitin	Cefuroxime	Cefotaxime	Ceftizoxime	Ceftriaxone	Ceftazidime	Cefepime	Cefadroxil	Cephalexin	Cefaclor/Loracarbef*	Cefprozil	Cefuroxime axetil	Cefixime	Ceftibuten	Cefpodox/Cefdinir/Cefditoren
	1st Gen	2nd Generation			3rd/4th Generation					1st Gen (Oral)		2nd Gen (Oral)			3rd Gen (Oral)		
GRAM-POSITIVE:																	
Strep, Group A,B,C,G	+	+	+	+	+	+	+	+	+	+	+	+	+	+	+	+	+
Strep. pneumoniae[1]	+	+	+	+	+	+	+	+[1]	+	+	+	+	+	+	+	±	+
Viridans strep	+	+	+	+	+	+	+	±[1]	+	+	+	+	0	+	+	0	+
Enterococcus faecalis	0	0	0	0	0	0	0	0	0	0	0	0	0	0	0	0	0
Staph. aureus (MSSA)	+	+	+	+	+	+	+	±	+	+	+	+	+	+	0	0	+
Staph. aureus (MRSA)	0	0	0	0	0	0	0	0	0	0	0	0	0	0	0	0	0
Staph. epidermidis	±	±	±	±	±	±	±	±	±	±	±	±	±	±	0	0	±
C. jeikeium	0	0	0	0	0	0	0	0		0	0	0	0	0	0	0	
L. monocytogenes	0	0	0	0	0	0	0	0	0	0	0	0	0	0	0	0	0
GRAM-NEGATIVE																	
N. gonorrhoeae	+	±	±	±	±	±	+	±	+	0	0	±	±	±	+	±	+
N. meningitidis	0	±	±	+	+	±	+	±	+	0	0	±	±	±	±	±	
M. catarrhalis	±	+	+	+	+	+	+	+	+	0	0	±	+	+	+	+	+
H. influenzae	+	+	+	+	+	+	+	+	+		0	+	+	+	+	+	+
E. coli	+	+	+	+	+	+	+	+	+	+	+	+	+	+	+	+	+
Klebsiella sp.	+	+	+	+	+	+	+	+	+	+	+	+	+	+	+	+	
Enterobacter sp.	0	±	0	±	+	+	+	+	+	0	0	0	0	0	0	±	0
Serratia sp.	0	+	0	0	+	+	+	+	+	0	0	0	0	0	±	±	0
Salmonella sp.					+	+	+	+	+	0	0				+	+	+
Shigella sp.					+	+	+	+		0	0				+	+	+
Proteus mirabilis	+	+	+	+	+	+	+	+	+	+	+	+	+	+	+	+	+
Proteus vulgaris	0	+	+	+	+	+	+	+	+	0	0	0	0	0	+	+	±
Providencia sp.	0	+	+	0	+	+	+	+	+	0	0	0	0	+	+	+	
Morganella sp.	0	+	+	±	+	+	+	+	+	0	0	0	0	±	0	0	0
C. freundii	0	0	0	0	0	0	0	+	+	0	0	0	0	0	0	0	0
C. diversus	0	±	±	±	+	+	+	+	+	0	0	0	0				+
Citrobacter sp.	0	±	±	±	+	+	+	+	+		0	±	0	±	+	+	+
Aeromonas sp.	0	+	±	+	+	+	+	+	+						+	+	
Acinetobacter sp.	0	0	0	0	+	+	+	+	±	0	0	0	0	0	0	0	
Ps. aeruginosa	0	0	0	0	±	±	±	+	+	0	0	0	0	0	0	0	0
B. (Ps.) cepacia§	0	0	0	0	±	±	±	+	+	0	0	0	0	0	0	+	
S. (X.) maltophilia§	0	0	0	0	0	0	0	±	0	0	0	0	0	0			
Y. enterocolitica	0	±	±	±	+	+	+	±	+						+	+	
Legionella sp.	0	0	0	0	0	0	0	0	0	0	0	0	0	0	0	0	0
P. multocida					+	+						0			+		+
H. ducreyi			+		+	+	+	+							+		
ANAEROBES:																	
Actinomyces						+	+										
Bacteroides fragilis	0	±[2]	+	0	0	±	0	0	0		0	0	0	0	0	0	
P. melaninogenica§		+	+	+	+	+	±	+	0				+	+	+	+	
Clostridium difficile			0		0	0			0								
Clostridium (not difficile)		+	+	+	+	+	+	+					+	+	0		
Peptostreptococcus sp.		+	+	+	+	+	+	+	+		+	+	+	+	+		

+ = usually effective clinically or >60% susceptible; ± = clinical trials lacking or 30–60% susceptible; 0 = not effective clinically or <30% susceptible; blank = data not available.

§ B. melaninogenicus → Prevotella melaninogenica, P. cepacia → Burkholderia cepacia, Xanthomonas → Stenotrophomonas

* A 1-carbacephem best classified as a cephalosporin

[1] Ceftaz 8–16 times less active than cefotax/ceftriax, effective only vs Pen-sens. strains (AAC 39:2193, 1995). Oral cefuroxime, cefprozil, cefpodoxime most active in vitro vs resistant S. pneumo (PIDJ 14:1037, 1995).

[2] Cefotetan is less active against B. ovatus, B. distasonis, B. thetaiotamicron

TABLE 4 (3)

Organisms	Gentamicin	Tobramycin	Amikacin	Netilmicin^NUS	Chloramphenicol	Clindamycin	Erythro/Dirithro	Azithromycin	Clarithromycin	Telithromycin	Doxycycline	Minocycline	Tigecycline	Vancomycin	Teicoplanin	Dalbavancin	Fusidic Acid^NUS	TMP-SMX	Trimethoprim	Nitrofurantoin	Fosfomycin	Rifampin	Metronidazole	Quinupristin-dalfopristin	Linezolid	Daptomycin	Colistimethate (Colistin)
GRAM-POSITIVE:																											
Strep Group A,B,C,G	0	0	0	0	+	+	+	+	+	+	±	+	+	+	+	+	±	+	+[1]	+		+	0	+	+	+	0
Strep. pneumoniae	0	0	0	0	+	+	+	+	+	+	+	+	+	+	+	+	±	+	+[1]	+	+	+	0	+	+	+	0
Enterococcus faecalis	S	S	S	S	±	0	0	0	0	±	0	0	+	+	+	+	+	+	+[1]	+	±	±	0	0	+	+	0
Enterococcus faecium	S	0	0	0	±	0	0	0	0	0	0	0	+	±	±	±		0	0	+	±	0	0	+	+	+	0
Staph.aureus (MSSA)	+	+	+	+	±	+	±	+	+	+	±	+	+	+	+	+	+	+	+	+	±	+	0	+	+	+	0
Staph.aureus (MRSA)	0	0	0	0	0	0	0	0	0	0	±	±	+	+	+	+	+	±	+	+	0	+	0	+	+	+	0
Staph. epidermidis	±	±	±	±	0	0	±	0	0	0	0	0	+	+	±	±	+	+	±			+	0	+	+	+	0
C. jeikeium	0	0	0	0	0	0	0	0	0	0	0	0	+	+	+	+	+	0	0	0		0		+	+	+	0
L. monocytogenes	S	S	S	S	+		+	+	+	+	+	+	+	+	+	+		+	+			+	0	+	+	+	0
GRAM-NEGATIVE:																											
N. gonorrhoeae	0	0	0	0	+	0	±	±	±		±	±	+				0	0	0	+	0	±	+	+	+	0	0
N. meningitidis	0	0	0	0	+	0	+	+			+	+	+	0	0	0		+	±	+		+	0	0	0	0	0
M. catarrhalis	+	+	+	+	+	0	+	+	+	+	+	+	+				+	+	+	0	±	+	0	±	±	0	
H. influenzae	+	+	+	+	+		+	±	+	+	+	+	+					±	±	+		+	0	±	±	0	
Aeromonas	0				+						+	+	+				0		+		+	0	0		0		
E. coli	+	+	+	+	+	0	0	0	0	0	0	0	+	0	0	0	0	+	0	+	+	+	+	0	0	0	0	0	+
Klebsiella sp.	+	+	+	+	±	0	0	0	0	0	±	±	+	0	0	0	0	+	0	±	±	0	0	0	0	0	+
Enterobacter sp.	+	+	+	+	0	0	0	0	0	0	0	0	+	0	0	0	0	±	0	±	±	0	0	0	0	0	+
Salmonella sp.					+	0	0	±	0	0	±	±	+	0	0	0	0	+	±	±	0	+	0	0	0	0	
Shigella sp.	+	+	+	+	0	0	±	0	0	0	±	±	+	0	0	0	0	±	±	+		0	0	0	0	0	
Serratia marcescens	+	+	+	+	0	0	0	0	0	0	0	0	+	0	0	0	0	±	0	±	±	0	0	0	0	0	
Proteus vulgaris	+	+	+	+	±	0	0	0	0	0	0	0	+	0	0	0	0	0	0	0	±	0	0	0	0	0	0
Acinetobacter sp.	0	+	0		0	0	0	0	0	0	±	±	+	0	0	0	0	±	0			0	0	0	0	0	0
Ps. aeruginosa	+	+	+	+	0	0	0	0	0	0	0	0	0	0	0	0	0	0	0	0	0	0	0	0	0	0	+
B. (Ps.) cepacia^§	0	0	0	0	+	0	0	0	0	0	0	±	±	0	0	0	0	+	+	0		0	0	0	0	0	0
S. (X.) maltophilia^§	0	0	0	0	+	0	0	0	0	0	0	0	0	0	0	0	0	+	0		0	0	0	0	0	0	
Y. enterocolitica	+	+	+		+	0	0	0	0	0	0	0						0		+		0	0	0	0	0	
F. tularensis	+				+						+							+				+	0	0	0	0	
Brucella sp.	+				+	0	0	0	0	0	+	+		0	0	0		+	+			+	0	0	0	0	
Legionella sp.							+	+	+	+	+	+						±	+			+	0		0	0	
H. ducreyi	±	±	±		+						+	+						0				+	0		0	0	
V. vulnificus					+						+	+						0				+	0		0	0	
MISC.:																											
Chlamydophilia sp.	0	0	0	0	+	±	+	+	+	+	+	+	+					0	0		0	+	0	+	+		
M. pneumoniae	0	0	0	0	+	0	+	+	+	+	+	+	+					0				0	+	0			
Rickettsia sp.	0	0	0	0	+		±			+	+	+		0		0	0	0				0					
Mycobacterium avium			+					+	+							0	0	0				0					
ANAEROBES:																											
Actinomyces	0	0	0	0	+	+	+	+	+			+	+	+		+	+		+				0				
Bacteroides fragilis^§	0	0	0	0	+	±	0	0	0		±	±	+	0		0	0		+	0		+	+		±		
P. melaninogenica^§	0	0	0	0	+	+		+	+		±	+	+	0		0	+					+	+				
Clostridium difficile	0	0	0	0	±									+	+	+							+	±	±		
Clostridium *(not difficile)**					+			±	+			+	+	+	+	+						+	+	+			
Peptostreptococcus sp.	0	0	0	0	+	+	±	±	±	+	+	+	+	+		+	+		+				+	+			

+ = usually effective clinically or >60% susceptible; ± = clinical trials lacking or 30–60% susceptible; 0 = not effective clinically or <30% susceptible; S = synergistic with penicillins (ampicillin); blank = data not available. Antimicrobials such as azithromycin have high tissue penetration and some such as clarithromycin are metabolized to more active compounds, hence in vivo activity may exceed in vitro activity.

Although active in vitro, TMP-SMX is not clinically effective for Group A strep pharyngitis or for infections due to E. faecalis.

B. melaninogenicus → Prevotella melaninogenica, P. cepacia → Burkholderia cepacia, Xanthomonas → Stenotrophomonas

* Vancomycin, metronidazole given po active vs C. difficile; IV vancomycin not effective

TABLE 5: TREATMENT OPTIONS FOR SELECTED HIGHLY RESISTANT BACTERIA (See page 2 for abbreviations)

ORGANISM/RESISTANCE	THERAPEUTIC OPTIONS		COMMENT[1]
E. faecalis. Resistant to:			
Vanco + strep/gentamicin (MIC >500 mcg per mL); β-lactamase neg. (JAC 40:161, 1997)	Penicillin G or AMP (systemic infections); Nitrofurantoin, fosfomycin (UTI only). Usually resistant to Synercid.		Non BL+ strains of E. faecalis resistant to penicillin and AMP described in Spain, but unknown (except BL+ strains) in U.S. and elsewhere (AAC 40:2420, 1996). Linezolid effective in 60–70% of cases (AnIM 138:135, 2003). Daptomycin, tigecycline active in vitro (JAC 52:123, 2003).
Penicillin (β-lactamase producers)	Vanco, AM-SB		Appear susceptible to AMP and penicillin by standard in vitro methods. Must use direct test for β-lactamase with chromogenic cephalosporin (nitrocefin) to identify. Rare since early 1990s.
E. faecium. Resistant to:			
Vanco and high levels (MIC >500 mcg per mL) of streptomycin and gentamicin	Penicillin G or AMP (systemic infections); fosfomycin, nitrofurantoin (UTI only)		For strains with pen/AMP MICs of >8 ≤64 mcg per mL, anecdotal evidence that high-dose (300 mg per kg per day) AMP rx may be effective. Daptomycin, tigecycline active in vitro (JAC 52:123, 2003).
Penicillin, AMP, vanco, & high-level resist. to streptomycin and gentamicin (NEJM 342:710, 2000)	Linezolid 600 mg po or IV q12h and quinu-dalfo 7.5 mg per kg IV q8h are bacteriostatic against most strains of E. faecium. Can try combinations of cell wall-active antibiotics with other agents (including FQ, chloramphenicol, RIF, or doxy). Chloramphenicol alone effective in some cases of bacteremia (Clin Micro Inf 7:17, 2001). Nitrofurantoin or fosfomycin may work for UTI.		For strains with Van B phenotype (vanco R, teico S), teicoplanin[NUS], preferably in combination with streptomycin or gentamicin (if not highly AG resistant), may be effective. Synercid roughly 70% effective in clinical trials (CID 30:790, 2000, & 33:1816, 2001). Linezolid shows similar efficacy. Comparable but somewhat lower (58% linezolid, 43% QD) response rates in cancer pts (JAC 53:646, 2004). Emergence of resistance with therapeutic failure may result in quinu-dalfo or linezolid (CID 30:790, 2000; Ln 357:1179, 2001). Nosocomial spread of linezolid-resistant E. faecium possible (NEJM 346:867, 2002). Daptomycin active in vitro against most strains (JAC 52:123, 2003). Tigecycline also active in vitro (Circulation 111:e394, 2005). **Infectious disease consultation imperative!**
S. aureus. Resistant to:			
Methicillin (health-care associated) (CID 32:108, 2001) **For community-acquired MRSA infections, see Table 6**	Vanco [for persistent bacteremia (≥7 days) on vanco or teicoplanin[NUS], see Table 6]	Alternatives: teicoplanin[NUS] SMX (test susceptibility first), minocycline & doxy (some strains), tigecycline (CID 41(Suppl.5):S303, 2005), or quinu-dalfo (CID 34:1481, 2002). Fusidic acid[NUS], fosfomycin, RIF may be active, use only in combination to prevent in vivo emergence of resistance. Staphyl-	daptomycin (AAC 49:770, 2005), linezolid (Chest 124:1789, 2003), dalbavancin (EMID 48:137, 2004), TMP- ococci (incl. CA-MRSA) with inducible MLSβ resistance may appear susceptible to clindamycin in vitro. Clinda therapy may result in therapeutic failure (CID 37:1257, 2003). Test for inducible resistance (double-disc "D test") before treating with clinda (J Clin Micro 42:2777, 2004). **Investigational drugs with activity against MRSA include** oritavancin (LY333328), telavancin, ceftobiprole.
Vanco, methicillin (VRMRSA) (NEJM 339:520, 1998; CID 32:108, 2001; MMWR 51:902, 2002; NEJM 348:1342, 2003)	Unknown; but even high-dose vanco may fail. Linezolid, quinu-dalfo, daptomycin active in vitro.		Most clinical isolates of VRMRSA have had only low levels (MIC ≤16 mcg per mL) of vanco resistance (MMWR 27:624, 1997; JAC 40:135, 1997). Some call these mosaic strains or GISA. Only anecdotal data on therapeutic regimens. Most susceptible to TMP-SMX, minocycline, doxycycline, RIF and AGs (CID 32:108, 2001). RIF should always be combined with a 2nd therapeutic agent to prevent emergence of RIF resistance during therapy. 4 clinical isolates of truly vancomycin-resistant (MIC >64) MRSA described. Organisms still susceptible to TMP-SMX, chloro, linezolid, minocycline, quinu-dalfo (MMWR 51:902, 2002; NEJM 348:1342, 2003).
S. epidermidis. Resistant to:			
Methicillin	Vanco (± RIF and gentamicin for prosthetic valve endocarditis)		
Methicillin, glycopeptides (AAC 49:770, 2005)	Quinu-dalfo (see comments on E. faecium), linezolid, daptomycin, & dalbavancin)		Vanco more active than teicoplanin[NUS] (Clin Micro Rev 8:585, 1995). New FQs (levofloxacin, gati-floxacin, moxifloxacin) active in vitro, but development of resistance is a potential problem.
S. pneumoniae. Resistant to:			
Penicillin G (MIC >0.1 ≤1.0)	Ceftriaxone or cefotaxime. High-dose penicillin (≥10 million units per day) or AMP (amox) likely effective for non-meningeal sites of infection (e.g., pneumonia), telithro		IMP, ERTA, cefepime, cefpodoxime, cefuroxime also active (IDCP 3:75, 1994). MER less active than IMP (AAC 38:898, 1994). Gati, gemi, levo, moxi also have good activity (AAC 38:898, 1994; DMID 31:45, 1998; Exp Opin Invest Drugs 8:123, 1999).
Penicillin G (MIC ≥2.0)	(Vanco ± RIF). Alternatives if non-meningeal infection: ceftriax/cefotax, high-dose AMP, ERTA, IMP, MER, or an active FQ: Gati, Gemi, Levo, Moxi, telithro		High-dose cefotaxime (300 mg per kg per day, max. 24 gm per day) effective in meningitis due to strains with cefotaxime MICs as high as 2 mcg per mL (AAC 40:218, 1996). Review: IDCP 6(Suppl.2):S21, 1997.
Penicillin, erythro, tetracycline, chloramphenicol, TMP-SMX	Vanco ± RIF; (Gati, Gemi, Levo, Moxi); telithro (non-meningeal infections)		60–80% of strains susceptible to clindamycin (DMID 25:201, 1996).
Acinetobacter baumannii. Resistant to: IMP, AP Ceph 3, AP Pen, APAG, FQ	AM-SB (CID 34:1425, 2002). Subactam alone is active against some A. baumannii (JAC 42:793, 1998)		6/8 patients with A. baumannii meningitis (7 organisms resistant to IMP) cured with AM/SB (CID 24: 932, 1997). Various combinations of FQs and AGs, IMP and AGs or RIF or AP Pens or AP Ceph 3s with AGs may show activity against **some** multiresistant strains (CID 36:1268, 2003). IV colistin also effective (CID 36:1111, 2003; JAC 54:1085, 2004). MER + subactam active in vitro & in vivo (JAC 53:393, 2004). Active in vitro: triple drug combinations of polymyxin B, IMP, & RIF (AAC 48:753, 2004) & tigecycline (CID 41:S315, 2005).

ORGANISM/RESISTANCE	THERAPEUTIC OPTIONS		COMMENT

Campylobacter jejuni. Resistant to: FQs	Erythro, azithro, clarithro, doxy, clindamycin		Resistance to **both** FQs & macrolides reported *(CID 22:868, 1996; EID 7:24, 2002, AAC 47:2358, 2003)*
Klebsiella pneumoniae (producing ESBL) **Resistant to:** Ceftazidime & other 3rd generation cepha- losporins *(see Table 10C)*, aztreonam	P Ceph 4, TC-CL, PIP-TZ show in vitro activity, but not proven entirely effective in animal models *(IJAA 8:37, 1997)*; some strains which hyperproduce ESBLs are primarily resistant to TC-CL and PIP-TZ *(J Clin Micro 34:358, 1996)*. Note: there are strains of ESBL-producing klebsiella sensitive in vitro to P Ceph 2, 3 but resistant to ceftazidime; infections with such strains do not respond to P Ceph 2 or 3 *(J Clin Micro 39:2206, 2001)*. FQ may be effective if susceptible. Note Klebsiella sp. with carbapenem resistance due to class A carbapenemase. Some of these organisms resistant to all antimicrobials except colistin *(CID 39:55, 2004)*		IMP, MER, ERTA *(CID 39:31, 2004)* *(See Comment)*
Pseudomonas aeruginosa. Resistant to: IMP, MER	CIP (check susceptibility), APAG (check susceptibility)		Many strains remain susceptible to aztreonam & ceftazidime or AP Pens *(JAC 36:1037, 1995)*. Combinations of (AP Pen & APAG) or (AP Ceph 3 + APAG) may show in vitro activity *(AAC 39:2411, 1995)*. IV colistin may have some utility *(CID 28:1008, 1999)*.

TABLE 6: SUGGESTED MANAGEMENT OF SUSPECTED OR CULTURE-POSITIVE COMMUNITY-ACQUIRED PHENOTYPE OF
METHICILLIN-RESISTANT S. AUREUS (CA-MRSA) INFECTIONS *(See page 2 for abbreviations)*

In the absence of definitive comparative efficacy studies, the Editors have generated the following guidelines. With the magnitude of the clinical problem and a number of new drugs, it is likely new data will require frequent revisions of the regimens suggested. Ref. *CID 40:562, 2005*

CLINICAL ILLNESS	ABSCESS, AFEBRILE; & IMMUNOCOMPETENT: OUTPATIENT CARE	ABSCESS(ES) WITH FEVER; OUTPATIENT CARE	VENTILATOR- ASSOCIATED PNEUMONIA	BACTEREMIA OR POSSIBLE ENDOCARDITIS OR BACTEREMIC SHOCK	BLOOD CULTURES DRAWN ON DAY 7 OF VANCO ARE POSITIVE (See footnote[1])
Management (for drug doses, see footnote)	TMP-SMX-DS or **doxycy- cline or minocycline** *(CID 40:1429, 2005)* **NOTE:** for abscesses <5 cm diameter, I&D only sufficient *(PID 23:123, 2004)*	(TMP-SMX-DS + **rifampin**) or **linezolid** IV or 1 dose of **dalbavancin** IV	**Vanco** or teico[NUS] IV or **linezolid** IV Ref.: *Chest 124:1632, 2003*	**Vanco** or teico[NUS] IV. If vanco allergy: **Daptomycin.** Could start with **nafcillin (or oxacillin) + vanco.** DC inactive drug when suscept. data available	Switch to **daptomycin. Quinupristin–dalfopristin** (Q-D) 2nd choice ± with **vanco.**[2] Linezolid ~70% effective in compassionate use trial *(JAC 50:1017, 2002)*. No strong data that adding **rifampin** helps. Adding **genta- micin** to **vanco** ↑ risk of nephrotoxicity with little evidence of enhanced efficacy. Could try **Gati, Levo,** or **Moxi** if isolate
	Culture abscess & maybe blood. I&D. Hot packs.	Culture abscess & I&D. Hot packs.	Need quant. cultures for diagnosis: e.g., protect- ed specimen brush	Blood cultures. Target trough level of vanco 15 (range 10-20) mcg per mL.	susceptible. In retrospective evaluation, linezolid & vanco equivalent efficacy—roughly 30% microbiologic failure with both drugs *(JAC, in press 10/2005)*.
Comments	If recurrent & post-rx decoloni- zation desired, see page 39	Close followup. Fever should resolve quickly post I&D. Rarely S pyogenes + MRSA: **TMP-SMX** not active vs S. pyogenes; **rifampin** active or add **Pen V-K**	Linezolid superior to vanco in retrospective subset analysis. Prospective study in progress.	Can't rely on **clinda** without in vitro documentation of ab- sence of inducible resistance *(CID 40:280, 2005)*. **TMP- SMX** IV of limited efficacy vs bacteremic S. aureus *(AnIM 117:390, 1992)*.	If MRSA resistant to **erythro**, likely that Q-D will have bacterio- static & not bactericidal activity. Interest in Q-D + vanco, but no data. Do not add **linezolid** to **vanco**; no benefit & may be antagonistic. Linezolid successful in compassionate use *(JAC 50:1017, 2002)* & in pts with reduced vanco in vitro suscept. *(CID 38:521, 2004)*. To date, no data for **dalbavancin** in vanco failures.

[1] Bacteremia may persist 7 days after starting vanco *(AnIM 115:674, 1991)*. Longer duration of bacteremia, greater likelihood of endocarditis *(JID 190:1140, 2004)*.
[2] Before switching, look for undrained abscess(es) &/or infected foreign body. Recheck vanco MIC to exclude intermediate or high-level vanco resistance.

Dalbavancin: 1000 mg IV, then 500 mg IV 8 days later. **Daptomycin:** 6 mg per kg IV q24h. **Doxycycline or minocycline:** 100 mg po bid. **Linezolid:** 600 mg po/IV bid (expensive). **Nafcillin or oxacillin:** 2
gm IV q4h. **Quinupristin-dalfopristin (Q-D):** 7.5 mg per /kg IV q8h via central line. **Rifampin:** Long serum half-life justifies dosing 600 mg po q24h; however, frequency of nausea less with 300 mg po bid.
TMP-SMX-DS: Standard dose 8–10 mg per kg per day. For 70 Kg person = 700 mg TMP component per day. TMP-SMX-DS contains 160 mg TMP. Hence, suggest **2** TMP-SMX-DS po bid *(J Am Acad Derm 50:854, 2004)*. 50% failure rate
with one TMP-SMX-DS bid *(J Am Acad Derm 50:854, 2004)*. **Vancomycin:** 1 gm IV q12h

TABLE 7: METHODS FOR PENICILLIN DESENSITIZATION [CID 35:26, 2002]
(See Table 10C, page 73, for TMP/SMX desensitization)

Perform in ICU setting. Discontinue all β-adrenergic antagonists. Have IV line, ECG and spirometer (CCTID 13:131, 1993). Once desensitized, rx must not lapse or risk of allergic reactions ↑. A history of Stevens-Johnson syndrome, exfoliative dermatitis, erythroderma are nearly absolute contraindications to desensitization (use only as an approach to IgE sensitivity).

Oral Route: If oral prep available and pt has functional GI tract, oral route is preferred. 1/3 pts will develop transient reaction during desensitization or treatment, usually mild.

Step *

	1	2	3	4	5	6	7	8	9	10	11	12	13	14
Drug (mg per mL)	0.5	0.5	0.5	0.5	0.5	0.5	0.5	5.0	5.0	5.0	50	50	50	50
Amount (mL)	0.1	0.2	0.4	0.8	1.6	3.2	6.4	1.2	2.4	4.8	1.0	2.0	4.0	8.0

* Interval between doses: 15 min. After Step 14, observe for 30 minutes, then 1.0 gm IV.

Parenteral Route:

Step **

	1	2	3	4	5	6	7	8	9	10	11	12	13	14	15	16	17
Drug (mg per mL)	0.1	0.1	0.1	0.1	1.0	1.0	1.0	10	10	10	100	100	100	100	1000	1000	1000
Amount (mL)	0.1	0.2	0.4	0.8	0.16	0.32	0.64	0.12	0.24	0.48	0.1	0.2	0.4	0.8	0.16	0.32	0.64

** Interval between doses: 15 min. After Step 17, observe for 30 minutes, then 1.0 gm IV. [Adapted from Sullivan, TJ. In Allergy: Principles and Practice, C.V. Mosby, 1993, p. 1726, with permission.]

TABLE 8: RISK CATEGORIES OF ANTIMICROBICS IN PREGNANCY

DRUG	FDA PREGNANCY RISK CATEGORIES
Antibacterial Agents	
Aminoglycosides:	
Amikacin, gentamicin, isepamicin[NUS], netilmicin[NUS], streptomycin & tobramycin	D
Beta Lactams	
Penicillins; pens + BLI; cephalosporins; aztreonam	B
Imipenem/cilastatin	C
Meropenem, ertapenem	B
Chloramphenicol	C
Clindamycin	B
Ciprofloxacin, oflox, levoflox, gemiflox, gatiflox, moxiflox	C
Colistin	C
Dalbavancin	C
Daptomycin	B
Fosfomycin	B
Linezolid	C
Macrolides:	
Erythromycins/azithromycin	B
Clarithromycin	C
Metronidazole	B
Nitrofurantoin	B
Rifaximin	C
Sulfonamides/trimethoprim	C
Telithromycin	C
Tetracyclines, tigecycline	D
Tinidazole	C
Vancomycin	C
Antifungal Agents: (CID 27:1151, 1998)	
Amphotericin B preparations	B
Anidulafungin	C
Caspofungin	C
Fluconazole, itraconazole, ketoconazole, flucytosine	C
Antifungal Agents: (continued)	
Micafungin	C
Terbinafine	B
Voriconazole	D
Antiparasitic Agents:	
Albendazole/mebendazole	C
Atovaquone/proguanil; atovaquone alone	C
Chloroquine, eflornithine	C
Ivermectin	C
Mefloquine	C
Miltefosine	X
Nitazoxanide	B
Pentamidine	C
Praziquantel	B
Pyrimethamine/pyrisulfadoxine	C
Quinidine	C
Quinine	X
Antimycobacterial Agents:	
Capreomycin	C
Clofazimine/cycloserine	"avoid"
Dapsone	C
Ethambutol	"safe"
Ethionamide	"do not use"
INH, pyrazinamide	C
Rifabutin	B
Rifampin	C
Thalidomide	X
Antiviral Agents:	
Abacavir	C
Acyclovir	B
Adefovir	C
Amantadine	C
Antiviral Agents: (continued)	
Atazanavir	B
Cidofovir	C
Delavirdine	C
Didanosine (ddI)	B
Efavirenz	D
Emtricitabine	B
Enfuvirtide	B
Entecavir	C
Famciclovir	B
Fosamprenavir	C
Foscarnet	C
Ganciclovir	C
Indinavir	C
Interferons	C
Lamivudine	C
Lopinavir/ritonavir	C
Nelfinavir	B
Nevirapine	C
Oseltamivir	C
Ribavirin	X
Rimantadine	C
Ritonavir	B
Saquinavir	B
Stavudine	C
Tenofovir	B
Tipranavir	C
Valacyclovir	B
Valganciclovir	C
Zalcitabine	C
Zanamivir	C
Zidovudine	C

* **FDA Pregnancy Categories: A**—studies in pregnant women, no risk; **B**—animal studies no risk, but human not adequate or animal toxicity but human studies no risk; **C**—animal studies show toxicity, human studies inadequate but benefit of use may exceed risk; **D**—evidence of human risk, but benefits may outweigh; **X**—fetal abnormalities in humans, risk > benefit

TABLE 9A: SELECTED PHARMACOLOGIC FEATURES OF ANTIMICROBIAL AGENTS

DRUG	DOSE, ROUTE OF ADMINISTRATION	FOR PO DOSING—Take Drug — WITH FOOD	WITHOUT FOOD[6]	WITH OR WITHOUT FOOD	% AB[1]	PEAK SERUM LEVEL mcg per mL[6]	PROTEIN BINDING, %	SERUM T½, HOURS[2]	BILIARY EXCRETION, %[3]	CSF[4]/BLOOD, %	CSF LEVEL POTENTIALLY THERAPEUTIC[5]
PENICILLINS: Natural											
Benzathine Pen G	1.2 million units IM					0.15					
Penicillin G	2 million units IV					20	65		500	5-10	Yes for Pen-sens. S. pneumo
Penicillin V	500 mg po		X		60-73	5-6	65	0.5			
PEN'ASE-RESISTANT PENICILLINS											
Clox/Diclox	500 mg po		X		50	10-15	95-98	0.5			
Nafcillin/Oxacillin	500 mg po		X		Erratic	10-15	90-94	0.5	>100/25	9-20	Yes-high-dose IV therapy
AMINOPENICILLINS											
Amoxicillin	250 mg po			X	75	4-5	17	1.2	100-3000	13-14	Yes
AM-CL	875/125 mg po	X		X		11.6/2.2	20/30	1.4/1.1	100-3000		
AM-CL-ER						17/2.1	18/25	1.3/1.0			
Ampicillin	2 gm IV					47	18-22	1.2	100-3000	13-14	Yes
AM-SB	3 gm IV					109-150	28/38	1.2			
ANTIPSEUDOMONAL PENICILLINS											
Indanyl carb.	382 mg po			X	35	6.5	50	1.0			
Piperacillin	4 gm IV					400	16-48	1.0	3000-6000	30	Not for P. aeruginosa; marginal for coliforms
PIP-TZ	3/.375 gm IV					209	16-48	1.0	>100		
Ticarcillin	3 gm IV					260	45	1.2		40	Not for P. aeruginosa, marginal for coliforms
TC-CL	3.1 gm IV					330	45/25	1.1			
CEPHALOSPORINS—1st Generation											
Cefadroxil	500 mg po			X	90	16	20	1.5	22		
Cefazolin	1 gm IV					188	73-87	1.9	29-300	1-4	No
Cephalexin	500 mg po			X	90	18-38	5-15	1.0	216		
CEPHALOSPORINS—2nd Generation											
Cefaclor	500 mg po		X		93	9.3	22-25	0.8	≥60		
Cefaclor-CD	500 mg po		X			8.4	22-25	0.8	≥60		
Cefotetan	1 gm IV					124	78-91	4.2	2-21		
Cefoxitin	1 gm IV					110	65-79	0.8	280		
Cefprozil	500 mg po			X	95	10.5	36	1.5			
Cefuroxime	1.5 gm IV					100	33-50	1.3	35-80	17-88	Yes
Cefuroxime axetil	250 mg po			X	52	4.1	50	1.5		3	±
Loracarbef			X		90	8	25	1.2			
CEPHALOSPORINS—3rd Generation											
Cefdinir	300 mg po			X	25	1.6	60-70	1.7			
Cefditoren pivoxil	400 mg po	X			16	4	88	1.6			

See page 63 for all footnotes; see page 2 for abbreviations

TABLE 9A (2)

DRUG	DOSE, ROUTE OF ADMINIS-TRATION	FOR PO DOSING—Take Drug			% AB[1]	PEAK SERUM LEVEL mcg per mL[6]	PROTEIN BINDING, %	SERUM T½, HOURS[2]	BILIARY EXCRETION, %[3]	CSF[4]/ BLOOD, %	CSF LEVEL POTENTIALLY THERAPEUTIC[5]
		WITH FOOD	WITHOUT FOOD[8]	WITH OR WITHOUT FOOD							
CEPHALOSPORINS—3rd Generation *(continued)*											
Cefixime	400 mg po			X	50	3–5	65	3.1	800		
Cefotaxime	1 gm IV					100	30–51	1.5	15–75	10	Yes
Cefpodoxime proxetil	200 mg po	X			46	2.9	40	2.3	115		
Ceftazidime	1 gm IV					60	<10	1.9	13–54	20–40	Yes
Ceftibuten	400 mg po		X		80	15	65	2.4	34–82		
Ceftizoxime	1 gm IV					132	30	1.7			
Ceftriaxone	1 gm IV					150	85–95	8	200–500	8–16	Yes
CEPHALOSPORIN—4th Generation											
Cefepime	2 gm IV					193	20	2.0	~5	10	Yes
CARBAPENEMS											
Ertapenem	1 gm IV					154	95	4	10	21	Yes
Imipenem	500 mg IV					40	15–25	1	minimal	8.5	+[9]
Meropenem	1 gm IV					49	2	1	3–300	Approx. 2	+
MONOBACTAM											
Aztreonam	1 gm IV					125	56	2	115–405	3–52	±
AMINOGLYCOSIDES											
Amikacin, gentamicin, kanamycin, tobramycin—see Table 10D, page 74, for dose & serum levels											
Neomycin	po				<3	0	0–10	2.5	10–60	0–30	No: intrathecal: 5–10 mg
FLUOROQUINOLONES[10]											
Ciprofloxacin	750 mg po			X	70	1.8–2.8	20–40	4	2800–4500	26	1 mcg per mL: inadequate for Strep. species (*CID 31:1131, 2000*).
	400 mg IV			X		4.6	20–40	4	2800–4500		
	500 mg ER po		X			1.6	20–40	6.6			
	1000 mg ER po		X			3.1	20–40	6.3			
Gatifloxacin	400 mg po/IV			X	96	4.2–4.6	20	7–8		36	
Gemifloxacin	320 mg po			X	71	0.7–2.6	55–73	7			
Levofloxacin	500 mg po/IV			X	98	5.7	24–38	7		30–50	
	750 mg po/IV			X	99	8.6	24–38	7			
Moxifloxacin	400 mg po/IV			X	89	4.5	50	10–14			
Ofloxacin	400 mg po/IV			X	98	4.6/6.2	32	9			
MACROLIDES, AZALIDES, LINCOSAMIDES, KETOLIDES											
Azithromycin	500 mg po			X	37	0.4	7–51	68	High		
	500 mg IV					3.6	7–51	12/68			
Azithromycin-ER	2 gm po		X		~30	0.8	7–50	59	6		
Clarithromycin	500 mg po			X	50	3–4	65–70	5–7	7000		
	ER—500 mg po	X			~50	2–3	65–70				

DRUG	DOSE, ROUTE OF ADMINISTRATION	FOR PO DOSING—Take Drug			% AB[1]	PEAK SERUM LEVEL mcg per mL[6]	PROTEIN BINDING, %	SERUM T½ HOURS[2]	BILIARY EXCRETION, %[3]	CSF[4]/BLOOD, %	CSF LEVEL POTENTIALLY THERAPEUTIC[5]
		WITH FOOD	WITHOUT FOOD[8]	WITH OR WITHOUT FOOD							
MACROLIDES, AZALIDES, LINCOSAMIDES, KETOLIDES *(continued)*											
Dirithromycin	500 mg po	X			10	0.4	15–30	8			
Erythromycin											
— Oral (various)	500 mg po		X		18–45	0.1–2	70–74	2–4			
— Lacto/gluecep	500 mg IV					3–4	70–74	2–4		2–13	No
Telithromycin	800 mg po				57	2.3	60–70	10	7		
Clindamycin	150 mg po			X	90	2.5	85–94	2.4	250–300		No
	600 mg IV			X		10	85–94	2.4	250–300		No
MISCELLANEOUS ANTIBACTERIALS											
Chloramphenicol	1 gm po			X	High	11–18	25–50	4.1		45–89	Yes
Colistin	150 mg IV					5–7.5	93	2–3	0		No
Dalbavancin	1 gm, then 0.5 gm IV on day 8					240	93	168			
Daptomycin	4–6 mg per kg IV					58–99	92	8–9			
Doxycycline	100 mg po			X		1.5–2.1	93	18	200–3200		No (26%)
Fosfomycin	3 gm po		X			26	<10	5.7			
Linezolid	600 mg po/IV			X	100	15–20	31	5		60–70	
Metronidazole	500 mg po/IV			X		20–25	20	6–14	100	45–89	
Minocycline	200 mg po			X		2.0–3.5	76	16	200–3200		
Polymyxin B	20,000 units per kg IV					1–8		4.3–6			No
Quinu-Dalfo	7.5 mg per kg IV					5		1.5			
Rifampin	600 mg po		X			4–32	80	2–5	10,000		
Rifaximin	200 mg po				<0.4	0.004–0.01		7–12			
Sulfamethoxazole (SMX)	2 gm po				70–90	50–120		8–15			
Trimethoprim (TMP)	100 mg po				80	1					
TMP-SMX-DS	160/800 mg po / 160/800 mg IV			X	85	1–2/40–60 9/105			100–200 40–70	50/40	Most meningococci resistant. Static vs coliforms
Tetracycline	250 mg po		X			1.5–2.2	71–89	6–12	200–3200		No (7%)
Tigecycline	50 mg IV q12h					0.63		42	138		
Vancomycin	1 gm IV					20–50	<10–55	4–6	50	7–14	Need high doses. See *Meningitis, Table 1, page 6*
ANTIFUNGALS											
Amphotericin B											
— Standard: 0.4–0.7 mg per kg IV						0.5–3.5		24		0	
— Ampho B lipid complex (ABLC): 5 mg per kg IV						1–2.5		24			
— Ampho B cholesteryl complex: 4 mg per kg IV						2.9		39			
— Liposomal ampho B: 5 mg per kg IV						58 ± 21		7–10/100			

TABLE 9A (4)

DRUG	DOSE, ROUTE OF ADMINISTRATION	FOR PO DOSING—Take Drug			% AB[1]	PEAK SERUM LEVEL mcg per mL[6]	PROTEIN BINDING, %	SERUM T½, HOURS[2]	BILIARY EXCRETION, %[3]	CSF[4]/ BLOOD, %	CSF LEVEL POTENTIALLY THERAPEUTIC[5]
		WITH FOOD	WITHOUT FOOD[8]	WITH OR WITHOUT FOOD							
ANTIFUNGALS (continued)											
Azoles											
Fluconazole	400 mg po/IV			X	90	6.7		20–50		50–94	Yes
	800 mg po/IV			X	90	Approx. 14		20–50			
Itraconazole	Oral soln 200 mg po		X		Low	0.3–0.7	99.8	35		0	
Voriconazole	200 mg po		X		96	3	58	6		22–100	Yes (CID 37:728, 2003)
Caspofungin	70 mg IV x1, then 50 mg IV qd					9.9	97	9–11			
Flucytosine	2.5 gm po			X	78–90	30–40		3–6		60–100	Yes
Micafungin	150 mg IV					5–16	>99	15–17			
ANTIMYCOBACTERIALS											
Ethambutol	25 mg per kg po	X			80	2–6	10–30	4		25–50	No
Isoniazid	300 mg po		X		100	3–5		0.7–4		90	Yes
Pyrazinamide	20–25 mg per kg po			X	95	30–50	5–10	10–16		100	Yes
Rifampin	600 mg po		X		70–90	4–32	80	1.5–5	10,000	7–56	Yes
Streptomycin	1 gm IV (see Table 10D, page 74)					25–50	0–10	2.5	10–60	0–30	No. Intrathecal: 5–10 mg
ANTIPARASITICS											
Albendazole	400 mg po	X				0.5–1.6	70				
Atovaquone suspension: 750 mg po					47	15	99.9	67		<1	No
Dapsone	100 mg po			X	100	1.1		10–50			
Ivermectin	12 mg po		X			0.05–0.08					
Mefloquine	1.25 gm po	X				0.5–1.2	98	13–24 **days**			
Nitazoxanide	200 mg po	X				3	99				
Proguanil[11]		X					75				
Pyrimethamine	25 mg po			X	"High"	0.1–0.3	87	96			
Praziquantel	20 mg per kg po	X			80	0.2–2.0		0.8–1.5			
Tinidazole	2 gm po	X			48		12	13	Chemically similar to metronidazole		
ANTIVIRAL DRUGS—NOT HIV											
Acyclovir	400 mg po			X	10–20	1.21	9–33	2.5–3.5			
Adefovir	10 mg po			X	59	0.02	≤4	7.5			
Entecavir	0.5 mg po		X		100	4.2 mg per mL	13	128–149			
Famciclovir	500 mg po			X	77	3–4	<20	2–3			
Foscarnet	60 mg per kg IV					155		4			No
Ganciclovir	5 mg per kg IV					8.3	1–2	3.5		<1	
Oseltamivir	75 mg po			X	75	0.65/3.5[12]	3	1–3			
Ribavirin	600 mg po			X	64	0.8		44			
Rimantadine	100 mg po			X		0.1–0.4	13–18	25			
Valacyclovir	1000 mg po			X	55	5.6		3			

TABLE 9A (3)

DRUG	DOSE, ROUTE OF ADMINIS-TRATION	FOR PO DOSING—Take Drug WITH FOOD	WITHOUT FOOD[8]	WITH OR WITHOUT FOOD	% AB[1]	PEAK SERUM LEVEL mcg per mL[6]	PROTEIN BINDING, %	INTRACELLULAR T½, HOURS[2]	SERUM T½, HOURS[2]	CYTOCHROME P450
ANTIVIRAL DRUGS—NOT HIV (continued)										
Valganciclovir	900 mg po	X			59	5.6	1-2	4	1.5	
ANTI-HIV VIRAL DRUGS										
Abacavir	600 mg po				83	3.0	50	20.6	1.5	
Amprenavir	1200 mg po			X	No data	6-9	90		7-11	Inhibitor
Atazanavir	400 mg po	X			"Good"	2.3	86		7	
Delavirdine	400 mg po			X	85	19 ± 11	98		5.8	Inhibitor
Didanosine	400 mg EC[13] po		X		30-40	?	<5	25-40	1.4	
Efavirenz	600 mg po		X		42	13 mcM	99		52-76	Inducer/Inhibitor
Emtricitabine	200 mg po			X	93	1.8	<4	39	10	
Enfuvirtide	90 mg sc				84	5	92		4	
Fosamprenavir	1400 mg po			X	No data	6	90	No data	7.7	Inducer/Inhibitor
Indinavir	800 mg po		X		65	12.6 mcM	60	18	1.2-2	Inhibitor
Lamivudine	300 mg po			X	86	2.6	<36		5-7	
Lopinavir	400 mg po			X	No data	9.6	98-99		5-6	Inhibitor
Nelfinavir	1250 mg po	X			20-80	3-4	98		3.5-5	Inhibitor
Nevirapine	200 mg po			X	>90	2	60		25-30	Inducer
Ritonavir	300 mg po	X			65	7.8	98-99		3-5	Potent inhibitor
Saquinavir	1000 mg po (with 100 mg ritonavir)	X			4	3.1	97		1-2	Inhibitor
Stavudine	100 mg XR[14] po			X	86	1.4	<5	3.5	1	
Tenofovir	300 mg po			X	39	0.12	<1-7	10->60	17	
Tipranavir	500 mg + 200 mg ritonavir	X			39	78-95 mcM	99.9		5.5-6	
Zalcitabine	0.75 mg po		X		85	0.03	<4	3	1.2	
Zidovudine	300 mg po		X		60	1-2	<38	11	0.5-3	

FOOTNOTES:

1 % absorbed under optimal conditions
2 Assumes CrCl >80 mL per min.
3 Peak concentration in bile/peak concentration in serum x 100.
4 If blank, no data.
5 CSF levels with inflammation
5 Judgment based on drug dose & organ susceptibility. CSF

6 concentration ideally ≥10 above MIC;
 Total drug; adjust for protein binding to determine free drug concentration.
7 For adult oral preps; not applicable for peds suspensions.
8 Food decreases rate and/or extent of absorption
9 Concern over seizure potential; see Table 10

10 Take all po FQs 2-4 hours before sucralfate or any multivalent cations: Ca^{++}, Fe^{++}, Zn^{++}
11 Given with atovaquone as Malarone for malaria prophylaxis.
12 Oseltamivir/oseltamivir carboxylate
13 EC = enteric coated
14 XR = extended release

TABLE 9B: PHARMACODYNAMICS OF ANTIBACTERIALS*

BACTERIAL KILLING/PERSISTENT EFFECT	DRUGS	THERAPY GOAL	PK/PD MEASUREMENT
Concentration-dependent/Prolonged persistent effect	Aminoglycosides; daptomycin; ketolides; quinolones	High peak serum concentration	24-hr AUC*/MIC
Time-dependent/No persistent effect	Penicillins; cephalosporins; carbapenems	Long duration of exposure	Time above MIC
Time-dependent/Moderate to long persistent effect	Clindamycin; erythro/azithro/clarithro; linezolid; tetracyclines; vancomycin	Enhanced amount of drug	24-hr AUC*/MIC

1 AUC = area under drug concentration curve

* Adapted from Craig, WA: IDC No. Amer 17:479, 2003

See page 2 for abbreviations

TABLE 10A
SELECTED ANTIBACTERIAL AGENTS—ADVERSE REACTIONS—OVERVIEW

Adverse reactions in individual patients represent all-or-none occurrences, even if rare. After selection of an agent, the physician should read the manufacturer's package insert [statements in the product labeling (package insert) must be approved by the FDA].

Numbers = frequency of occurrence (%); + = occurs, incidence not available; ++ = significant adverse reaction; 0 = not reported; R = rare, defined as <1%. NOTE: Important reactions in bold print. A blank means no data found.

ADVERSE REACTIONS	Penicillin G,V	Dicloxacillin	Nafcillin	Oxacillin	Amoxicillin	Amox-Clav	Ampicillin	Amp-Sub	Piperacillin	Pip-Taz	Ticarcillin	Ticar-Clav	Ertapenem	Imipenem	Meropenem	Aztreonam	Amikacin / Gentamicin / Kanamycin / Netilmicin[NUS] / Tobramycin	Linezolid	Telithromycin
Rx stopped due to AE						2–4.4			3.2	3.2					1.2	<1			
Local, phlebitis	+		++	+				3	4	1	3		4	3	1	4			
Hypersensitivity	+													3	3				
Fever	+	+	+	+	+	+	+	+	+	2	+	+	+	+		2	+		+
Rash	**3**	**4**	**4**	**4**	**5**	**3**	**5**	**2**	**1**	**4**	**3**	**2**	+	+	+	**2**			
Photosensitivity	0	0	0	0	0	0	0	0	0	0	0	0		0			+		
Anaphylaxis	R	0	R	R	0	R	R	+	0	0	+	+		+			+		
Serum sickness	4								+	+	+	+		+			+		
Hematologic																			
+ Coombs	3	0	R	R	+	0	+	0	+	+	0	+		2	+		R		
Neutropenia	R	0	+	R	+	+	+	+	6	+	0	+		+			+	1.1	
Eosinophilia	+	+	22	22	2	+	22	22	+	+	+	+	1	+		8			
Thrombocyto-penia	R	0	R	R	R	R	R	R	+	+	R	R		+	+	+		3–10 (see 10C)	
↑ PT/PTT	R	0	+	0	+	0	+	0	+	+	+	+			R	R			
GI																			
Nausea/vomiting		+	0	0	2	3	2	+	+	7	+	1	3	2	4	R		3/1	7/2
Diarrhea		+	0	0	5	9	10	2	2	11	3	1	6	2	5	R		4	10
C. difficile colitis		R	R	R	R	+	R	+	+	+	+	+		+		+		+	+
Hepatic, LFTs	R	R	0	+	R	+	R	6	+	+	0	+	6	4	4	2		1.3	
Hepatic failure	0	0	0	0	0	0	0	0	0	0	0	0		0					
Renal: ↑ BUN, Cr	R	0	0	0	R	0	R	0	+	+	0	0		+	0	0	5–25[1]		
CNS																			
Headache	R	0	R	R	0	+	R	R	R	8	R	R	2	+	3	+		2	2
Confusion	R	0	R	R	0	0	R	R	R	R	R	R		+		+		+	
Seizures	R	0	0	+	0	R	R	0	0	R	R	+	See footnote[2]			+			
Special Senses																			
Ototoxicity	0	0	0	0	0	0	0	0	0	0	0	0		R		0	3–14[1]		
Vestibular	0	0	0	0	0	0	0	0	0	0	0	0		0		0	4–6[1]		
Cardiac																			
Dysrhythmias	R	0		0	0	0	0	0	0	0	0	0		0		+			
Miscellaneous, Unique (Table 10C)	+	+	+	+	+	+	+	+	+	+	+	+	+	+		+			+
Drug/drug inter-actions, common (Table 22)	0	0	0	0	0	0	0	0	0	0	0	0		0		0	+	+	+

[1] Varies with criteria used

[2] **All β-lactams in high concentration can cause seizures** (JAC 45:5, 2000). In rabbit, IMP 10 times more neurotoxic than benzylpenicillin (JAC 22:687, 1988). In clinical trial of IMP for pediatric meningitis, trial stopped due to seizures in 7/25 IMP recipients; hard to interpret as purulent meningitis causes seizures (PIDJ 10:122, 1991). Risk with IMP less with careful attention to dosage (Epilepsia 42:1590, 2001).
  Postulated mechanism: Drug binding to GABA$_A$ receptor. IMP binds with greater affinity than MER. Package insert, percent seizures: ERTA 0.5, IMP 0.4, MER 0.7. However, in 3 clinical trials of MER for bacterial meningitis, no drug-related seizures (Scand J Inf Dis 31:3, 1999; Drug Safety 22:191, 2000). In febrile neutropenic cancer pts, IMP-related seizures reported at 2% (CID 32:381, 2001; Peds Hem Onc 17:585, 2000).

TABLE 10A (2)

CEPHALOSPORINS/CEPHAMYCINS

ADVERSE REACTIONS	Cefazolin	Cefotetan	Cefoxitin	Cefuroxime	Cefotaxime	Ceftazidime	Ceftizoxime	Ceftriaxone	Cefepime	Cefpirome[NUS]	Cefaclor/Cef.ER[1]/Loracarb	Cefadroxil	Cefdinir	Cefixime	Cefpodoxime	Cefprozil	Ceftibuten	Cefditoren pivoxil	Cefuroxime axetil	Cephalexin
Rx stopped due to AE									1.5		3				2.7	2	2	2	2.2	
Local, phlebitis	+	R	R	2	5	1	4	2	1											
Hypersensitivity	5	1				2			+		2									
Fever	+	+	+			R	+	R		+	+				R	+			R	R
Rash	+		2	R	2	2	2	2	2	1	1	+	R	1	1	1	R	R	R	1
Photosensitivity	0	0	0	0	0	R	0	0												
Anaphylaxis	R	+				R					R				R				R	
Serum sickness											≤0.5[2]	+								+
Hematologic																				
+ Coombs	3	+	2	R	6	4			14	3	R							R	R	+
Neutropenia	+		2	R	+	1	+	2	1		+	+	R	R	R	2		R		3
Eosinophilia		+	3	7	1	8	4	6	1				R	R	3	2	5	R	1	9
Thrombocytopenia	+				+	+			+		2				R	R	+	R		
↑ PT/PTT		++	+		+	+	+	+	+											
GI			2								3		3	13		6				2
Nausea/vomiting		1		R	R			R	1	+	2				7	4	4	2	6/1	3
Diarrhea		4		R	1	1		3	1	+	1–4		15	16	7	3	3	1.4	4	
C. difficile colitis	+	+	+	+	+	+	+	+	+	+	+	+	+	+	+	+	+	+	+	+
Hepatic, ↑ LFTs	+	1	3	4	1	6	4	3	+	+	3	+	1	R	4	2	R	R	2	+
Hepatic failure	0	0	0	0	0	0	0	0	0	0										
Renal: ↑ BUN, Cr	+		3			R		1	+		+		R	+	4	R	R	R		+
CNS																				
Headache	0					1		R	2		3		2		1	R	R	2	R	+
Confusion	0										+				R					+
Seizures	0																			
Special Senses																				
Ototoxicity	0	0	0		0	0	0	0			0	0	0	0	0	0	0		0	0
Vestibular	0	0	0		0	0	0	0			0	0	0	0	0	0	0		0	0
Cardiac																				
Dysrhythmias	0	0	0		0	0	0	0			0	0		0	0	0	0		0	0
Miscellaneous, Unique (Table 10C)								+			+[2]								+	
Drug/drug interactions, common (Table 22)	0	0	0	0	0	0	0	0			0	0		0	0	0	0		0	0

[1] Cefaclor extended release tablets

[2] Serum sickness requires biotransformation of parent drug plus inherited defect in metabolism of reactive intermediates (Ped Pharm & Therap 125:805, 1994)

* See note at head of table, page 64

TABLE 10A (3)

ADVERSE REACTIONS (AE)	MACROLIDES — Azithromycin, Reg. & ER²	Clarithromycin, Reg. & ER²	Erythromycin	QUINOLONES — Ciprofloxacin/Cipro XR	Gatifloxacin	Gemifloxacin	Levofloxacin	Moxifloxacin	Ofloxacin	OTHER AGENTS — Chloramphenicol	Clindamycin	Colistimethate (Colistin)	Daptomycin	Metronidazole	Quinupristin-dalfopristin	Rifampin	Tetracycline/Doxy/Mino	Tigecycline	TMP-SMX	Vancomycin
Rx stopped due to AE	1	3		3.5	2.9	2.2	4	3.8	4				2.8					5		
Local, phlebitis					5						+		6	++			+	2		13
Hypersensitivity																1		R	++	8
Fever				R	R		R			+	+	+	2			+	+	7	+	1
Rash	R		+	3	R	1–22⁴	1.7	R	2	+	+	+	4	+	R		+	2.4	+	3
Photosensitivity	R			R	R	R	R	R	R				4				+	+	+	0
Anaphylaxis			+	R		R	R		R											R
Serum sickness											+									
Hematologic				R													R			
Neutropenia	R	1		R	R				1	+	+			+			+		+	2
Eosinophilia				R					1		+						+		+	+
Thrombocytopenia	R	R		R						+	+				R		+		+	+
↑ PT/PTT		1																4		0
GI			++															3		
Nausea/vomiting	3	3³	25	5	8/<3	2.7	7/2	7/2	7		+	+	6.3	12		+		30/20	+	+
Diarrhea	5	3–6	8	2	4	3.6	1.2	6	4	+	7		5	+		+		13	3	
C. difficile colitis		+	+	R	R	R	R		R	++	+					R		+		+
Hepatic, LFTs	R	R	+	2	R	1.5	+		2		+				2	+	+	4		0
Hepatic failure	0	0														+	+			0
Renal ↑ BUN, Cr	+	4		1					R	0		R				+	+	2	+	5
CNS												++								
Dizziness, lightheadedness				R	3	0.8	2.5	3	3									3.5		
Headache	R	2		1	4	1.2	5.4	2		+	+		5	+			+		+	
Confusion			+	+				R	2	+				+	+				+	
Seizures			+	+			+		R					+						
Special senses — Ototoxicity	+		+	0					0											R
Vestibular																	21⁵			
Cardiac — Dysrhythmias			+	R	+¹	+¹	+¹	+¹	+¹	R										0
Miscellaneous, Unique (Table 10C)	+		+	+	+	+	+	+	+	+	+	+	+	+	+	+	+	+	+	+
Drug/drug interactions, common (Table 22)	+	+	+	+	+	+	+	+	+							+	++	+	+	+

¹ Fluoroquinolones as class assoc. **with QT$_c$ prolongation**. Ref.: CID 34:861, 2002.
² Regular and extended-release formulations
³ Less GI upset/abnormal taste with ER formulation
⁴ **Highest frequency:** females <40 years of age after 14 days of rx
⁵ Minocycline has 21% vestibular toxicity

TABLE 10B: ANTIMICROBIAL AGENTS ASSOCIATED WITH PHOTOSENSITIVITY

The following drugs are known to cause photosensitivity in some individuals. There is no intent to indicate relative frequency or severity of reactions.
Source: 2005 Drug Topics Red Book, Medical Economics, Montvale, NJ. Listed in alphabetical order:
Amantadine, azithromycin, benznidazole, ciprofloxacin, clofazimine, dapsone, doxycycline, erythromycin ethyl succinate, flucytosine, ganciclovir, griseofulvin, interferons, levofloxacin, lomefloxacin, ofloxacin, pefloxacin, pyrazinamide, saquinavir, sulfonamides, tetracyclines, tigecycline, tretinoins, trimethoprim, voriconazole

* See note at head of table, page 64

CLASS, AGENT, GENERIC NAME (TRADE NAME)	USUAL ADULT DOSAGE* (Cost$)	ADVERSE REACTIONS, COMMENTS (See Table 10A for Summary)
		Most common adverse reactions are hypersensitivity. Anaphylaxis in up to 0.05%, 5–10% fatal. Commercially available skin test antigen (penicilloyl polylysine) does not predict anaphylactic reactions. Hematologic, renal, CNS (seizures) reactions usually seen with high dose (>20 million units per day) and renal failure. With procaine pen G and benzathine pen G, an immediate but transient (5–30 min. after injection) toxic reaction with bizarre behavior and neurologic reactions can occur (Hoignes syndrome). Coombs test positive hemolytic anemias are rare but typically severe; in contrast, the Coombs test is often positive with cephalosporin therapy, but clinically significant hemolysis is rare. Penicillin allergy ref.: *JAMA* 278:1895, 1997
NATURAL PENICILLINS		
Benzathine penicillin G (Bicillin L-A)	**600,000–1.2 million units IM q2–4 wks** Cost: 1.2 million units $47	
Penicillin G	**Low: 600,000–1.2 million units IM per day** **High: ≥20 million units IV q24h(=12 gm) per day** Cost: 5 million units $42	
Penicillin V	**0.25–0.5 gm po bid, tid, qid before meals & at bedtime** Cost: 500 mg G $0.39	
PENICILLINASE-RESISTANT PENICILLINS		
Dicloxacillin (Dynapen)	**0.125–0.5 gm po q6h ac.** Cost: 500 mg G $0.20	Blood levels ~2 times greater than cloxacillin. Acute hemorrhagic cystitis reported. Acute abdominal pain with GI bleeding in patient on high dose also reported.
Flucloxacillin[aus] (Floxapen, Lutropin, Staphcil)	**0.25–0.5 gm po q6h**	In Australia, cholestatic hepatitis [women predominate, age >65, rx onset 3 weeks from starting rx (*Ln* 339:679, 1992)]. 16 deaths since 1980; recommendation: use only in severe infection (*Ln* 344:676, 1994).
Nafcillin (Unipen, Natcil)	**1–2 gm IV/IM q4h.** Cost: 2 gm IV $20.11	Extravasation can result in tissue necrosis. With dosages of 200–300 mg per kg per day hypokalemia may occur.
Oxacillin (Prostaphlin)	**1–2 gm IV/IM q4h.** Cost: 2 gm IV $20.11	**Reversible neutropenia (over 10% with ≥21-day rx, occasionally WBC <1000 per mm³).** **Hepatic dysfunction with ≥12 gm per day.** LFTs usually ↑2–24 days after the start of rx, reversible. In children, more rash and liver toxicity with oxacillin as compared to nafcillin (*CID* 34:50, 2002).
AMINOPENICILLINS		
Amoxicillin (Amoxil, Polymox)	**250 mg–1 gm po tid** Cost: 500 mg G $0.13, NB $0.55 Peds ES susp.: 600/42.9 per 5 mL. Dose: 90/6.4 mg per kg div bid. Cost: 75 mL $42.65 For adult formulations, see Comments	IV available in UK, Europe. IV amoxicillin rapidly converted to ampicillin. Rash with infectious mono—see Ampicillin. 500–875 mg po bid listed in past; may be inadequate due to ↑ resistance.
Amoxicillin-clavulanate (Augmentin) AM-CL extra-strength peds suspension (ES-600) AM-CL-ER—extended release adult tabs	See Comment for adult products/cost	With bid regimen, less clavulanate & less diarrhea. Clavulanate assoc. with rare reversible cholestatic hepatitis, esp. men >60 yrs, on rx >2 weeks (*ArM* 156:1327, 1996). 2 cases anaphylactic reaction to clavulanic acid (*J All Clin Immun* 95:748, 1995). **Comparison adult Augmentin product dosage regimens:** Augmentin 500/125 1 tab po tid Augmentin 875/125 1 tab po bid Augmentin-XR 1000/62.5 2 tabs po bid Cost for 10 days rx: $114 $101 $120
Ampicillin (Principen)	**0.25–0.5 gm po q6h.** Cost: 500 mg po G $0.30 **150–200 mg per kg IV per day.** Cost: 1 gm IV G $10.36	A maculopapular rash occurs (not urticaria), **not true penicillin allergy,** in 65–100% pts with infectious mono, 90% with chronic lymphocytic leukemia, and 15–20% with allopurinol therapy.
Ampicillin-sulbactam (Unasyn)	**1.5–3 gm IV q6h.** Cost: 3 gm NB $14.15 (see Comment)	Supplied in vials: ampicillin 1 gm, sulbactam 0.5 gm or amp 2 gm, sulbactam 1 gm. Antibiotic is not active vs pseudomonas. Total daily dose sulbactam ≤4 gm.
ANTIPSEUDOMONAL PENICILLINS NOTE: Platelet dysfunction may occur with any of the antipseudomonal penicillins, esp. in renal failure patients.		
Piperacillin (Pipracil) (Canada only)	**3–4 gm IV q4–6h (200–300 mg per kg per day up to 500 mg per kg per day). For urinary tract infection: 2** [1.85 mEq Na⁺ per gm gm IV q6h.] Cost: 3 gm NB $12.52	
Piperacillin-tazobactam (Zosyn)	**3.375 gm IV q6h.** Cost: 3.375 gm NB $17.56 **4.5 gm q8h available** 4.5 gm NB $21.81 For P. aeruginosa: 4.5 gm IV q6h + tobra	Supplied as: piperacillin 3 gm + tazobactam (TZ) 0.375 gm. TZ similar to clavulanate; more active than subbactam as β-lactamase inhibitor. Has ↑ activity over pip alone vs gram-negatives and anaerobes. PIP-TZ 3.375 gm q6h as monotherapy **not adequate for serious pseudomonas infections. For empiric or specific treatment of P. aeruginosa dose is 4.5 gm IV q6h + tobramycin.** Rx longer than 10 d. may ↑ risk of neutropenia (*CID* 37:1568, 2003). Piperacillin can cause false-pos. test for galactomannan—a test for invasive aspergillosis.
Ticarcillin disodium (Ticar)	**3 gm IV q4–6h.** Cost: 3.0 gm NB $12.38	Coagulation abnormalities common with large doses, interferes with platelet function, ↑ bleeding times; may be clinically significant in pts with renal failure. (4.5 mEq Na⁺ per gm)
Ticarcillin-clavulanate (Timentin)	**3.1 gm IV q4–6h.** Cost: 3.1 gm NB $15.37	Supplied in vials: ticarcillin 3 gm, clavulanate 0.1 gm per vial. 4.5–5 mEq Na⁺ per gm. Diarrhea due to clavulanate. Rare reversible cholestatic hepatitis secondary to clavulanate (*ArM* 156:1327, 1996).

(See page 2 for abbreviations)
* NOTE: all dosage recommendations are for adults (unless otherwise indicated) & assume normal renal function. $ Cost = average wholesale price from 2005 DRUG TOPICS RED BOOK, Medical Economics

TABLE 10C (2)

CLASS, AGENT, GENERIC NAME (TRADE NAME)	USUAL ADULT DOSAGE* (Cost§)	ADVERSE REACTIONS, COMMENTS (See Table 10A for Summary)
CARBAPENEMS. NOTE: In pts with pen allergy, 11% had allergic reaction after imipenem or meropenem (CID 38:1102, 2004); 9% in a 2nd study (JAC 54:1155, 2004).		
Ertapenem (Invanz)	1 gm IV/IM q24h. Cost: 1 gm $51.39	Lidocaine diluent for IM use; ask about lidocaine allergy.
Imipenem + cilastatin (Primaxin)	0.5 gm IV q6h: for P. aeruginosa: 1 gm q6-8h (see Comment). Cost: 500 mg NB $32.64	For moderate or severe infection due to P. aeruginosa, dosage can be increased to 3 or 4 gm per day div. q8h or q6h. Pharmacokinetic studies suggest that continuous infusion of carbapenems may be more efficacious & safer (J Clin Pharm 43:1116, 2003; AAC 49:1881, 2005). For seizure comment, see footnote 2, Table 10A, page 64.
Meropenem (Merrem)	0.5–1 gm IV q8h. Up to 2 gm IV q8h for meningitis. Cost: 1 gm NB $60	For seizure incidence comment, see Table 10A, page 64. Comments: Does not require a dehydropeptidase inhibitor (cilastatin). Activity vs aerobic gm-neg. slightly ↑ over IMP, activity vs staph & strep slightly ↓; anaerobes = to IMP. B. ovatus, B. distasonis more resistant to meropenem.
MONOBACTAMS		
Aztreonam (Azactam)	1 gm q8h–2 gm IV q6h. Cost: $23.30	Can be used in pts with allergy to penicillins/cephalosporins. Animal data and a letter raise concern about cross-reactivity with ceftazidime (Rev Int Dis 7:613, 1985); side-chains of aztreonam and ceftazidime are identical.
CEPHALOSPORINS (1st parenteral, then oral drugs).	**NOTE:** Prospective data demonstrate correlation between use of cephalosporins (esp. 3rd generation) and ↑ risk of C. difficile toxin-induced diarrhea. May also ↑ risk of colonization with vancomycin-resistant enterococci. **For cross-allergenicity, see Oral, next page.**	
1st Generation, Parenteral		
Cefazolin (Ancef, Kefzol)	0.25 gm q8h–1.5 gm IV/IM q6h. Cost: 1 gm G $1.20, NB $5.59	Do not give into lateral ventricles—seizures!
2nd Generation, Parenteral		
Cefotetan (Cefotan)	1–3 gm IV/IM q12h. (Max. dose not >6 gm q24h). Cost: 1 gm NB $14	Increasing resistance of B. fragilis, Prevotella bivius, Prevotella disiens (most common in pelvic infections). Ref.: CID 35(Suppl.1):S126, 2002. Methylthiotetrazole (MTT) side chain can inhibit vitamin K activation.
Cefoxitin (Mefoxin)	1 gm–3 gm IV/IM q4h. Cost: 1 gm G $11.23, NB $15.29	In vitro may induce ↑ β-lactamase, esp. in Enterobacter sp.
Cefuroxime (Kefurox, Ceftin, Zinacef)	0.75–1.5 gm IV/IM q8h. Cost: 1.5 gm IV G $13.46	More stable vs staphylococcal β-lactamase than cefazolin.
3rd Generation, Parenteral—Use of P Ceph 3 drugs correlates with incidence of C. difficile toxin diarrhea, perhaps due to cephalosporin resistance of C. difficile (CID 38:646, 2004).		
Cefoperazone-sulbactamAUS (Sulperazon)	Usual dose 1–2 gm IV q12h; should use 2–3 gm IV q6h	Investigational in U.S. In SE Asia & elsewhere, used to treat intra-abdominal, biliary, & gyn. infections. Other uses due to broad spectrum of activity. Possible clotting problem due to side-chain. For dose logic: JAC 15:136, 1985
Cefotaxime (Claforan)	1 gm q8–12h to 2 gm q4h. Cost: 2 gm G $22, NB $26.38 [Maximum daily dose: 12 gm]	
Ceftazidime (Fortaz, Tazicef)	1–2 gm IV/IM q8–12h. Cost: 2 gm NB $28.93–47.78	Excessive use may result in ↑ incidence of C. difficile-assoc. diarrhea and/or selection of vancomycin-resistant E. faecium. Ceftaz is susceptible to extended-spectrum cephalosporinases (CID 27:76 & 81, 1998).
Ceftizoxime (Cefizox)	1 gm q8–12h to 4 gm IV q8h. Cost: 2 gm NB $24.64 [Maximum daily dose: 12 gm]	
Ceftriaxone (Rocephin)	Commonly used IV dosage in adults: < Age 65: 2 gm once daily > Age 65: 1 gm once daily Purulent meningitis: 2 gm q12h. Can give IM in 1% lidocaine. Cost: 1 gm NB $51.16	Dosage: 2 gm IV q24h gives better tissue levels than 1 gm q12h (overcomes protein binding) (see footnote1). "Pseudocholelithiasis" 2° to sludge in gallbladder by ultrasound (50%), symptomatic (9%) (NEJM 322:1821, 1990). More likely with ≥2 gm per day with pt on total parenteral nutrition and not eating (AnIM 115:712, 1991). Clinical significance still unclear but has led to cholecystectomy (JID 17:356, 1995) and gallstone pancreatitis (Ln 17:662, 1998).
4th Generation, Parenteral		
Cefepime (Maxipime)	1–2 gm IV q12h. Cost: 2 gm NB $36.59	Active vs P. aeruginosa and many strains of Enterobacter, serratia, C. freundii resistant to ceftazidime, cefotaxime, aztreonam (CID 20:56, 1995). More active vs S. aureus than 3rd generation cephalosporins.
Cefpirome AUS (HR 810)	1–2 gm IV q12h	Similar to cefepime: ↑ activity vs enterobacteriaceae; P. aeruginosa, Gm + organisms. Anaerobes: less active than cefoxitin, more active than cefotax or ceftaz.

1 The age-related dosing of ceftriaxone is based on unpublished pharmacokinetic data that show an age-related reduction in hepatic clearance of ceftriaxone; hence, there is possible underdosing in younger pts, therefore the suggested 2 gm per day dose.

(See page 2 for abbreviations)

TABLE 10C (3)

CLASS, AGENT, GENERIC NAME (TRADE NAME)	USUAL ADULT DOSAGE* (Cost§)	ADVERSE REACTIONS, COMMENTS (See Table 10A for Summary)
CEPHALOSPORINS (continued)		
Oral Cephalosporins		The oral cephalosporins are generally safe. **Patients with a history of IgE-mediated allergic reactions to a penicillin (e.g., anaphylaxis, angioneurotic edema, immediate urticaria) should not receive a cephalosporin.** If the history is a "measles-like" rash to a penicillin, available data suggest a 5–10% risk of rash in such patients; there is no enhanced risk of anaphylaxis. Cephalosporin skin tests, if available, predictive of reaction (AnIM 141:16, 2004).
1st Generation, Oral		
Cefadroxil (Duricef)	0.5–1 gm po q12h. Cost: 0.5 gm G $2.48, NB $8.68	Any of the cephalosporins can result in **C. difficile** toxin-mediated diarrhea/enterocolitis.
Cephalexin (Keflex, Keftab, generic)	0.25–0.5 gm po q6h. Cost: 0.5 gm G $0.44, NB $3.23–4.85	The reported frequency of diarrhea/non-C. difficile toxin diarrhea is summarized in Table 10A.
2nd Generation, Oral		There are few drug-specific adverse effects, e.g.:
Cefaclor (Ceclor)	0.25–0.5 gm po q8h. Cost: 0.25 gm G $0.66, NB $2.40	**Cefaclor:** Serum sickness-like reaction 0.1–0.5%—arthralgia, rash, erythema multiforme but no adenopathy, proteinuria or demonstrable immune complexes. Anecdotal reports of similar reaction to loracarbef. Appear due to mixture of drug biotransformation and genetic susceptibility (Ped Pharm & Therap 125:805, 1994).
Cefaclor-ER (Ceclor CD)	0.375–0.5 gm po q12h. Cost: 0.5 gm $3.50	
Cefprozil (Cefzil)	0.25–0.5 gm po q12h. Cost: 0.5 gm NB $9.10	
Cefuroxime axetil po (Ceftin)	0.125–0.5 gm po q12h. Cost: 0.5 gm NB $10.95	**Cefdinir:** Drug-iron complex causes red stools in roughly 1% of pts.
Loracarbef (Lorabid)	0.4 gm po q12h. Cost: 0.4 gm NB $6.37	**Cefditoren pivoxil:** Hydrolysis yields pivalate. Pivalate absorbed (70%) & becomes pivaloylcarnitine which is renally excreted; 39–63% ↓ **in serum carnitine concentrations.** Carnitine involved in fatty acid (FA) metabolism & FA transport into mitochondria. Effect transient & reversible. No clinical events documented to date (Med Lett 44:5, 2002). Also contains caseinate (milk protein); **avoid if milk allergy** (not same as lactose intolerance). Need gastric acid for optimal absorption.
3rd Generation, Oral		
Cefdinir (Omnicef)	300 mg po q12h or 600 mg q24h. Cost: 300 mg $4.75	
Cefditoren pivoxil (Spectracef)	200–400 mg po bid. Cost: 200 mg $2.08	
Cefixime (Suprax)	0.4 gm po q12–24h. Cost: 0.4 gm NB $10.26	**Cefpodoxime:** There are rare reports of acute liver injury, bloody diarrhea, pulmonary infiltrates with eosinophilia.
Cefpodoxime proxetil (Vantin)	0.1–0.2 gm po q12h. Cost: 0.2 gm G $4.44, NB $6.22	**Cefixime:** Now available from Lupin Pharmaceuticals.
Ceftibuten (Cedax)	0.4 gm po q24h. Cost: 0.4 gm NB $9.10	**Cephalexin:** Can cause false-neg. urine dipstick test for leukocytes.
AMINOGLYCOSIDES AND RELATED ANTIBIOTICS—See Table 10D, page 74, and Table 17, page 134		
GLYCOPEPTIDES		
Dalbavancin (Trade name pending)	1 gm IV, then 0.5 gm IV on day 8. No cost data.	Semi-synthetic lipoglycopeptide with very long serum half-life. As of 8/05, FDA approval pending. So far, 2 published clinical trials (CID 40:374, 2005 & 37:1298, 2003). No serious AEs. Drug fever described in 18% of a small patient sample.
Teicoplanin^AUS (Targocid)	**For septic arthritis—maintenance dose 12 mg per kg per day.**	**S.** **aureus endocarditis—trough serum levels >20 mcg per mL required (12 mg per kg q12h times 3 loading dose, then 12 mg per kg q24h).** Hypersensitivity: fever (at 3 mg per kg 2.2%, at 24 mg per kg 8.2%), skin reactions 2.4%. Marked ↓ platelets (high dose ≥15 mg per kg per day). Red neck syndrome less common than with vancomycin.
Vancomycin (Vancocin)	15 mg per kg IV q12h; 125 mg po q6h; intrathecal 5–10 mg q48–72h. Cost: 1 gm IV G $6, NB $20.35. Oral "Pulvule" 125 mg Cost $9.15 For other uses, **see Comment.** One report of safety & efficacy of once-daily vanco, 30 mg per kg (JAC 49:155, 2002).	**Measure serum levels** if: planned dose ≥2 gm per day, rapidly changing renal function, chronic renal failure, or on hemodialysis. Target levels: peak 20–50 mcg per mL, trough 5–10 mcg per mL. Rapid infusion (over <1 hr) can cause non-specific histamine release manifest as angioneurotic edema, flushed skin ("red neck syndrome"), or hypotension. Can continue vanco but infuse over 1–2 hrs. **Ototoxicity and nephrotoxicity now rare** unless vanco given with an aminoglycoside; aminoglycoside amplifies the risk of nephrotoxicity. Neutropenia, rash occur. Rarely, association with linear IgA bullous dermatosis (CID 38:442, 2004). **Intrathecal vanco** occ. used for meningitis and/or ventriculitis/shunt infections. **Initial** dosing ranges from 5–10 mg per day (infants) to 10–20 mg per day (children/adults) adjusted to achieve trough CSF conc. of 10–20 mcg per mL (AnPharmacotherapy 27:912, 1993). **Critically ill pts:** Safe & reasonable to give loading dose of 25 mg per kg at 500 mg per hr (JAC 47:246, 2001).

(See page 2 for abbreviations)
* NOTE: all dosage recommendations are for adults (unless otherwise indicated) & assume normal renal function.   § Cost = average wholesale price from 2005 DRUG TOPICS RED BOOK, Medical Economics

TABLE 10C (4)

CLASS, AGENT, GENERIC NAME (TRADE NAME)	USUAL ADULT DOSAGE* (Cost$)		ADVERSE REACTIONS, COMMENTS (See Table 10A for Summary)
CHLORAMPHENICOL, CLINDAMYCIN(S), ERYTHROMYCIN GROUP, KETOLIDES, OXAZOLIDINONES, QUINUPRISTIN-DALFOPRISTIN (SYNERCID)			
Chloramphenicol (Chloromycetin)	0.25–1 gm po/IV q6h to max. of 4 gm per day. Cost: 1 gm IV $22.75; po $6.60	No oral drug distributed in U.S. Hematologic (↓ RBC −1/3 pts, aplastic anemia 1:21,600 courses). Gray baby syndrome in premature infants, anaphylactoid reactions, optic atrophy or neuropathy (very rare), digital paresthesias, minor disulfiram-like reactions.	
Clindamycin (Cleocin)	0.15–0.45 gm po q6h. 600–900 mg IV/IM q8h. Cost: 300 mg po NB $5.71, G $3.76. 600 mg IV NB $7.29, G $4.31	**Lincomycin** (Lincocin)	Based on number of exposed pts, these drugs are the most frequent cause of **C. difficile toxin-mediated diarrhea**. In most severe form can cause pseudomembranous colitis/toxic megacolon.
Erythromycin Group (Review drug interactions before use)			**Motilin** is gastric hormone that activates duodenal/jejunal receptors to initiate peristalsis. Erythro (E) and E esters, both po and IV, activate motilin receptors and cause uncoordinated peristalsis with resultant 20–25% incidence of anorexia, nausea or vomiting (Gut 33:397, 1992). Less binding and GI distress with azithromycin/clarithromycin.
Azithromycin (Zithromax) **Azithromycin ER** (ZMax)	**po preps:** Tabs 250 & 600 mg. Peds suspension: 100 & 200 mg per 5 mL. Adult ER suspension: 2 gm. Dose varies with indication, e.g., see Table 1, Acute otitis media (page 9), acute exac. chronic bronchitis (page 28), Comm.-acq. pneumonia (pages 29–30), & sinusitis (page 36). Cost: 250 mg G $7.53, NB $8.30. IV: 0.5 gm per day. Cost: $32.		Systemic erythro in 1st 2 wks of life associated with **infantile hypertrophic pyloric stenosis** (J Ped 139:380, 2001). Frequent **drug-drug interactions:** see Table 22, page 148. Major concern is cardiac QT_c interval on EKG. **Prolonged QT_c:** Mutations in 6 genes (LQT 1–6) produce abnormal cardiac K^+/Na^+ channels. Variable penetrance: no symptoms, repeated syncope, to sudden death. ↑ **risk if female & QT_c >500 msec! Risk amplified by drugs** [macrolides, antiarrhythmics, & drug-drug interactions (see FCs pages 71–72 for list)]. Can result in torsades de pointes (ventricular tachycardia) and/or cardiac arrest. Refs.: NEJM 348:1837 & 1866; 2003; 351:1053 & 1089, 2004; www.qtdrugs.org
Base and esters (Erythrocin, Ilosone) IV name: E. lactobionate	0.25 gm q6h–0.5 gm po/IV q6h: 15–20 mg per kg up to 4 gm q24h. Infuse over 30 or more minutes. Cost: po 250 mg base G $0.18, stearate $0.18, estolate $0.31; ESS 400 $0.23. IV 1 gm NB $7.73		Cholestatic hepatitis in approx. 1:1000 adults (not children) given E estolate. **Transient reversible tinnitus or deafness** with ≥4 gm per day of erythro IV in pts with renal or hepatic impairment. Reported with ≥600 mg per day of azithro (CID 24:76, 1997). Dosages of oral erythro preparations expressed as base equivalents. With differences in absorption/biotransformation, variable amounts of erythro esters required to achieve same free erythro serum level. e.g., 400 mg E ethyl succinate = 250 mg E base.
Clarithromycin (Biaxin) or clarithro extended release (Biaxin XL)	0.5 gm po q12h. Cost: 500 mg $5. **Extended release: Two 0.5 gm tabs po per day.** Cost: 500 mg ER $4.93		**Dirithromycin** available as once-daily macrolide. **Very low serum levels; do not use if potential for bacteremic disease.**
Dirithromycin (Dynabac)	0.5 gm po q24h. Cost: 250 mg $4.25		
Ketolide **Telithromycin** (Ketek) (Med Lett 46:66, 2004)	Two 400 mg tabs po q24h. 400 mg tabs. Cost: 400 mg $5.53 300 mg tabs available		1st ketolide (similar to erythro). **Common:** diarrhea 10%, nausea 7%, vomiting 2.4%. **Uncommon: blurred vision** 2° slow accommodation, occurs in 1% (women 2%); may cause exacerbation of **myasthenia gravis**. Potential QT_c prolongation. Several **drug-drug interactions** (Table 22, pages 150–151).
Linezolid (Zyvox)	**PO or IV dose: 600 mg q12h all indications except 400 mg q12h for uncomplicated skin infections.** Available as 400 & 600 mg tabs, oral suspension (100 mg per 5 mL), & IV solution. 600 mg po $65; 600 mg IV $82.		**Reversible myelosuppression:** thrombocytopenia, anemia, & neutropenia reported. Most often after >2 wks of therapy. Not sure of incidence of thrombocytopenia after 2 wks of rx: 7/20 osteomyelitic pts; 5/7 pts treated with vanco & then linezolid. Refs.: CID 37:1609, 2003 & 38:1058 & 1065, 2004. **Other reported serious adverse effects:** Lactic acidosis (N/V, low HCO₃); toxic neuropathy reported after prolonged therapy (peripheral neuropathy LnID 4:528, 2004 & optic neuropathy JAC 53:1114, 2004; Am J Ophthal 139:1114, 2005). **Inhibitor of monoamine oxidase:** risk of severe hypertension if taken with foods rich in tyramine. Be careful with drugs containing pseudoephedrine, phenylpropanolamine or if taking SSRIs. **Serotonin syndrome** (fever, agitation, mental status changes, tremors) reported (CID 36:1197, 2003 & 37:1274, 2003).
Quinupristin + dalfopristin (Synercid) (CID 36:473, 2003)	**7.5 mg per kg IV q8h via central line** Cost: 350 mg–150 mg $122		Venous irritation (5%); none with central venous line. Asymptomatic ↑ in unconjugated bilirubin. **Arthralgia** 2%–50% (CID 36:476, 2003). **Drug-drug interactions:** Cyclosporine, nifedipine, midazolam, many more—see Table 22.

¹ **SSRI** = selective serotonin reuptake inhibitors, e.g., fluoxetine (Prozac). (See page 2 for abbreviations).

* NOTE: all dosage recommendations are for adults (unless otherwise indicated) & assume normal renal function. $ Cost = average wholesale price from 2005 DRUG TOPICS RED BOOK, Medical Economics

TABLE 10C (5)

CLASS, AGENT, GENERIC NAME (TRADE NAME)	USUAL ADULT DOSAGE* (Cost$)	ADVERSE REACTIONS, COMMENTS (See Table 10A for Summary)
TETRACYCLINES (Mayo Clin Proc 74:727, 1999)		
Doxycycline (Vibramycin, Doryx, Monodox, Adoxa)	**0.1 gm po/IV q12h** Cost: 100 mg po G $0.08–0.11, NB $5.10; 100 mg IV NB $14.16	Similar to other tetracyclines. ↑ nausea on empty stomach. Erosive esophagitis, esp. if taken at bedtime. Phototoxicity + but less than with tetracycline. Deposition in teeth less. Can be used in patients with renal failure. *Comments:* Effective in treatment and prophylaxis for malaria, leptospirosis, typhus fevers.
Minocycline (Minocin, Dynacin)	**0.1 gm po q12h.** Cost: 100 mg G $1.80, NB $3.88	Similar to other tetracyclines. **Vestibular symptoms** (30–90% in some groups, none in others): vertigo 33%, ataxia 43%, nausea 50%, vomiting 3%, women more frequently than men. Hypersensitivity pneumonitis, reversible, ~34 cases reported (*BMJ* 310:1520, 1995). *Comments:* More effective than other tetracyclines vs staph and in prophylaxis of meningococcal disease. P. acnes: many resistant to other tetracyclines, not to mino. Active vs Nocardia asteroides, Mycobacterium marinum.
Tetracycline, Oxytetracycline (Sumycin) (*CID* 36:462, 2003)	**0.25–0.5 gm po q6h, 0.5–1 gm IV q12h** Cost: 250 mg po $0.06	GI (oxy 19%, tetra 4), anaphylactoid reaction (rare), deposition in teeth, negative N balance, hepatotoxicity, enamel agenesis, pseudotumor cerebri/encephalopathy. Outdated drug: Fanconi syndrome. *See drug-drug interactions, Table 22.* **Contraindicated in pregnancy, hepatotoxicity in mother, transplacental to fetus.** *Comments:* IV dosage over 2.0 gm per day may be associated with fatal hepatotoxicity. False-neg. urine dipstick for leukocytes.
Tigecycline (Tygacil)	**100 mg IV initially, then 50 mg IV q12h.** Cost: 50 mg $55.18	**If severe liver dis. (Child Pugh C):** 100 mg IV initially, then 25 mg IV q12h	Derivative of tetracycline. High incidence of nausea (25%) & vomiting (20%) but only 1% of pts discontinued therapy due to an adverse event. Pregnancy Category D. Do not use in children under age 18. Like other tetracyclines, may cause photosensitivity, pseudotumor cerebri, pancreatitis, & a catabolic state (elevated BUN).
FLUOROQUINOLONES (FQs)		
Ciprofloxacin (Cipro) and **Ciprofloxacin-extended release** (Cipro XR)	**500–750 mg po bid. Urinary tract infection: 250 mg bid po or Cipro XR 500 mg q24h Parenteral** rx 200–400 mg IV q12h. Cost: 500 mg po $5.80, Cipro XR 500 mg $8.66, 400 mg IV $30	**Children:** No FQ approved for use under age 16 based on joint cartilage injury in immature animals. Articular SEs in children est. at 2–3% (*LnID* 3:537, 2003). **CNS toxicity:** Poorly understood. Varies from mild (lightheadedness) to moderate (confusion) to severe (seizures). May be aggravated by NSAIDs. **Gemi skin rash:** Macular rash after 8–10 d. of rx. Frequency highest females, < age 40, treated 14 d. (22.6%). In men, < age 40, treated 14 d. frequency 7.7%. Mechanism unclear. Indication to DC therapy.
Gatifloxacin (Tequin)	**200–400 mg IV/po q24h** Cost: 400 mg po $9.84, 400 mg IV $38.20	**Hypoglycemia/hyperglycemia** (*Med Lett* 45:64, 2003): Data based on case reports only. Various FQs ↑ insulin release in rats. No known drug-drug interactions; most pts reported have type 2 diabetes; no interaction with oral hypoglycemic drugs found. No data to allow comparative frequency between FQs.
Gemifloxacin (Factive)	**320 mg po q24h.** Cost: 320 mg $18.78	**Opiate screen false-positives.** FQs can cause **false-positive urine assay for opiates** (*JAMA* 286:3115, 2001; *AnPharmacotherapy* 38:1525, 2004).
Levofloxacin (Levaquin)	**250–750 mg, po/IV q24h** Cost: 750 mg po $21, 750 mg IV $58	**QTc (corrected QT) interval prolongation:** See Table 10B, page 66. ↑ QTc (>500 msec or >60 msec from baseline) is considered possible with any FQ. ↑ QTc can lead to torsades de pointes and ventricular fibrillation. Risk low with current marketed drugs). Risk ↑ in women, ↓ K+, ↓ Mg++, bradycardia. (Refs.: *NEJM* 348: 1837 & 1866, 2003). Major problem is ↑ risk with concomitant drugs.
Moxifloxacin (Avelox)	**400 mg po/IV q24h** Cost: 400 mg po $10, IV $44	**Photosensitivity.** See Table 10B, page 66

(continued on next page)

(See page 2 for abbreviations)
* NOTE: all dosage recommendations are for adults (unless otherwise indicated) & assume normal renal function. $ Cost = average wholesale price from 2005 *Drug Topics Red Book, Medical Economics*

TABLE 10C (6)

CLASS, AGENT, GENERIC NAME (TRADE NAME)	USUAL ADULT DOSAGE* (Cost$)	ADVERSE REACTIONS, COMMENTS (See Table 10A for Summary)
FLUOROQUINOLONES (FQs) (continued)		
Ofloxacin (Floxin)	200–400 mg po bid. Cost: 400 mg po $6.80	*(continued from previous page)*

Avoid concomitant drugs with potential to prolong QT$_c$:

Antiarrhythmics:	Anti-Infectives:	CNS Drugs	Misc.
Amiodarone	Clarithro	Fluoxetine	Salmeterol
Disopyramide	Erythro	Sertraline	Naratriptan
Dofetilide	Foscarnet	Tricyclics	Sumatriptan
Flecainide	Mefloquine	Venlafaxine	Dolasetron
Ibutilide	Pentamidine	Haloperidol	Droperidol
Procainamide	**Anti-Hypertensives:**	Phenothiazines	Fosphenytoin
Quinidine	Bepridil	Pimozide	Indapamide
Sotalol	Isradipine	Quetiapine	Tamoxifen
	Nicardipine	Ziprasidone	Tizanidine
	Moexipril	Risperidone	

Updates online: www.qtdrugs.org; www.torsades.org.

Tendinopathy: Over age 60, approx. 2–6% of all Achilles tendon ruptures attributable to use of FQ (AIM 163:1801, 2003). ↑ risk with concomitant steroid or renal disease (CID 36:1404, 2003).

CLASS, AGENT, GENERIC NAME (TRADE NAME)	USUAL ADULT DOSAGE* (Cost$)	ADVERSE REACTIONS, COMMENTS (See Table 10A for Summary)
POLYMYXINS		
Polymyxin B (Poly-Rx)	Rarely used parenterally in U.S. Use colistin for parenteral therapy	Used as/for: bladder irrigation, intrathecal, ophthalmic. Source: Bedford Labs, Bedford, OH
Polymyxin E = colistin Colistin sulfate used po or topical. IV form is colistimethate (Coly-Mycin M) (CID 40:1333, 2005)	1 mg colistin = 12,500 units. U.S.: 2.5–5 mg per kg per day div. in 2–4 equal doses. Cost: 150 mg IV $64.34 U.K.: > 60 kg: 80–160 mg q8h < 60 kg: 4–6 mg per kg per day div. q8h	**Inhalation dose:** 80 mg q12h. **Intrathecal:** not standardized. Reports range from 1.6 mg to 20 mg intraventricularly; usually 10 mg. **Nephrotoxicity** (tubular necrosis): Reports vary from 14–20%. Reversible. **Neurotoxicity** (frequency?): Vertigo, facial paresthesia, abnormal vision, confusion, ataxia, & neuromuscular blockade → respiratory failure. Dose-dependent. In cystic fibrosis pts, 29% experienced paresthesia, ataxia or both.
MISCELLANEOUS AGENTS		
Daptomycin (Cubicin) (Med Lett 46:11, 2004; CID 38:994, 2004)	**Skin/soft tissue: 4 mg per kg IV q24h** **Bacteremia/endocarditis: 6 mg per kg IV q24h** (see Comment). Cost 500 mg $171.	FDA approved skin/soft tissue infections. Bacteremia/endocarditis trials ongoing. **Potential muscle toxicity:** At 4 mg per kg per day, ↑ CPK in 2.8% dapto pts & 1.8% comparator-treated pts. In very small study, no CPK ↑ in pts taking a statin drug given daptomycin (manufacturer suggests stopping statins during dapto rx)
Fosfomycin (Monurol)	3 gm with water po times 1 dose. Cost $38	Diarrhea in 9% compared to 6% of pts given nitrofurantoin and 2.3% given TMP-SMX.
Fusidic acid[NUS] (Fucidin)	500 mg po/IV tid (Leo Laboratories, Denmark)	Mild GI, occ. skin rash, jaundice (17% with IV, 6% with po). (None in CSF, <1% in urine.)
Immune globulin IV therapy	**Dosage, frequency vary with the indication.** At least 7 manufacturers. Cost for 10–12 gm ranges from $500–$1100.	Reported adverse effects range from 1–15%. Fever, headache, myalgia, N/V relate to rate of infusion, mild, & self-limited. **More serious:** anaphylactoid reactions, thromboemboli, aseptic meningitis, & renal injury in 6.7% (QJM 93:751, 2000).
Methenamine hippurate (Hiprex, Urex)	**1 gm po q6h.** Cost: 1 gm $1.23 1 gm = 480 mg methenamine	Nausea and vomiting, skin rash or dysuria. Overall ~3%. Methenamine requires (pH ≤5) urine to liberate formaldehyde. Useful in suppressive therapy after infecting organisms cleared; do not use for pyelonephritis. **Comment:** Do not force fluids; may dilute formaldehyde. Of no value in pts with chronic Foley. If urine pH >5.0, co-administer ascorbic acid (1–2
Methenamine mandelate (Mandelamine)	**1 gm po q6h (480 mg methenamine)**. Cost: 1 gm NB $0.29	gm q4h) to acidify the urine; cranberry juice (1200–4000 mL per day) has been used, results ±.

(See page 2 for abbreviations)
* NOTE: all dosage recommendations are for adults (unless otherwise indicated) & assume normal renal function. $ Cost = average wholesale price from 2005 Drug Topics RED BOOK, Medical Economics

TABLE 10C (7)

CLASS, AGENT, GENERIC NAME (TRADE NAME)	USUAL ADULT DOSAGE* (Cost§)	ADVERSE REACTIONS, COMMENTS (See Table 10A for Summary)
MISCELLANEOUS AGENTS (continued)		
Metronidazole (Flagyl) Ref.: Mayo Clin Proc 74:825, 1999	**Anaerobic infections:** usually IV, 7.5 mg per kg (~500 mg) q6h (not to exceed 4 gm q24h). With long $T\frac{1}{2}$, can use IV at 15 mg per kg IV15 mg per kg. **Oral dose: 500 mg qid.** Cost: 500 mg tab G $0.21, NB $4.56; 500 mg IV G $2.80, NB $26.16; 70 gm vaginal gel $63.24. Ext. release 750 mg $9.50	Can be given rectally (enema or suppository). In pts with **decompensated liver disease** (manifest by ≥2 L of ascites, encephalopathy, ↑ prothrombin time, ↓ serum albumin) **↑½ prolonged; unless dose ↓ by approx. ½, side-effects ↑.** Absorbed into serum from vaginal gel. **Neurol.:** headache, rare paresthesias or peripheral neuropathy, ataxia, seizures, aseptic meningitis; report of reversible metro-induced cerebellar lesions (NEJM 346:68, 2002). **Avoid alcohol during & 48 hrs after (disulfiram-like reaction).** Very dark urine (common but harmless). Skin: urticaria. Mutagenic in Ames test. Tumorigenic in animals (high dose over lifetime). No evidence of risk in man. No teratogenicity.
Mupirocin (Bactroban)	**Skin cream or ointment 2%: Apply tid times 10 days.** Cost: 15 gm $31.48. **Nasal ointment 2%: apply bid times 5 days.** Cost: 22 gm NB $49.90, G $40.23	Skin cream: itch, burning, stinging 1–1.5%; Nasal: headache 9%, rhinitis 6%, respiratory congestion 5%
Nitrofurantoin macrocrystals (Macrodantin, Furadantin)	**100 mg po q6h.** Cost: 100 mg G $1.21, NB $2.44. **Dose for long-term UTI suppression: 50–100 mg at bedtime**	Absorption ↑ with meals. Increased activity in acid urine, much reduced at pH 8 or over. Not effective in endstage renal disease (JAC 33(Suppl. A):121, 1994). Nausea and vomiting, hypersensitivity, peripheral neuropathy. Pulmonary reactions (with chronic rx): acute ARDS type, **chronic desquamative interstitial pneumonia with fibrosis.** Intrahepatic cholestasis & **hepatitis** similar to chronic active hepatitis. Hemolytic anemia in G6PD deficiency. **Contraindicated in renal failure.** Should not be used in infants <1 month of age.
monohydrate/macrocrystals (Macrobid)	**100 mg po bid** times 3 days. Cost: 100 mg $2.44	Efficacy of Macrobid 100 mg bid = Macrodantin 50 mg qid. Adverse effects 5.6%, less nausea than with Macrodantin.
Rifaximin (Xifaxan)	**200 mg tab po tid** times 3 days. Cost: 200 mg $3.60	For traveler's diarrhea. In general, adverse events equal to or less than placebo.
Sulfonamides [e.g., sulfisoxazole (Gantrisin), sulfamethoxazole (Gantanol)]	**Sulfisoxazole** (Gantrisin) peds suspension: Cost: 500 mg per 5 mL: 480 mL $46.02	**Short-acting are best:** high urine concentration and good solubility at acid pH. More active in alkaline urine. **Allergic reactions:** skin rash, drug fever, pruritus, photosensitization. Periarteritis nodosa & SLE. Stevens-Johnson syndrome, serum sickness syndrome, myocarditis. Neurotoxicity (psychosis, neuritis) hepatic toxicity. Blood dyscrasias, usually agranulocytosis. Crystalluria. Nausea & vomiting, headache, dizziness, lassitude, mental depression, acidosis, sulfhemoglobin. Hemolytic anemia in G6PD deficient & unstable hemoglobins (Hb Zürich). Do not use in newborn infants or in women near term. ↑ frequency of kernicterus (binds to albumin, blocking binding of bilirubin to albumin).
Tinidazole (Tindamax)	**2 gm po** times 1 with food. Cost: 2 gm $18.24	**Adverse reactions:** metallic taste 3.7%, nausea 3.2%, anorexia/vomiting 1.5%. All higher with multi-day dosing.
Trimethoprim (Trimpex, Proloprim, and others)	**100 mg po q12h or 200 mg po q24h.** Cost: 100 mg NB $0.90, G $0.15	Creatinine side-effects are rash and pruritus. Rash in 3% pts at 100 mg bid; 6.7% at 200 mg q24h. Rare reports of photosensitivity, exfoliative dermatitis, Stevens-Johnson syndrome, toxic epidermal necrosis, and aseptic meningitis (CID 19:431, 1994). Check drug interaction with phenytoin. Increases serum K⁺ (see TMP-SMX Comments). TMP can ↑ homocysteine blood levels (Ln 352:1827, 1998).
Trimethoprim (TMP)-Sulfamethoxazole (SMX) (Bactrim, Septra) Single-strength (SS) is 80 TMP/400 SMX, double-strength (DS) 160 TMP/800 SMX Ref.: ArIM 163:402, 2003	**Standard po rx (UTI, otitis media): 1 DS tab bid.** P. **carinii: see Table 13, page 98. IV rx (base on TMP component):** standard 8–10 mg per kg per day divided q6h, q8h, or q12h. **For shigellosis: 2.5 mg per kg IV q6h.** Cost: 160/800 po G $0.15, NB $2; 160/800 IV G $11.21 **Rapid Oral TMP-SMX Desensitization:** Hour / Dose TMP/SMX/(mg) 0 / 0.004/0.02 1 / 0.04/0.2 2 / 0.4/2 Hour / Dose TMP/SMX (mg) 3 / 4/20 4 / 40/200 5 / 160/180	Adverse reactions in 10%: GI: nausea, vomiting, anorexia. Skin: Rash, urticaria, photosensitivity. More serious (~1–10%): Stevens-Johnson syndrome & toxic epidermal necrosis. Skin reactions may represent toxic metabolites of SMX rather than allergy (AnPharmacotherapy 32:381, 1998). Daily ascorbic acid 0.5–1.0 mg may promote detoxification (JAIDS 36:1041, 2004). TMP competes with creatinine for tubular secretion; serum creatinine can ↑; TMP also blocks distal renal tubule secretion of K⁺. ↑ serum K⁺ in 21% of pts (AnIM 124:316, 1996). TMP-SMX contains sulfites and may trigger asthma in sulfite-sensitive pts. Frequent drug cause thrombocytopenia (AnIM 129:886, 1998). TMP suspected etiology of aseptic meningitis (CID 19:431, 1994). **Comment:** Perform in hospital or clinic. Use oral suspension [40 mg TMP/ 200 mg SMX per 5 mL (tsp)]. Take 6 oz water after each dose. Corticosteroids, anti-histaminics NOT used. Refs.: CID 20:849, 1995; AIDS 5:311, 1991

(See page 2 for abbreviations)

* NOTE: all dosage recommendations are for adults (unless otherwise indicated) & assume normal renal function.   § Cost = average wholesale price from 2005 DRUG TOPICS RED BOOK, Medical Economic

TABLE 10D
AMINOGLYCOSIDE ONCE-DAILY AND MULTIPLE DAILY DOSING REGIMENS
(See Table 17, page 134, if estimated creatinine clearance <90 mL per min.)

General: Dosage given as both once-daily (OD) and multiple daily dose (MDD) regimens.
Pertinent formulae: (1) Estimated creatinine clearance (CrCl): $\frac{(140 - age)(ideal\ body\ weight\ in\ kg)}{(72)(serum\ creatinine)}$ = CrCl for men in ml per min; multiply answer times 0.85 for CrCl of women

(2) Ideal body weight (IBW)—Females: 45.5 kg + 2.3 kg per inch over 5' = weight in kg
Males: 50 kg + 2.3 kg per inch over 5' = weight in kg

(3) Obesity adjustment: use if actual dosing weight (ABW) is ≥30% above IBW. To calculate adjusted dosing weight in kg: IBW + 0.4(ABW–IBW) = adjusted weight (CID 25:112, 1997)

DRUG	MDD AND OD IV REGIMENS/ TARGETED PEAK (P) AND TROUGH (T) SERUM LEVELS	COST§ Name Brand (NB), Generic (G)	COMMENTS For more data on once-daily dosing, see AJM 105:182, 1998, and Table 17, page 134
Gentamicin (Garamycin), **Tobramycin** (Nebcin)	MDD: 2 mg per kg load, then 1.7 mg per kg q8h P 4–10 mcg/ml, T 1–2 mcg per ml -------- OD: 5.1 (7 if critically ill) mg per kg q24h P 16–24 mcg per ml, T <1 mcg per ml	Gentamicin: 80 mg $5.75, Tobramycin: 80 mg NB $7.28, G $4.20	**All aminoglycosides have potential to cause tubular necrosis and renal failure, deafness due to cochlear toxicity, vertigo due to damage to vestibular organs, and rarely neuromuscular blockade.** Risk minimal with oral or topical application due to small % absorption unless tissues altered by disease. Risk of nephrotoxicity ↑ with concomitant administration of cyclosporine, vancomycin, ampho B, radiocontrast. Risk of nephrotoxicity ↓ by concomitant AP Pen and perhaps by once-daily dosing method (especially if baseline renal function normal). In general, same factors influence risk of ototoxicity. **NOTE: There is no known method to eliminate risk of aminoglycoside nephro/ototoxicity. Proper rx attempts to ↓ the % risk.** The clinical trial data of OD aminoglycosides have been reviewed extensively by meta-analysis (CID 24:816, 1997). **Serum levels:** Collect serum for a peak serum level (PSL) exactly 1 hr after the start of the infusion of the 3rd dose. In critically ill pts, it is reasonable to measure the PSL after the 1st dose as well as later doses as volume of distribution and renal function may change rapidly. Other dosing methods and references: For once-daily 7 mg per kg per day of gentamicin—Hartford Hospital method, see AAC 39:650, 1995.
Kanamycin (Kantrex), **Amikacin** (Amikin), Streptomycin	MDD: 7.5 mg per kg q12h P 15–30 mcg per ml, T 5–10 mcg per ml -------- OD: 15 mg per kg q24h P 56–64 mcg per ml, T <1 mcg per ml	Kanamycin: 1 gm $9.60 Amikacin: 500 mg NB $34.26, G $7.80 Streptomycin: 1 gm $9.75	
Netilmicin^NUS	MDD: 2 mg per kg q8h P 4–10 mcg per ml, T 1–2 mcg per ml -------- OD: 6.5 mg per kg q24h P 22–30 mcg per ml, T <1 mcg per ml		
Isepamicin^NUS	Only OD: Severe infections 15 mg per kg q24h, less severe 8 mg per kg q24h		
Spectinomycin (Trobicin)	2 gm IM times 1—gonococcal infections	2 gm NB $34.06	
Neomycin—oral	Prophylaxis GI surgery: 1 gm po times 3 with erythro, see Table 15B, page 125 For hepatic coma: 4–12 gm per day po	500 mg G $1.24	

Tobramycin—inhaled (Tobi): See Cystic fibrosis, Table 1, page 32. Adverse effects few: transient voice alteration (13%) and transient tinnitus (3%). Cost: 300 mg $57.23

Paromomycin—oral: See Entamoeba and Cryptosporidia, Table 13, page 95. Cost: 250 mg $2.72

---
[1] Estimated CrCl invalid if serum creatinine <0.6 mg per dL. Consultation suggested.
§ Cost = average wholesale price from 2005 Drug Topics Red Book, Medical Economics.

TABLE 11A: TREATMENT OF FUNGAL, ACTINOMYCOTIC, AND NOCARDIAL INFECTIONS—ANTIMICROBIAL AGENTS OF CHOICE*
(See Table 11B for Amphotericin B Preparations and Adverse Effects)

TYPE OF INFECTION/ORGANISM/ SITE OF INFECTION	ANTIMICROBIAL AGENTS OF CHOICE		COMMENTS
	PRIMARY	ALTERNATIVE	
Actinomycosis (A. israelii most common, also A. naeslundii, A. viscosus, A. odontolyticus, A. meyeri, A. gerencseriae) Cervicofacial, pulmonary, abdominal, cerebral, & rarely pericarditis Classically abdominal actino presents as interabdominal & pubic mass abscess, fistula tract. May mimic cancer (World J Gastro 11:1722, 2005). Fine needle aspirate of cervicofacial actino established dx in 15 pts in Spain (Med Oral Patol Oral Ciro Bucal 9:467, 2004).	**Ampicillin** 50 mg per kg per day IV times 4-6 wks, then 0.5 gm **amoxicillin** po tid **OR** **Penicillin G** 10–20 million units per day IV times 4-6 wks, then **penicillin V** 2-4 gm per day po. Duration individualized; esp. with surgical debulking, total duration 3–6 mos. usually adequate for thoracic & abdominal & 3–6 wks for cervicofacial (CID 38:444, 2004).	**Doxycycline or ceftriaxone** or **clindamycin or erythromycin** **Chloramphenicol** 12.5–15 mg per kg IV/po q6h recommended for CNS infection in pen-allergic pts.	Tuboovarian abscesses may complicate IUDs. Removal of IUD is primary rx. With abscesses, inflammatory mass or fistulae, surgery often required. While penicillin G and ampicillin IV have been effective, with home IV therapy, agents given q24h, e.g., ceftriaxone, are more practical (CID 19:161, 1994). Surgery may be necessary for hemoptysis (An Thor Surg 74:185, 2002).
Aspergillosis (A. fumigatus most common, also A. flavus and others) (CID 30:696, 2000)			
Allergic bronchopulmonary aspergillosis (ABPA) ABPA found in 1–2% of pts with asthma & 1–15% with cystic fibrosis [CID 37 (Suppl.3):37, 2003]. Clinical manifestations: wheezing, pulmonary infiltrates, bronchiectasis & fibrosis. Airway colonization assoc. with ↑ blood eosinophils, ↑ serum IgE, ↑ specific serum antibodies.	Acute asthma attacks associated with ABPA: ↑ **Corticosteroids**	Rx of ABPA: **itraconazole**[1] 200 mg po q24h times16 wks or longer (Allergy 60:1004, 2005)	In 2 PRCTs, itra ↓ number of exacerbations requiring corticosteroids (p <0.03), improved immunological markers (eosinophils in sputum & ↓ serum IgE levels), & in 1 study improved lung function & exercise tolerance (NEJM 342:756, 2000; Cochrane Database Syst Rev 3:CD001108, 2004).
Allergic fungal sinusitis: relapsing chronic sinusitis; nasal polyps without bony invasion; asthma, eczema or allergic rhinitis; ↑ IgE levels and isolation of Aspergillus sp. or other dematiaceous sp. (Alternaria, Cladosporium, etc.)	**Rx controversial:** systemic corticosteroids + surgical debridement (80% respond if 2/3 relapse) (Otolaryn Head Neck Surg 131:704, 2004)	For failures ↑ **itra**[1] 200 mg po bid times12 mos. (CID 31: 203, 2000). Flucon nasal spray benefited 12/16 pts (ENT J 83: 692, 2004).	
Aspergilloma (fungus ball) (J Resp Dis 23:300, 2002)	**Itraconazole** (po) benefit reported sporadically (J Am Acad Derm 23:607, 1990).		Aspergillus may complicate pulmonary sequestration (Eur J Cardio Thor Surg 27:28, 2005).
Invasive, pulmonary (IPA) or extrapulmonary: (See COID 18:314, 2005) Post-transplantation and post-chemotherapy in neutropenic pts (PMN <500 per mm³) but may also present with neutrophil recovery (Mycopathologia 159:181, 2005). Most common pneumonia in transplant recipients. Usually a late (≥100 days) complication in allogeneic bone marrow & liver transplantation: median survival 36 days, but **overall mortality rates vary from 78–94%** (CID 36:46, 2003). May complicate COPD when corticosteroids used (Clin Micro Inf 11:427, 2005). **Typical x-ray/CT lung lesions** (halo sign, cavitation, or mycotic lung sequestration) have 90% positive predictive value for invasive pulmonary aspergillosis in pts with hematologic malignancies (CID 31:859, 2000). An immunologic test that detects circulating galactomannan is available for dx of invasive aspergillosis. A recent article reviews the strengths & weaknesses of the test [CID 41(Suppl. 6):S381, 2005].	**Voriconazole** 6 mg per kg IV q12h on day 1; then either 4 mg per kg IV q12h or (200 mg po q12h for body weight ≥40 kg, but 100 mg po q12h for body weight <40 kg) **Lipid-based ampho B** as effective and less nephrotoxic than standard ampho B **but much more expensive** (see footnote³ for dosages). Some authorities now prefer lipid-based ampho B over standard ampho B as initial rx (CID 32: 415, 2003). **OR** **Ampho B** (see footnote², page 76): Rapid increase to 1 mg per kg (1–1.25 mg per kg if neutropenic) IV q24h. Total dose of 2–2.5 gm rec. by some but data to support this lacking. **OR Combination rx: Vori** (dosage above) **+ caspo** (dosage below) are currently preferred initial treatment in many bone marrow transplant units, esp. in pts receiving high doses of corticosteroids (Abstracts in Heme & Onc 8:11, 2005).	**Voriconazole** more effective than ampho B in randomized trial of 277 immunosuppressed pts with IPA. 53% responded vs 32% rx with ampho B. Overall survival better (71 vs 58%) (NEJM 347: 408, 2002). Appears particularly advantageous in cerebral aspergillosis (CID 39:603, 2004) & as salvage therapy in those with refractory infection (Eur J Haematol 73:50, 2004). 40% of 31 pts survived with vori alone. Vori reported satisfactory results in 11/20 pts with bone involvement (18 for salvage), follow-up average of 3 mos. (CID 40:1141, 2005). **Ampho B overall success rate 34–42%** (CID 32:358, 2001) in pulmonary aspergillosis in pts rx ≥14 days. Success dependent on underlying disease: 83% heart/kidney transplants, 54% pulmonary leukemia pts, 33% bone marrow transplant, 20% liver transplant (CID 23: 608, 1996). 44% of 398 pts receiving **ampho B lipid complex (ABLC)** were cured or improved & 21% stabilized; most had failed to respond or poor antifungal rx (CID 40:S392, 2005). **A. terreus infections particularly resistant to ampho B: in 83 cases, 73.4% mortality with ampho B rx vs 55.8% with voriconazole rx (p <0.01)** (CID 39:192, 2004). **Use vori!** **Caspofungin:** Among 83 pts with IPA included in the primary (MITT) analysis, 37 (45%) had favorable responses following salvage rx with caspo monotherapy. In pts necessary >7 days of caspo monotherapy, 56% (37/66) responded favorably (CID 39:1563, 2004). Response in compassionate use program 44% (J Inf 50:196, 2005). Minimal toxicity reported (Transpl Inf Dis 7:25, 2006). **Micafungin:** 57% clinical response in an open-label study of "deep-seated" infections (Scand J Inf Dis 36:72, 2004). **Combination therapy:** To date no controlled patient trials, and they are needed (CID 39:803, 2004). No antagonism between triazoles (vori & itra), echinocandins (caspo), & ampho B. Synergy *(continued on next page)*

(continued on next page)

---

[1] Oral solution preferred to tablets because of ↑ absorption (see Table 11B, page 83).
[2] **PRCTs** = Prospective randomized controlled trials
[3] **Dosages: ABLC** 5 mg per kg per day IV over 2 hrs.; **ABCC** 3–4 mg per kg per day IV given as 1 mg per kg per hr, **liposomal Ampho B** 3–5 mg per kg per day IV given over 1-2 hrs.

* See page 2 for abbreviations. All dosage recommendations are for adults (unless otherwise indicated) and assume normal renal function

TABLE 11A (2)

TYPE OF INFECTION/ORGANISM/ SITE OF INFECTION	ANTIMICROBIAL AGENTS OF CHOICE		COMMENTS
	PRIMARY	ALTERNATIVE	

Aspergillosis/invasive, pulmonary (IPA) or extrapulmonary *(continued)*

(continued from previous page) 2005). **False-pos. tests consistently found in serum from pts receiving PIP-TZ & AM-CL** (*J Clin Micro* 43:2548, 2005). Concomitant antifungal rx may also ↓ sensitivity (*CID 40:1762, 2005). (MiraVista: 1-866-647-2847)

Alternative: Caspofungin 70 mg IV on day 1, then 50 mg IV q24h (reduce to 35 mg with moderate hepatic insufficiency). For all regimens: if response good may switch to oral **vori** after 2–3 wks *(See previous page)*

Micafungin[NFDA] 150 mg IV q24h

(continued from previous page) demonstrated vs aspergillus in vitro &/or animal models between triazoles & caspo (*AAC 47:1416, 2003*) & ampho B plus caspo (*AAC 46:245 & 2564, 2002; JID 187:1834, 2003*). Some failures to show synergy (*JAC 56:166, 2005*).

In retrospective evaluation of bone marrow transplant pts with IPA who failed ampho B, vori + caspo superior to vori alone (*CID 39:797, 2004*).

Resistance: A. fumigatus isolates from stem cell transplants showed ↓ susceptibility to vori, caspo, & some to ampho B.

Blastomycosis (*CID 30:679, 2000*) (Blastomyces dermatitidis) Cutaneous, pulmonary or extrapulmonary For blood/urine antigen, call 1-866-647-2847

Itraconazole[2] oral solution 200–400 mg per day x 6 mos. **OR Ampho B**[3] 0.7–1 mg per kg per day to a total dose of ≥1.5 gm for very sick pts

Fluconazole 400–800 mg per day for at least 6 mos. 85% + effective for non-life-threatening disease (*CID 25:200, 1997*)

Itra: in patients treated for ≥2 months, 95% cure (*AJM 93: 489, 1992*). Ampho B successful in >90% (*CID 22:S102, 1996*). Vori not successful in rx of 1 pt with cerebral blastomycosis (*CID 40:e69, 2005*).

Candidiasis: A decrease in C. albicans & increase in non-albicans species continues. The latter show ↓ susceptibility to antifungal agents (esp. fluconazole). These changes predominantly in immuno-compromised pts wherein antifungal prophylaxis (esp. fluconazole) is widely used (*JCM 43:2729, 2005; COID 18:490, 2005*). In vitro susceptibility testing for antifungal drugs has not undergone in vivo validation studies; clinical outcome often more dependent on host factors (*AJM 112:380, 2002*). Susceptibility profiles help select empiric antifungal rx. The table summarizes current published reports of frequency of candida isolates, & interpretation as in vitro **(S = susceptible)**, may require dose escalation **(S-DD = susceptible with dose escalation)**, or is likely to be ineffective **(R = resistant)** (*Ln 359:1135, 2002*). **S-I = less activity in vitro but clinically effective:** only rare failures reported (*IDSA Guidelines, 2004: CID 38:161, 2004*). In vitro testing for caspo not standardized. In clinical studies of candida infections, MIC did not correlate with treatment outcome following caspofungin therapy (*AAC 49:3616, 2005*).

	% of Candida Isolates[†]	Risk Factors	% Sensitive In Vitro[†]							Rx if species known
			Fluconazole	Itraconazole	Voriconazole	Ampho B	Caspofungin	Micafungin/ Anidulafungin		
C. albicans	45–63	HIV/AIDS, surgery	97% (S)	93% (S)	99% (S)	>95% (S)	S	S		Flu,[§] caspo, or ampho B
C. glabrata	12–24	Heme malignancies, azole prophylaxis	85–90% (S-DD)	50% (R)	92% (S-I)	>95% (S-I)	S	S		Caspo, ampho B, or vori
C. parapsilosis	11–29	Azole prophylaxis, neonates, foreign bodies	99% (S)	4% (S-DD)	99% (S)	>95% (S)	S-I	S-I		Flu, caspo, or ampho B
C. tropicalis	6–19	Neutropenia	98% (S)	58% (S)	99% (S)	>95% (S)	S	S		Flu, caspo, or ampho B
C. krusei	1–5	Heme malignancies, azole prophylaxis	5% (R)	69% (S)	99% (S-I)	>95% (S-I)	S	S		Caspo, ampho B, or vori[¶]
C. guilliermondi	1	Azole prophylaxis, previous ampho rx	>95% (S)	? (S)	>95% (S)	? (R)	S	S		Flu, caspo, or vori
C. lusitaniae	1	Previous ampho rx	>95% (S)	? (S)	>95% (S)	? (R)	S	S		Flu, caspo, or vori

[†] *Inf Med 21:S17, 2004*   [§] If patient had prior heavy basal exposure, use ampho B or caspo (*CID 35:1073, 2002; 36:1497, 2003*)   [¶] *JAC 55:188, 2005*

Bloodstream: clinically stable with or without venous catheter *(IDSA Guidelines: CID 38:161, 2004)*
- **All positive blood cultures require therapy!**
- Remove & replace venous catheter ("not over a wire") (*CID 36:1221, 2003; Scand J Inf Dis 37:111, 2005; J Clin Micro 43:1829, 2005*), esp. in non-neutropenic: mortality 21% vs 4% if catheter not removed.
- Ophthalmologic exam recommended for all pts with candidemia.
- Treat for 2 wks after last pos. blood culture & resolution of signs & symptoms of infection

Fluconazole ≥6 mg per kg per day or 400 mg q24h IV or po times 7 days then po for 14 days after last +ve blood culture **OR Caspofungin** 70 mg IV on day 1 followed by 50 mg IV q24h (reduce to 35 mg IV q24h with moderate hepatic insufficiency). Would use in place of flu in those heavily pretreated with azoles (i.e., flu or itra prophylaxis) **OR** *(continued on next page)*

In pts who fail to respond or deteriorate, higher doses of either drug may be used (**ampho B** 8–1 mg per kg per day IV or **flucon** 800 mg per day IV or po). **Be sure catheter is removed.**

or

Voriconazole: 6 mg per kg IV q12h times 2 doses, then maintenance doses of 3 mg per kg IV q12h or 200 mg po q12h, after at least 3 days of IV therapy *(continued on next page)*

Observational studies suggest flu & ampho B are similarly effective in neutropenic pts (*IDSA Guidelines, 2003*). A randomized study (277 pts, 10% were neutropenic) found caspofungin equivalent to ampho B (0.6–1 mg per kg per day) for invasive candidiasis. For candidemia 71.7% rx with caspo vs 62.8% with ampho B had successful outcomes but caspo had significantly less toxicity (*NEJM 347:2020, 2002*). Caspo had 70% favorable response vs 56% for ampho B in 58 cancer pts with candidemia (*J Inf 50:443, 2005*). In 119 pts with candidemia, micafungin effective in 88% with new infection, 76% with *(continued on next page)*

---

[1] Hydration before and after infusion with 500 cc saline has been shown to reduce renal toxicity.
[2] **Oral solution preferred to tablets because of ↑ absorption** *(see Table 11B, page 83)*.

See page 2 for abbreviations. All dosage recommendations are for adults (unless otherwise indicated) and assume normal renal function

TYPE OF INFECTION/ORGANISM/ SITE OF INFECTION	ANTIMICROBIAL AGENTS OF CHOICE		COMMENTS
	PRIMARY	ALTERNATIVE	

Candidiasis: Bloodstream: clinically stable with or without venous catheter *(continued)*

	(continued from previous page)	*(continued from previous page)*	*(continued from previous page)*
	Micafungin 50 mg IV q24h for C. albicans, 100 mg IV q24h for non-albicans candida **OR** **Ampho B** 0.6 mg per kg IV q24h, total dose 5–7 mg per kg or lipid-based ampho B[1]	**Anidulafungin** 200 mg IV times 1, then 100 mg q24h (no dosage adjustments for renal or hepatic insufficiency) *(Pending FDA label)*	reinfection *(Eur J Clin Inf Dis, in press).* Preliminary data from a randomized double-blind study (n=245) suggests anidula-fungin was superior to flu for invasive candidiasis/candidemia. Global response (clinical + micro) at end of IV rx, 75.6% rx with anidula vs 60.2% with flu had successful outcomes. Tolerability was comparable *(ICAAC 2005; IDSA 2005, #259).*

Bloodstream: unstable, deteriorating ± neutropenia OR stable disseminated (pulmonary, eye, hepatosplenic) *(IDSA Guidelines: CID 38:161, 2004)* For endophthalmitis, see below	**Ampho B** 0.8–1 mg per kg per day IV ±5FC 37.5[2] mg per kg po q6h or **lipid-based ampho B** (ABLC) 5 mg per kg per day **OR** **Fluconazole** 400–800 mg per day (or >6 mg per kg per day) IV q24h. If start ampho B, switch to flucon 400 mg po q24h times 14 days after last positive blood culture, resolution of neutropenia & disappearance of signs/symptoms of candidal infection **OR** **Combination of fluconazole** 800 mg per day + **ampho** B 0.7 mg per kg per day for first 5–6 days, then switch to flu 400 mg per day po	**Voriconazole.** 6 mg per kg IV q12h times 2 doses, then maintenance doses of 3 mg per kg IV q12h or 200 mg po q12h, after at least 3 days of IV therapy. or **Caspofungin** 70 mg IV on day 1 followed by 50 mg IV q24h (reduce to 35 mg IV q24h with moderate hepatic insufficiency)	In a randomized trial of 219 pts with non-neutropenic candidemia, fluconazole (800 mg per day) + ampho B (0.7 mg per kg per day for the 1st 5 days) was slightly better than flu alone: Primary analysis, success rate on day 30 was 69% vs 57% (p=.08) respectively, overall success rate 69% vs 56% (p=.045). clearance of fungemia 94% vs 83% (p=.02), & renal toxicity in combination greater (23% vs 3%, p <.001) *(CID 36:1221, 2003).* Given difficulty with interpretation of this study, the editors reserve combination of flu + ampho B for only the sickest candidemic patient. Voriconazole may have a role in this clinical setting.

Cutaneous *(including paronychia, Table 1, page 21)*	Apply topical **ampho B, clotrimazole, econazole, miconazole,** or **nystatin** 3–4 times daily for 7–14 days of **ketoconazole** 400 mg po once daily times 14 days. **Ciclopirox olamine** 1% cream/lotion. Apply topically bid times 7–14 days.		Cost (30 gm tube cream): Clo $13. Eco $28. Mic $50. Nys $4.

Endocarditis Causes: C. albicans 24%, non-albicans Candida sp. 24%, Aspergillus sp. 24%, others 27% *(CID 32:50, 2001)* Surgery may not always be required *(Scand J Inf Dis 32:86, 2000 & 37:320, 2005).*	(**Ampho B** 0.6 mg per day IV for 7 days, then 0.8 mg per kg IV every other day or **lipid-based ampho B** 3–5 mg per kg per day) Continue 6–8 weeks after surgery + **surgical resection**	**Fluconazole** 200–400 mg per day for chronic suppression may be of value when valve cannot be replaced *(Chest 122:302, 2002)* + Surgical resection	Cic $19

Endophthalmitis *(IDSA Guidelines: CID 38:161, 2004)* • Occurs in 10% of candidemia *(PIDJ 23:635, 2004),* thus ophthalmological consult for all pts • Diagnosis: typical white exudates on retinal exam and/or isolation by vitrectomy	[**Ampho B** or **lipid-based ampho B** (ABLC 4.5 mg per kg per day)] **OR fluconazole** 400 mg per day IV or po either as initial rx or follow-up after ampho B. Role of intravitreal ampho B not well defined but commonly used in pts with substantial vision loss *(CID 27:1130, 1998).* Treat 6–12 weeks.		**Adjust flucyt dose and interval to produce serum levels: peak 70–80 mg per L, trough 30–40 mg per L.** **Caspofungin** cidal vs candida, several reports of cure *(CID 39:1094-e70-3, 2004; CID 40:e-72, 2005).* Cure of refractory candidal meningitis with caspo *(J Clin Micro 42:5950, 2004).* Treatment results mixed in small series: Fluconazole *(CID 20:657, 1995),* ABLC *(J Infl 40:92, 2000),* and vitrectomy *(CID 27:1130, 1998).* Vori successful alone or with caspo *(Korean J Ophthal 19:73, 2005; Am J Ophthal 139:135, 2005).*

Oral (thrush)—not AIDS patient *(See below for vaginitis)*	**Fluconazole** 200 mg single dose or 100 mg per day po times 14 days or **Itraconazole** oral solution 200 mg q24h without food times 7 days.	**Nystatin pastilles** (200,000 units) lozenge qid, 500,000 units (swish & swallow) qid or 2 (500,000 units) tabs tid for 14 days **OR Clotrimazole** 1 troche (10 mg) 5 times per day times 14 days.	Maintenance not required in non-AIDS pts. Usually improves in 3–4 days, longer rx ↓ relapse. Fluconazole-resistant C. krusei fungemia reported in flucon-rx pts *(NEJM 325:1315, 1991).*

[1] ABLC or liposomal ampho B recommended for pts intolerant of or refractory to ampho B, i.e., failure of 500 mg ampho B, initial renal insufficiency (creatinine >2.5 mg per dL or CrCl <25 mL per min), a sig. ↑ in serum Cr (to >2.5 mg per dL for adults or 1.5 mg per dL for children) or severe acute administration-related toxicity *(CID 26:1383, 1998).* Since efficacy similar and toxicity less, some now recommend lipid-based preps in place of ampho B as initial rx *(CID 32:415, 2003).*

[2] Some experts reduce dose of 5FC to 25 mg per kg q6h

See page 2 for abbreviations. All dosage recommendations are for adults (unless otherwise indicated) and assume normal renal function

TABLE 11A (4)

TYPE OF INFECTION/ORGANISM/ SITE OF INFECTION	ANTIMICROBIAL AGENTS OF CHOICE		COMMENTS
	PRIMARY	**ALTERNATIVE**	

Candidiasis (continued)

AIDS patient

Stomatitis, esophagitis

HAART has resulted in dramatic ↓ in prevalence of oropharyngeal & esophageal candidiasis & ↓ in refractory disease. [MMWR 53(RR-15):97, 2004] Oral candidiasis is a strong clinical marker of immune failure in pts receiving HAART (AIDS Pt Care STDs 19:70, 2005).

	PRIMARY	**ALTERNATIVE**	**COMMENTS**
	Oropharyngeal, initial episodes (7–14 day rx): • **Fluconazole** 100 mg po q24h; or • **itraconazole** oral solution 200 mg po q24h; or • **clotrimazole** troches 10 mg po 5 times per day; or • **nystatin** suspension 4–6 mL q6h or 1–2 flavored pastilles 4–5 times per day.	**Fluconazole-refractory oropharyngeal:** • **Itra** oral solution ≥200 mg po q24h; or • **ampho B** suspension 100 mg per mL[NUS] 1 mL po q6h; or • **ampho B** 0.3 mg per kg IV q24h	**Fluconazole-refractory disease remains uncommon** (4% in ACTG 816) & is seen in pts with low CD4 counts (<50 per mm³). **Flu** superior to oral suspension of **nystatin** (CID 24:1204, 1997). **Itra** 100 mg po bid times 14 days achieved clinical response in 41/74 (55%) pts unresponsive to flu (AIDS Res Hum Retrovir 15:1413, 1999). **Ampho B oral suspension** gave 42.6% response rate in 54 pts refractory to flu, but 70% of those relapsed (AIDS 14:845, 2000). For esophagitis, **caspofungin** as effective as **ampho B IV** but less toxic (CID 33:1529, 2001; AAC 46:451, 2002; JAIDS 31:183, 2002). Also as effective as flucon with similar toxicity profile (AJM 113:294, 2002). **Voriconazole** as effective as **fluconazole** for esophagitis (CID 33:1447, 2001). **Micafungin** 100 mg or 150 mg IV per day equal to flu 200 mg per day (CID 39:842, 2004; Aliment Pharmacol 21:899, 2005). **Anidulafungin** 100 mg IV day 1 followed by 50 mg per day = to flu 200 mg on day 1 followed by 100 mg per day in 494 pts. cure rate 97% vs 98.8% (CID 39:770, 2004). Pending FDA labeling.
	Esophageal (14–21 days): • **Flucon** 100 mg (up to 400 mg) po or IV q24h; or • **itra** oral solution 200 mg po q24h; or • **vori** 200 mg po q12h; or • **caspofungin** 50 mg IV q24h; or • **micafungin** 150 IV q24h or 300 mg every other day.	**Fluconazole-refractory esophageal:** • **Caspofungin** 50 mg IV q24h; or • **vori** 200 mg po q12h; or • **ampho B** 0.3–0.7 mg per kg IV q24h; or • **ampho liposomal** 3–5 mg per kg IV q24h or **ampho lipid complex** 5 mg per kg IV q24h.	
Post-treatment chronic suppression (secondary prophylaxis) for recurrent infection. Authors would dc if CD4 count ↑ (>200 per mm³).	Suppressive rx generally not recommended unless pts have frequent or severe recurrences. • **Oropharyngeal: fluconazole** or **itraconazole** oral solution may be considered. • **Vulvovaginal:** daily **topical azole** for recurrent cases. • **Esophageal: fluconazole** 100–200 mg q24h. Chronic or prolonged use of azoles might promote development of resistance.		Fluconazole 200 mg q24h does reduce risk of candida esophagitis & cryptococcosis (NEJM 332:700, 1995). Disadvantages: Concern of enhanced risk of emergence of fluconazole (azole)-resistant Candida species.
Peritonitis (Chronic Ambulatory Peritoneal Dialysis) See Table 19, page 139	**Fluconazole** 400 mg q24h times 2–3 wks or **caspofungin** 70 mg IV on day 1 followed by 50 mg IV q24h for 14 days	**Ampho B**, continuous IP dosing at 1.5 mg per L of dialysis fluid times 4–6 weeks	Remove cath immediately or if no clinical improvement in 4–7 days. In 1 study, all 8 pts with candida peritonitis who received caspo responded favorably (as compared to 7/8 pts on ampho B) (NEJM 347:2020, 2002).
Urinary: Candiduria • Usually colonization of urinary catheter, a benign event • Rarely may be source of dissemination if pt has obstructive uropathy or marker of acute hematogenous dissemination Persistent candiduria in immunocompromised pt warrants ultrasound or CT of kidneys	**Remove urinary catheter or stent:** 40% will clear but only 20% if replaced (CID 30:14, 2000). Antifungal rx not indicated unless pt has symptoms of UTI, neutropenic, low birth-weight infant, has renal allograft or is undergoing urologic manipulation. Then: **fluconazole** 200 mg per day po or IV times 7–14 days OR **ampho B** 0.5 mg per kg per day IV times 7–14 days		**Fluconazole:** In a placebo-controlled trial, candiduria was cleared more rapidly in pts treated with flucon 200 mg per day times 14 days; 2 weeks after completion, clearance was not different than placebo group (CID 30:15, 2000). **Bladder washout** with ampho B not recommended; will not treat upper tract infection. 5FC may be of value in non-albicans UTI but resistance develops rapidly. **Caspofungin** was effective in clearing candiduria in 12 pts (most with candidemia) but urine levels low (IDSA 2003, Abst. 735). **NOTE:** Vori not in urine in active form
Vaginitis—Non-AIDS patients. Review article: MMWR 51(RR-6), 2002. (Candida vaginitis in AIDS patients: see Stomatitis, vaginitis above). (See Table 1, page 19)			
Sporadic/infrequent	**Intravaginal:** Multiple **imidazoles** with 85–95% cure rates. See footnote[1] **Oral: Fluconazole** 150 mg po times 1 **OR itraconazole** 200 mg po bid times 1 day ** For over-the-counter preparations, see below in footnote[1]		**In general, oral & vaginal rx are similarly effective.** Rx aided by avoiding tight clothing, e.g., pantyhose. Oral drugs ↓ rectal candida & may ↓ relapses. **Ampho B** vaginal 50 mg suppository effective in non-albicans candida infection when other rx failed (Am J Ob Gyn 192:2009 & 2012, 2005).
Chronic recurrent (5–8%) ≥4 episodes per yr Ref.: NEJM 351:876, 2004	**Fluconazole** 150 mg po times 3 & then 150 mg po q wk		After 6 mos. >90% free of disease vs 36% of 173 receiving placebo. By 6 mos. off rx, 42.9% free of disease vs 21.9% who received placebo (p <0.001). Significance: NEJM 351:2554, 2004. Only 76.9% cured 1 mo. following 3-day rx with itra (Mycosis 48:165, 2005).

[1] **Butoconazole** 2% cream (5 gm) q24h at bedtime times 3 days**; or 2% cream SR 5 gm times1; or **clotrimazole** 100 mg vaginal tabs (2 at bedtime times 3 days) or 1% cream (5 gm) at bedtime times 7 days (14 days may ↑ cure rate) or 100 mg vaginal tab times 7 days or 500 mg vaginal tab times 1; or **miconazole** 200 mg vaginal suppos. (1 at bedtime times 3 days**) or 100 mg vaginal suppos. q24h times 7 days or 2% cream (5 gm) at bedtime times 7 days; or **terconazole** 80 mg vaginal tab (1 at bedtime times 3 days) or 0.4% cream (5 gm) at bedtime times 7 days or 0.8% cream 5 gm intravaginal q24h times 3 days; or **tioconazole** 6.5% vag. ointment times 1 dose**. ** = over-the-counter product

TABLE 11A (5)

TYPE OF INFECTION/ORGANISM/ SITE OF INFECTION	ANTIMICROBIAL AGENTS OF CHOICE		COMMENTS
	PRIMARY	ALTERNATIVE	
Chromoblastomycosis (*J Am Acad Derm* 44:585, 2001) (Cladosporium or Fonsecaea). Cutaneous (usually feet, legs); raised scaly lesions, most common in tropical areas	If lesions small and few, **surgical excision or cryosurgery with liquid nitrogen** (*Int J Dermatol* 42:408, 2003). If lesions chronic, extensive, burrowing: **itraconazole**.	**Itraconazole** 100 mg po q24h times 18 months (or until response).[NFDA-I] Fluconazole experience disappointing.	**13/13 patients rx itra responded** (*CID* 15:553, 1992). **Terbinafine**[NFDA-I] impressive in 35 pts rx for 12 mos. (800 mg per day)—86% mycologic cures (*J Derm Treat* 9:S29, 1998). In 4 pts resistance to itra developed on rx with 2 clinical failures (*Mycosis* 47:216, 2004). 5/6 responded to **posaconazole** (*Drugs* 65:1560, 2005)
Coccidioidomycosis (Coccidioides immitis) (*ID Clin No.Amer* 17:41, 2003; *Medicine* 83:149, 2004); (IDSA Guidelines 2005: *CID* 41:1217, 2005)			
Primary pulmonary (San Joaquin or Valley Fever): Pts low risk persistence/complication.	**Antifungal rx not generally recommended.** Treat if fever, wt loss and/or fatigue do not resolve within several wks to 2 months (see below).	Uncomplicated pulmonary in normal host. Influenza-like illness of 1–2 wks duration.	
Primary pulmonary in pts with ↑ risk for complications or dissemination. Rx indicated: • Immunosuppressive disease, AIDS, post-transplantation, hematological malignancies (*AnIM* 165:113, 2005), or therapies (steroids, TNF-α antagonists) (*Arth Rheum* 50:1959, 2004) • Pregnancy in 3rd trimester. • Diabetes • CF antibody >1:16 • ↑ pulmonary infiltrates • Dissemination (identification of spherules or culture of organism from ulcer, joint effusion, pus from abscess or bone bx, etc.)	**Mild to moderate severity:** **Itraconazole** solution 200 mg po or IV bid OR **Fluconazole** 400 mg po q24h for 3–12 months **Locally severe or disseminated disease:** **Ampho B** 0.6–1 mg per kg per day times 7 days then 0.8 mg per kg every other day. Total dose 2.5 gm or more, followed by **itra** or **flu** **Consultation with specialist recommended:** surgery may be required.		**Ampho B cure rate 50–70%. Responses to azoles are similar. Itra** may have slight advantage, esp. in soft tissue infection. Relapse rates after rx 40%. Relapse rate ↑ if ↑ CF titer ≥1:256 (RR = 4.7) (*CID* 25:1205, 1997). Following CF titers after completion of rx important; rising titers warrant readministration of rx (*CID* 25:1211, 1997). In an RDBS[3] of 198 pts with progressive non-meningeal cocci, 57% responded to flu vs 72% to itra (p=0.05). (*AnIM* 133:676, 2000). **Vori** effective in 1 case of widely disseminated cocci (*CID* 39:e74, 2004). **Posaconazole**, oral suspension 800 mg per day successful in 5/6 pts with refractory non-meningeal cocci (*CID* 40:1770, 2005) & 11/16 cases successful reported overall (*Drugs* 65:1559, 2005).
Meningitis: occurs in 1/3 to 1/2 of pts with disseminated coccidioidomycosis			
Adult	**Fluconazole** 400–800 mg po q24h indefinitely	**Ampho B** IV as for pulmonary (above) + 0.1–0.3 mg daily intrathecal (intraventricular) via reservoir device. **OR itra** 400–800 mg q24h **OR voriconazole** (see Comment) **OR caspo** (see Comment)	**80% relapse rate, continue flucon indefinitely. Voriconazole** successful in high doses (6 mg per kg IV q12h) followed by oral suppression (400 mg po q12h) (*CID* 36:1619, 2003; *AAC* 48: 2341, 2004). **Caspofungin** also used (*JAC* 54:292, 2004) & failed in another case (*CID* 39:879, 2004).
Child	**Fluconazole** (po) (Pediatric dose not established, 6 mg per kg q24h used)		
Cryptococcosis (*CID* 30:710, 2000). Excellent review: *Brit Med Bull* 72:99, 2005			
Non-meningeal (non-AIDS) Risk 57% in organ transplant (*Transpl Inf Dis* 4:183, 2002 & 7:26, 2005) & those receiving other forms of immunosuppressive agents (alemtuzumab—*Transplant Proc* 37:934, 2005)	**Fluconazole** 400 mg po per day IV wks to 6 mos **For more severe disease: Ampho B** 0.5–0.8 mg per kg per day IV till response then change to **fluconazole** 400 mg po q24h for 8–10-week course	**Itraconazole** 200–400 mg solution q24h for 6–12 mos OR **Ampho B** 0.3 mg per kg per day IV + **flucytosine** 37.5 mg per kg[1] po qid times 6 wks.	**Flucon alone 90% effective for meningeal and non-meningeal forms.** Fluconazole as effective as ampho B (*CID* 32:E145, 2001). Addition of **interferon-γ** (IFN-γ-Ib 50 mcg per M[2] subcut. 3 times per wk times 9 wks) to liposomal ampho B assoc. with response in pt failing antifungal rx (*CID* 38: 910, 2004).
Meningitis (non-AIDS)	**Ampho B** 0.5–0.8 mg per kg per day IV + **flucytosine** 37.5 mg per kg[1] po q6h until pt afebrile and cultures negative (~6 weeks) (*NEJM* 301:126, 1979), then stop ampho B/flucyt, start **fluconazole** 200 mg po q24h (*AnIM* 113:183, 1990) **OR Fluconazole** 400 mg po q24h times 8–10 weeks (less severely ill patient). Some recommend flu for 2 yrs to reduce relapse late (*CID* 28:297, 1999).		**Fluconazole alone used successfully**, comparative clinical trials lacking (*NEJM* 330:263, 1994). Hydrocephalus may be successfully rx with VP[2] or VA[2] shunting (*CID* 28:629, 1999); poor response if pts in coma (*CID* 37:673, 2003).
HIV+/AIDS: Cryptococcemia and/or Meningitis Treatment (see *CID* 30:710, 2000) ↓ in era of HAART (*Neurol* 56:257, 2001; *CID* 36:789, 2003) but still common when pt presents with AIDS & HIV status unknown (*AIDS* 18:555, 2004). (continued on next page)	**Ampho B** 0.7 mg per kg IV q24h + **flucytosine** 25 mg per kg po q24h[1] (continued on next page)	[**Fluconazole** 400–800 mg po or IV q24h for less severe disease **or** **Itra** 400 mg po q24h times 8 wks (continued on next page)	If normal mental status, >20 cells per mm[3] CSF, and CSF crypto antigen <1:1024, flucon alone is reasonable (*CID* 22:322, 1996). Serum cryptococcal antigen useful in dx (95% sens); no help in monitoring therapy. (continued on next page)

[1] Some experts would reduce to 25 mg per kg q6h
[2] **VP** = ventriculoperitoneal. **VA** = ventriculoatrial. **RDBS** = randomized double-blind study
[3] **Flucytosine** = 5-FC

See page 2 for abbreviations. All dosage recommendations are for adults (unless otherwise indicated) and assume normal renal function

TABLE 11A (6)

TYPE OF INFECTION/ORGANISM/ SITE OF INFECTION	ANTIMICROBIAL AGENTS OF CHOICE		COMMENTS
	PRIMARY	ALTERNATIVE	

Cryptococcosis/HIV+/AIDS: Cryptococcemia and/or Meningitis/Treatment (continued)

(continued from previous page) With HAART, symptoms of acute meningitis may return: Immune Reconstitution Inflammatory Syndrome (IRIS). In 1 study of 59 cryptomeningitis (CM) pts started on HAART, 18 (30%) IRIS or 17.9 events per 100 pt years. Symptoms included return of meningeal symptoms, with ↑ CSF pressure, ↑ WBC & glucose level vs pts with CM, but cultures were negative. Median time to symptoms following HAART was 30 days, but pts who received HAART within 30 days of dx & rx of CM were more likely to develop IRIS (RR 1-73 p=0.03) (CID 40:1049, 2005). In some ↑ ICP may be sustained (J Inf 51:165, 2005). Therefore, delaying HAART >30 days after rx for CM would seem prudent albeit in 1 study, most clinicians initiate ART after 2 wks (AIDS 19:535, 2005).	(continued from previous page) q6h times 2 wks **or** Liposomal amphotericin B 4 mg per kg IV q24h + flucytosine 25 mg per kg po q6h times 2 wks] **Then** Consolidation therapy: Fluconazole 400 mg po q24h to complete a 10-week course or until CSF culture sterile, then suppression (see below) Start Highly Active Antiretroviral Therapy (HAART) if possible.	(continued from previous page) Fluconazole 400–800 mg po or IV q24h + fluctosine 25 mg per kg po q6h times 4–6 wks **or** Ampho B 0.7 mg per kg IV q24h times 2 wks] Itraconazole 200 mg po bid if flu intolerant or failure	(continued from previous page) If ↑ CSF pressure, lower with CSF removal (CID 38:134, 2004). If frequent LPs not possible, ventriculoperitoneal shunts an option (Surg Neurol 63:529 & 531, 2005). Higher levels assoc. with bone marrow toxicity. Itraconazole does not penetrate CSF (CID 22:329, 1996). Ampho B + 5FC treatment: 29/236 pts died within 1st 2 wks & 62 (26%) by 10 wks; only 129 (55%) were alive & culture-neg. at 10 wks (CID 28:82, 1999). In 64 pts, ampho + 5FC ↓ crypto CFUs more rapidly than ampho + flu or combination of all 3 drugs (p <0.001) (Ln 363:1764, 2004). Successful outcomes were observed in 14/29 (48%) subjects with cryptococcal meningitis treated with posaconazole (JAC 56:745, 2005). Must monitor 5-FC levels: peak 70-80 mg per L, trough 30–40 mg per L.

Suppression (chronic maintenance therapy)

Discontinuation of antifungal rx considered if pts asymptomatic, with CD4 >100–200 per mm³ for ≥6 months (www.hivatis.org). Must have culture-neg. CSF.	Fluconazole 200 mg po q24h	Itraconazole 200 mg po q24h	Itraconazole not as effective as fluconazole. 13/57 (23%) pts relapsed vs 2/51 (4%) receiving fluconazole (p=0.006) (CID 28:291, 1999).

Dermatophytosis (See Superficial fungal infections, Ln 364:1173, 2004)

Onychomycosis (Tinea unguium) [Derm Ther 17:517, 2004; Brit J Derm 148:402, 2003; Am J Clin Derm 5:225, 2004; Cutis 74:516, 2004]

A topical nail lacquer (ciclopirox) approved but cure in only 5–9% after 48 wks (Med Lett 42:51, 2000) but ↑ to 50% cure in another study (Cutis 73:81, 2004). May enhance oral rx (Cutis 74:55, 2004; J Eur Acad Dermato Venereol 19:21, 2005).

Terbinafine appears to be most cost-effective rx (Manag Care 12:47, 2003; Manag Care Interface 18:55, 2005). Overall cure rates from randomized controlled trials is 76% (J Drugs Derm 4:302, 2005).

Fingernail Rx Options:
Terbinafine[1] 250 mg po q24h times 4 wks for tonsurans, 4–8 wks for Microsporum canis[NFDA-I] or

Itraconazole[2] 200 mg po q24h times 3 mos. or

Itraconazole[2] 200 mg po bid times 1 wk per mo. times 2 mos. or

Fluconazole 150–300 mg po q wk times 3–6 mos.

NOTE: For side-effects, see footnotes **1 & 2**

Toenail Rx Options:
Terbinafine[1] 250 mg po q24h [children <20 kg: 67.5 mg per day, 20–40 kg: 125 mg per day, >40 kg: 250 mg per day] times 12 wks (76% effective) or

Itraconazole[2] 200 mg po q24h times 3 mos (59% effective) or

Itraconazole[2] 200 mg po q24h times 1 wk per mo. times 3–4 mos (63% effective)[NFDA-I] or

Fluconazole 150–300 mg po q wk times 6–12 mos (48% effective)[NFDA-I] [Data reflect cure rate from meta-analysis of all randomized controlled trials (Brit J Derm 150:537, 2004]

Tinea capitis ("ringworm") (Trichophyton tonsurans, Microsporum canis, N. America: other sp. elsewhere) (PIDJ 18:191, 1999)

Terbinafine[1] 250 mg po q24h times 4 wks for tonsurans, 4–8 wks for Microsporum canis[NFDA-I]. Children 125 mg (>6–12 mg per kg per day) q24h. (COID 17:97, 2004; Exp Opin Pharm Ther 5:219, 2004; J Eur Acad Dermatol Venereol 18:155, 2004).	Itraconazole[2] 3–5 mg per kg per day for 30 days[NFDA-I] Fluconazole 8 mg per kg q wk times 8-12 wks.[NFDA-I] Cap at 150 mg q wk for adults Griseofulvin: adults 500 mg po q24h times 4–6 wks, children 10–20 mg per kg per day until hair regrows, usually 6–8 wks.	Terbinafine[1] 250 mg po q24h [children <20 kg: 67.5 mg per day, 20–40 kg: 125 mg per day, >40 kg: 250 mg per day] times 12 wks (76% effective)

All agents with similar cure rates (60-100%) in clinical studies (Ped Derm 17:304, 2000). Griseofulvin considered drug of choice by some although concerns for resistance and toxicities. Addition of topical ketoconazole or selenium sulfate shampoo reduces transmissibility (Int J Dermatol 39:261, 2000)

Tinea corporis, cruris, or pedis (Trichophyton rubrum, T. mentagrophytes, Epidermophyton floccosum) "Athlete's foot, jock itch," and ringworm

Terbinafine 250 mg po q24h times 2 wks[NFDA-I] OR ketoconazole 200 mg po q24h times 4 wks OR fluconazole 150 mg po 1 time per wk for 2–4 wks[1] OR Griseofulvin: adults 500 mg po q24h times 4–6 wks, children 10–20 mg per kg per day. Duration: 2–4 wks for corporis, 4–8 wks for pedis.	**Topical rx:** Generally applied 2 times per day. Available as creams, ointments, sprays, by prescription & "over the counter". Apply 2 times per day for 2–3 wks. See footnote³ for names and prices. Recommend: Lotrimin Ultra or Lamisil AT, contain butenafine & terbinafine—both are fungicidal

Keto oft too effective in severe recalcitrant infection. Follow for hepatotoxicity. Terbinafine: 87% achieved mycological cure in double-blind study (32 pts) (J Med Assn Thai 76:388, 1993; Brit J Derm 130(S43):22, 1994) and fluconazole 78% (J Am Acad Derm 40:531, 1999).

---

¹ **Serious but rare cases of hepatic failure** have been reported in pts receiving terbinafine & should not be used in those with chronic or active liver disease. (See Table 11B, page 83). Suggest checking ALT & AST before prescribing (Am J Health Sys Pharm 58:1076, 2001).

² Use of itraconazole has been associated with myocardial dysfunction and with onset of congestive heart failure (see Ln 357:1766, 2001).

³ Drug name (trade name) & wholesale price for 15 gm. All are applied to affected area bid. **Prescription drugs:** butenafine (Mentax) $40, ciclopirox (Loprox) $23, clotrimazole (Lotrimin $19, Mycelex $11). (continued at bottom of next page)

See page 2 for abbreviations. All dosage recommendations are for adults (unless otherwise indicated) and assume normal renal function

TABLE 11A (7)

TYPE OF INFECTION/ORGANISM/ SITE OF INFECTION	ANTIMICROBIAL AGENTS OF CHOICE		COMMENTS
	PRIMARY	ALTERNATIVE	

Dermatophytosis *(continued)*

Tinea versicolor (Malassezia furfur or Pityrosporum orbiculare) Rule out erythrasma—*see Table 1, page 40*	**Ketoconazole** (400 mg po single dose)[NFDA-1] or (200 mg q24h times 7 days), or (2% cream applied 1 time q24h times 2 wks)	**Fluconazole** 400 mg po single dose or **Itraconazole** 400 mg po q24h times 3–7 days	Keto (po) times 1 97% effective in 1 study. Another alternative: Selenium sulfide (Selsun), 2.5% lotion, apply as lather, leave on 10 min then wash off, 1 time per day times 7 day or 3–5 times per week times 2–4 weeks
Fusariosis Infections in eye, skin, sinus & disseminated diseases— 1 in transplant & cancer pts *(Clin Micro Inf 10:499 & 567, 2004; COID 17:527, 2004)*	**Voriconazole** 6 mg per kg IV q12h times 1, then either (4 mg per kg q12h) or (200 mg po q12h for body weight ≥40 kg, but 100 mg po q12h for body weight <40 kg)	**Ampho B** 1–1.2 mg per kg or lipid-associated ampho B	Voriconazole successful in 9/21: 4 eye, 2 bloodstream, 2 sinus & 1 skin *(CID 35:909, 2002; 36:1122, 2003; 37:311, 2003).*

Histoplasmosis (Histoplasma capsulatum): *See CID 30:688, 2000; ID Clin No. Amer 17:1, 2003.* Best diagnostic test 2nd generation is urinary, serum, or CSF histoplasma antigen: MiraVista Diagnostics (1-866-647-2847).

Immunocompetent patient: Pulmonary, localized, disseminated Definition of severe—Temp >39.5°C, Karnofsky <60, albumin <3 gm per dL, hepatic enzymes >5 times normal, WBC <500, platelets <50,000, creatinine >6 mg per dL	**Minimal disease: No rx** **Moderate: Itraconazole** 200 mg per day solution po for 9 months. If life-threatening 200 mg po tid times 3 days, then 200 mg po bid until response.[1] If IV rx necessary: Dose 200 mg IV bid times 4 doses followed by 200 mg IV q24h *(see Table 11B).* **Severe, including meningitis: Liposomal ampho B** 3 mg per kg per day IV times 7 days, then 0.8 mg per kg every other day IV up to 1 gm, then switch to **itra** 200 mg po per day for 9 months. **Itra not recommended for meningitis.** *(See CID 38:463, 2004)*		With ≥2 months itra rx, 86% success in chronic pulmonary & extrapulmonary *(AJM 93:489, 1992).* Meningitis is difficult to rx & no prospective studies. **Liposomal ampho B** recommended because of ↑ CSF levels vs ampho B. Histo antigen in CSF should fall to undetectable levels before rx dc *(see CID 40:844, 2005).* **Flu less effective than itra.**
Immunocompromised patient (AIDS) *(CID 30:688, 2000, & 32:1215, 2001)* Risk factors for death: dyspnea, platelet count <100,000 per mm³ & LDH >2 times upper limit normal *(CID 38:134, 2004).* In 1 study suppression was safely dc after 12 mos. of antifungal rx & 6 mos. of HAART with CD4 >150: 0 relapses after 2 yrs follow-up in 32 pts *(CID 38:1485, 2004).*	**Primary prophylaxis:** Consider for pts from endemic area with CD4 <150 per mcL. If used: itraconazole 200 mg po q24h. **Severe disseminated:** **Acute phase** (3–10 days or until clinically improved): • **Ampho B** 0.7 mg per kg IV q24h; or • **liposomal ampho B** 4 mg per kg IV q24h **Continuation phase** (12 wks): **Itra** 200 mg po q12h **Less severe disseminated:** **Itra** 200 mg po q8h times 3 days, then 200 mg po q12h times 12 wks **Meningitis:** **Ampho B or liposomal ampho B** times 12–16 wks **Suppression:** Insufficient data to rec. dc with ↑ CD4 from HAART but probably OK—**Itraconazole** 200 mg po q24h indefinitely	**Severe disseminated:** **Acute phase: Itra** 400 mg IV q24h **Continuation phase:** • **Itra** oral solution 200 mg po q12h; or • **flucon** 800 mg po q24h. **Mild disseminated:** **Fluconazole** 800 mg po q24h **Amphotericin B** 1 mg per kg IV weekly or biweekly indefinitely	Acute pulmonary histoplasmosis among HIV-1 infected pts with CD4 counts >500 per mm³ might require no rx. **Liposomal ampho B** superior at 2 wks vs ampho B (88% vs 64% clinical success) in 81 pts with ↓ nephrotoxicity (97% vs 37%) *(AnIM 137:105, 2002)* **Itra (ACTG 120) 50/59 (85%) pts responded,** cleared fungemia with only 5% toxicity. Avoid rifampin, reduces itra serum concentration *(AJM 98:336, 1995).* Mortality 12.5% in 110 cases of disseminated histo + AIDS receiving ampho B up to 1 gm followed by itra in Panama *(CID 40:1199, 2005).* **Itra best drug for suppression at 200 mg q24h** but 3/46 had probable hepatic toxicity *(J AIDS & HR 16:100, 1997).* Flu less effective than itra & induces flu resistance *(CID 33:1910, 2001).* There are no prospective studies addressing the management of CNS histoplasmosis *(CID 40:844, 2005).*

Madura foot *(See Nocardia & Scedosporium, below)*

---

econazole (Spectazole) $22, ketoconazole (Nizoral) $22, miconazole (Monistat-Derm) $21, naftifine (Naftin) $27, oxiconazole (Oxistat) $26, sulconazole (Exelderm) $13, terconazole (Terazol) $30, sertaconazole (Ertaczo) $47. **Non-prescription (over-the-counter):** Tolnaftate (Tinactin) $5, Ting or Tolnate $2), undecylenic acid (Cruex $5, Desenex $5), Lotrimin 1% 12 gm $6.17, Lamisil AT 1%, 12 gm $6.79.

[1] **Oral solution preferred to tablets because of ↑ absorption** *(see Table 11B, page 83).*

See page 2 for abbreviations. All dosage recommendations are for adults (unless otherwise indicated) and assume normal renal function

TABLE 11A (8)

TYPE OF INFECTION/ORGANISM/ SITE OF INFECTION	ANTIMICROBIAL AGENTS OF CHOICE		COMMENTS
	PRIMARY	ALTERNATIVE	
Mucormycosis (Zygomycosis—Rhizopus, Rhizomucor, Mucor, Absidia) (CID 41:521, 2005) Rhinocerebral, pulmonary (AnM 159:1301, 1999) Key to successful rx: early dx with symptoms suggestive of sinusitis (or lateral facial pain or numbness); think mucor with symptoms suggestive of sinusitis, &/or black eschars, onset unilateral blindness in immunocompromised or diabetic pt (J Otolaryn 34:166, 2005). Rapidly fatal without rx. Dx by culture of tissue or stain: wide ribbon-like, non-septated with variation in diameter & right angle branching (CID 17:517, 2004).	**Ampho B**: Increase rapidly to 0.8–1.5 mg per kg per day IV; when improving, then every other day. Total dose usually 2.5–3 gm. **or** **Lipid-based Ampho B or Posaconazole** 200 mg qid (when available will be drug of choice)		Cure dependent on: (1) surgical debridement, (2) rx of hyperglycemia, correction of neutropenia, or reduction in immunosuppression; (3) antifungal rx: liposomal amphotericin (J Clin Micro 43:2012, 2005) longterm or **posaconazole** (FDA approval pending)—striking improvement reported. 54–70% overall success in refractory zygomycosis vs 25% or less with amphotericin or lipid ampho B (Drugs 65:1553, 2005).
Nocardiosis (N. asteroides & N. brasiliensis). Culture & sensitivities may be valuable in refractory cases: Reference Labs, R.J. Wallace (903) 877-7680 or CDC (404) 639-3158 (IDCP 8.27, 1999)	**TMP-SMX**: 5–10 mg per kg per day of TMP & 25–50 mg per kg per day of SMX in 2–4 div. doses per day IV	**Sulfisoxazole** 2 gm po qid or **minocycline** 100–200 mg po bid	**Linezolid** 300–600 mg po bid times 3–24 mos. successful in 6/6 pts, 4 with disseminated disease of whom 2 had brain abscesses (CID 36: 313, 2003; Eur J Neurol 12:536, 2005).
Cutaneous and lymphocutaneous (sporotrichoid)	**TMP-SMX**: Initially 15 mg per kg per day of TMP & 75 mg per kg per day of SMX IV or po, div. in 2–4 doses. After 3–4 wks, ↓ dose to 10 mg per kg per day TMP in 2–4 doses po. Do serum level (see Comment)		Survival improved when sulfa-containing regimen used (Medicine 68:38, 1999). **Prosthetic valve endocarditis** with N. asteroides cured with IMP + amikacin times 2 mos. followed by TMP-SMX times 4 mos. (AJM 115:330, 2003).
Pulmonary, disseminated, brain abscess Duration of rx generally 3 mos. for immunocompetent host (38%), & 6 mos. for immunocompromised (62% organ transplant, malignancy, chronic lung disease, diabetes, ETOH use, steroid rx, AIDS, & infliximab rx (Canad Med J 171:1063, 2004).		**IMP** 500 mg IV q6h) + **amikacin** 7.5 mg per kg IV q12h) times 3–4 wks & then po regimen	Measure sulfonamide blood levels: Peak of 100–150 mcg per mL 2 hrs post-po dose. Increasing sulfa resistance—recommend sensitivity testing (Eur J Clin Micro Inf Dis 24:142, 2005; AAC 48:832, 2004).
Lobomycosis (keloidal blastomycosis)/ P. loboi	Surgical excision, clofazimine or ampho B		
Paracoccidioidomycosis (South American blastomycosis)/P. brasiliensis	**Itraconazole** 200 mg per day po times 6 months or **Ketoconazole** 400 mg per day po for 6–18 months.	**Ampho B** 0.4–0.5 mg per kg per day IV to total dose of 1.5–2.5 gm. or **sulfonamides** (dose: see Comment)	Improvement in >90% pts on itra or keto. NFDA4 **Sulfa**: 4–6 gm per day for weeks, then 500 mg per day for 3–5 yrs also used (CID 74 (Suppl.):S-68, 1992). Low-dose itra (50–100 mg per day), keto (200–400 mg per day) & sulfadiazine (up to 6 mg per day) showed similar clinical responses in 4–6 mos. in a randomized study (Med Mycol 40: 411, 2002). HIV+: TMP-SMX suppressive rx indefinitely (CID 21:1275, 1995).
Penicilliosis (Penicillium marneffei): Common disseminated fungal infection in AIDS pts in SE Asia (esp. Thailand & Vietnam) (CID 24:1080, 1997; Intl J Inf Dis 3:48, 1998)	**Ampho B** 0.5–1 mg per kg per day times 2 wks followed by **itraconazole** 400 mg per day for 10 wks followed by 200 mg per day po **indefinitely for HIV-infected pts** (CID 26:1107, 1998). See Comment	**Itra** 200 mg po tid times 3 days, then 200 mg po bid times 12 wks, then 200 mg po q24h.¹ (IV if unable to take po) For less sick patients	3rd most common OI in AIDS pts in SE Asia following TBc and cryptococcal meningitis. Prolonged fever, lymphadenopathy, hepatomegaly. Skin nodules are umbilicated (mimic cryptococcal infection or molluscum contagiosum). In AIDS pts, suppression with itra effective in **preventing relapses** (NEJM 339:1739, 1998).
Phaeohyphomycosis (black molds/ dematiaceous fungi) (See CID 41:521, 2005) Sinuses, skin, bone & joint, brain abscess, endocarditis **Species: Scedosporium prolificans** (Australia & Spain—J Chemother 15:S16, 2003), Bipolaris, Wangiella, Curvularia, Exophiala, Phialemonium, Scytalidium, Alternaria	Surgery + itraconazole 400 mg per day po, duration not defined, probably 6 months NFDA4	**Voriconazole** has in vitro activity, but clinical experience limited vs S. prolificans (COID 17:527, 2004). **Itraconazole + terbinafine** synergistic against S. prolificans (AAC 44:470, 2000). No clinical data but combination could show ↑ toxicity (see Table 11B, page 85).	Notoriously resistant to antifungal rx including amphotericin & azoles (CID 34:909, 2002). Mortality >80%. Posaconazole successful in case of brain abscess (CID 34:648, 2002). Accounted for 10% of mycelial infections post-transplant (CID 37:221, 2003).
Scedosporium apiospermum (Pseudallescheria boydii) (not considered a true dematiaceous mold) (Medicine 81:333, 2002) Skin, subcutaneous (Madura foot), brain abscess, recurrent meningitis. May appear after near-drowning incidents.	**Voriconazole** 6 mg per kg IV q12h on day 1, then either (4 mg per kg IV q12h) or (200 mg po q12h for body weight ≥40 kg, but 100 mg po q12h for body weight <40 kg) (PIDJ 21:240, 2002)	Surgery + **itraconazole** 200 mg po bid until clinically well NFDA4 (Many species now resistant or refractory to itra) or **Miconazole** NUS 600 mg IV q8h	Notoriously resistant to antifungal drugs including amphotericin. In vitro voriconazole more active than itra (J Clin Micro 39: 954, 2001). Case reports of successful rx of disseminated and CNS disease with voriconazole (Clin Micro Inf 9:750, 2003; EJCMID 22:408, 2003).

¹ **Oral solution preferred to tablets because of ↑ absorption** (see Table 11B, page 85).

See page 2 for abbreviations. All dosage recommendations are for adults (unless otherwise indicated) and assume normal renal function

TABLE 11A (9)

TYPE OF INFECTION/ORGANISM/ SITE OF INFECTION	ANTIMICROBIAL AGENTS OF CHOICE		COMMENTS
	PRIMARY	ALTERNATIVE	
Sporotrichosis (CID 36:34, 2003; ID Clin No. Amer 17:59, 2003; Derm Ther 17: 523, 2004)			
Cutaneous/Lymphonodular	**Itraconazole** 100–200 mg per day po times 6 mos. (then 200 mg po bid long-term[1] for HIV-infected pts[NFDA1])	**Fluconazole** 400 mg po q24h times 6 mos **or** Sat. soln. potassium iodide (**SSKI**) (1 gm of KI in 1 mL of H₂O). Start with 5–10 drops tid, gradually ↑ to 40–50 drops tid for 3–6 mos. Take after meals.	Itra ref.: CID 17:210, 1993. Some authorities use ampho B as primary therapy. Ampho B resistant strains reported (AJM 95: 279, 1993). Itra rx for up to 24 months effective in multifocal osteoarticular infection (CID 23: 394, 1996). SSKI side-effects: nausea, rash, fever, metallic taste, salivary gland swelling.
Extracutaneous: Osteoarticular, pulmonary, disseminated, meningeal	**Osteoarticular, pulmonary: itraconazole 300 mg po bid times 6-12 mos., Disseminated, meningeal: Ampho B** 0.5 mg per kg per day to then 200 mg po bid (long-term for HIV-infected pts)	(IV if unable to take po)	total of 1–2 gm, followed by **itra** 200 mg bid or **flu** 800 mg q24h

TABLE 11B: ANTIFUNGAL DRUGS: ADVERSE EFFECTS, COMMENTS, COST

DRUG NAME, GENERIC (TRADE)/ USUAL DOSAGE/COST*	ADVERSE EFFECTS/COMMENTS
Non-lipid amphotericin B deoxycholate (Fungizone): 0.3–1 mg per kg per day as single infusion 50 mg $36.55 Mixing ampho B with lipid emulsion results in precipitation and is discouraged (Am J Hlth Pharm 52:1463, 1995)	**Admin.:** Ampho B is a colloidal suspension that must be prepared in electrolyte-free D5W at 0.1 mg per mL to avoid precipitation. No need to protect drug suspensions from light. Ampho B infusions cause chills/fever, myalgia, anorexia, nausea, rarely hemodynamic collapse/hypotension. Postulated due to proinflammatory cytokines but does not appear to be histamine release (Pharmacol 23:966, 2003). Manufacturer recommends a test dose of 1 mg, but often not done (1st few mL of 1st dose is a test dose). Duration of infusion usually 4 or more hrs. No difference found in 1- vs 4-hr infusions (AAC 34:1402, 1992) except chills/fever occurred sooner with 1-hr infusion. Febrile reactions decrease with repeated doses. Rare pulmonary reactions (severe dyspnea and focal infiltrates suggesting pulmonary edema) associated with rapid infusion (CID 33:75, 2001). Severe rigors respond to meperidine (25–50 mg IV). Premedication with acetaminophen, diphenhydramine, hydrocortisone (1000 units) and heparin (25–50 mg) had no influence on rigors/fever (CID 70:755, 1995). If cytokine postulate correct, NSAIDs or high-dose steroids may prove efficacious but their use may risk worsening infection under rx of proven infection (i.e., NSAIDs). Clinical side effects ↓ with ↑ age (CID 26:334, 1998). **Toxicity:** Major concern is nephrotoxicity (15% of 102 pts surveyed, CID 26:334, 1998). Manifest initially by kaliuresis and hypokalemia, then fall in serum bicarbonate (may proceed to renal tubular acidosis),↓ in renal erythropoietin and anemia, ↑ BUN/serum creatinine. Hypomagnesemia may occur. Can reduce risk of renal injury by **(a) pre- and post-infusion hydration with 500 mL saline (if clinical status will allow salt load)**, **(b)** avoidance of other nephrotoxins, e.g. radiocontrast, aminoglycosides, cis-platinum, (c) use of lipid prep of ampho B. Use of low-dose dopamine did not significantly reduce renal toxicity (AAC 42:3703, 1998). In a single randomized controlled trial of 80 neutropenic pts with refractory fever & suspected or proven invasive fungal infection, **infused over 4 hrs.** Continuous infusion produced less nephrotoxicity [26% ↑ in max. serum Cr (p=0.005)], a reduction in fever, chills & vomiting (p <0.02– 0.97 mg per kg per day amphotericin **continuously infused over a 24-hr period** was compared to the classical **rapid infusion** of 0.95 mg per kg per day 0.0003) & appeared as effective as rapid infusion but in very few proven fungal infections (7 & 3, respectively) (BMJ 322:1, 2001). Continuous infusion also allows a dramatic ↑ in administered dosage without sig. toxicity (CID 36:943, 2003). It is disturbing that these exciting observations have not led to controlled trials examining antifungal efficacy in rx of life-threatening fungal infections (CID 36:952, 2003). Await trials of efficacy in larger number of proven fungal infections!
Lipid-based ampho B products:[2] **Amphotericin B lipid complex (ABLC) (Abelcet):** 5 mg per kg per day as single infusion 100 mg IV $240	**Admin.:** Consists of ampho B complexed with 2 lipid bilayer ribbons. Compared to standard ampho B, larger volume of distribution, rapid blood clearance and high tissue concentrations (liver, spleen, lung). Dosage: **5 mg per kg once daily.** infuse at 2.5 mg per kg per hr; adult and ped. dose the same. Do NOT use an in-line filter. Do not dilute with saline or mix with other drugs or electrolytes.[3] **Toxicity:** Fever and chills in 14–18%; nausea 9%, vomiting 8%, serum creatinine ↑ in 11%; renal failure 5%; anemia 4%; ↓ K 5%; rash 4%. A fatal case of fat embolism reported following ABLC infusion (Exp Mol Path 177:246, 2004).

[1] **Oral solution preferred to tablets because of ↑ absorption** (see Table 11B, page 85).
[2] Published data from patients intolerant of or refractory to conventional ampho B deoxycholate (Amp B d). **None of the lipid ampho B preps has shown superior efficacy compared to ampho B in prospective trials (except liposomal ampho B was more effective vs ampho B in rx of disseminated histoplasmosis at 2 wks** (AnIM 137:105, 2002; CID 37:415, 2003). **Dosage equivalency has not been established** (CID 36:1500, 2003). Nephrotoxicity ↓ with all lipid ampho B preps (NEJM 340:764, 1999).
[3] Comparisons between Abelcet & AmBisome suggest higher infusion-assoc. toxicity (rigors) & febrile episodes with Abelcet (70% vs 36%) but a higher frequency of mild hepatic toxicity with AmBisome (59% vs 38%, p=0.05). Mild elevations in serum creatinine were observed in 1/3 of both (BJ Hemat 103:198, 1998; Focus on Fungal Inf #9, 1999; Bone Marrow Tx 20:39, 1997; CID 26:1383, 1998).

* From 2005 Drug Topics Red Book, Medical Economics Data and Hospital Formulary Pricing Guide. **Price is average wholesale price (AWP).**
See page 2 for abbreviations. All dosage recommendations are for adults (unless otherwise indicated) and assume normal renal function

84

TABLE 11B (2)

DRUG NAME, GENERIC (TRADE)/ USUAL DOSAGE/COST*	ADVERSE EFFECTS/COMMENTS
Liposomal amphotericin B (L-AmB, AmBisome): 1–5 mg per kg per day as single infusion. 50 mg $188	**Admin.:** Consists of vesicular bilayer liposome with ampho B intercalated within the membrane. Dosage: **3–5 mg per kg per day** IV as single dose infused over a period of approx. 120 min. If well tolerated, infusion time can be reduced to 60 min. *(see footnote 3, page 83)* 1 mg per kg per day was as effective as 4 mg per kg per day (6 mos. survival rates 43% vs 37%, respectively) in pts with invasive aspergillosis complicating bone marrow transplant and/or neutropenia from malignancy *(CID 27:1406, 1998).* Tolerated well in elderly pts *(J Inf 50:277, 2005).* **Major toxicity:** Generally less than ampho B. Nephrotoxicity 18.7% vs 33.7% for ampho B, chills 47% vs 75%, nausea 39.7% vs 38.7%, vomiting 31.8% vs 43.9%, rash 24% for both, ↓ Ca 18.4% vs 20.9%, ↓ K 20.4% vs 25.6%, ↓ Mg 20.4% vs 25.6%. Acute infusion-related reactions are common with liposomal ampho B, 20–40%. 86% occurred within 5 min. of infusion, including chest pain, dyspnea & hypoxia or severe abdominal, flank or leg pain; 14% developed flushing & urticaria near the end of 4-hr infusion. All responded to diphenhydramine (1 mg per kg) & interruption of L-AmB infusion. These reactions may be due to complement activation by the liposome *(CID 36:1213, 2003).*
Amphotericin B cholesteryl complex (amphotericin B colloidal dispersion, ABCD, Amphotec): 3–4 mg per kg per day as single infusion. 100 mg $160	**Admin.:** Consists of ampho B deoxycholate stabilized with cholesteryl sulfate resulting in a disc-shaped colloidal complex. Compared to standard ampho B, larger volume of distribution, rapid blood clearance, high tissue concentrations. Dosage: Initial dose for adults & children: **3–4 mg per kg per day.** If necessary, can ↑ to 6 mg per kg per day. Dilute in D5W & infuse at 1 mg per kg per hr. Do NOT use in-line filter. **Toxicity:** Chills 50%, fever 33%, ↑ serum creatinine 12–20%, ↓ Ca 6%, ↓ K 17%. Hepatotoxicity more common (incidence 1.5) in bone marrow transplant pts than ampho B (inc. 0.78/100 pt days) *(CID 41:301, 2005)* & ↑ with continuing rx.
Caspofungin (Cancidas) 70 mg IV on day 1 followed by 50 mg IV q24h (reduce to 35 mg IV q24h with moderate hepatic insufficiency) 70 mg $424.44; 50 mg $329.47 or $8485.26 for 21-day course	An echinocandin which inhibits synthesis of β-(1,3)-D-glucan. Fungicidal against candida (MIC <2 mcg per mL). Active against aspergillus (MIC 0.4–2.7 mcg per mL). Interestingly, in some preclinical studies very high drug concentrations found to be less effective *(AAC 48:3407, 2004),* but this has not been demonstrated clinically. Approved indications for caspo include: empirical rx for febrile, neutropenic pts; rx of candidemia, candida intra-abdominal abscesses, peritonitis, & pleural space infections; esophageal candidiasis; & invasive aspergillosis in pts refractory to or intolerant of other therapies. Serum levels on rx: dosages = peak 12, trough 1.3 (24 hrs) mcg per mL. **Toxicity:** remarkably non-toxic *(Mycosis 48:227, 2005; Neph Dial Transplant, July 5, 2005).* Only 2% of 263 pts in double-blind trial for drug-related adverse event *(Transpl Inf Dis 1:25, 2002).* 14% had ↑ transaminases (similar to triazoles). Most common adverse effect: pruritus at infusion site & headache, fever, chills, vomiting, & diarrhea associated with infusion. ↑ serum creatinine in 8% on caspo vs 21% short-course ampho B in 422 pts with candidemia *(Ln, Oct. 12, 2005, online).* Drug metabolized in liver & dosage ↓ to 35 mg in moderate to severe hepatic failure. Class C for pregnancy (embryotoxic in rats & rabbits). See Table 22, page 146 for drug-drug interactions, esp. cyclosporine (hepatic toxicity) & tacrolimus (drug level monitoring recommended). Reversible thrombocytopenia reported *(Pharmacother 24:1408, 2004).*
Micafungin (Mycamine) 50 mg per day for prophylaxis post-bone marrow stem cell transplant; $95 per day 150 mg IV per day for rx: $280.50 per day for esophageal candidiasis; 100 mg IV q24h for candidemia (50 mg vials): $5890.30 for 150 mg IV q24h for 21 days *(Med Lett 47:52, 2005)*	The 2nd echinocandin approved by the FDA (March 2005) for rx of esophageal candidiasis & for prophylaxis against candida infections in HSCT recipients. Active against most strains of candida sp. & aspergillus sp. including those resistant to fluconazole such as C. glabrata & C. krusei. No antagonism seen when combined with other antifungal drugs & occ. synergism with ampho B *(AAC 49:2994, 2004).* No dosage adjustment for severe renal failure or moderate hepatic impairment. Watch for drug-drug interactions with sirolimus or nifedipine. Micafungin is well tolerated & common adverse events include nausea 7.8%, vomiting 2.4%, & headache 2.4%. Transient ↑ LFTs, BUN, creatinine reported; rare cases of significant hepatitis & renal insufficiency *(package insert for micafungin)*
Anidulafungin 200 mg IV on day 1 followed by 100 mg per day IV *(FDA approval pending)*; for esophageal candidiasis 100 mg IV times 1, then 50 mg IV q24h (no cost data available)	An echinocandin with antifungal activity (cidal) against candida sp. & aspergillus sp. including ampho B- & triazole-resistant strains. Effective in clinical trials of esophageal candidiasis & in 1 trial was superior to fluconazole in rx of invasive candidiasis/candidemia in 245 pts (75.6% vs 60.2%) *(ICAAC 2005).* Like other echinocandins, remarkably non-toxic; most common side-effects: nausea, vomiting, ↓ Mg, ↓ K & headache in 11–13% of pts. No dose adjustments for renal or hepatic insufficiency *(see Table 22).*
Fluconazole (Diflucan) 100 mg tabs NB $9.80, G $1.73 150 mg tabs NB $16, G $7 200 mg tabs NB $16, G $1 400 mg IV NB $170, G $152 Oral suspension: 50 mg per 5 mL, $40/35 mL bottle—NB	IV=oral dose because of excellent bioavailability. **Pharmacology:** absorbed po, water solubility enables IV. Peak serum levels *(see Table 9, page 62).* T½ 30 hrs (range 20–50 hrs). 12% protein bound. **CSF levels 50–90% of serum in normals.** No effect on mammalian steroid metabolism. **Drug-drug interactions common, see Table 22.** Side-effects overall 16% [more common in HIV+ pts (21%)]. Nausea 3.7%, headache 1.9%, skin rash 1.8%, abdominal pain 1.7%, vomiting 1.7%, diarrhea 1.5%, ↑ SGOT 20%. Alopecia (scalp, pubic crest) in 12–20% pts on >400 mg po q24h after median of 3 months (reversible in approx. 6 mos.) *(AnIM 123:354, 1995).* Rare: severe hepatotoxicity *(CID 41:301, 2005),* exfoliative dermatitis. Anaphylaxis *(BMJ 302:1341, 1991).* Ref.: *NEJM 330:263, 1994*
Flucytosine (Ancobon) 500 mg cap $9	AEs: Overall 30%. GI 6% (diarrhea, anorexia, nausea, vomiting); hematologic 22% [leukopenia, thrombocytopenia, when serum level >100 mcg per mL (esp. in azotemic pts)]; hepatotoxicity (asymptomatic ↑ SGOT, reversible); skin rash 7%; aplastic anemia (rare–2 or 3 cases). False ↑ in serum creatinine on EKTACHEM analyzer. *(JAC 26:171, 2000)*
Griseofulvin (Fulvicin, Grifulvin, Grisactin) 500 mg G $3.45, susp 125 mg per mL: 120 mL $52	Photosensitivity, urticaria, GI upset, fatigue, leukopenia (rare). Interferes with warfarin drugs. Increases blood and urine porphyrins, should not be used in patients with porphyria. Minor disulfiram-like reactions. Exacerbation of systemic lupus erythematosus.
Imidazoles, topical For vaginal and/or skin use	Not recommended in 1st trimester of pregnancy. Local reactions: 0.5–1.5%: dyspareunia, mild vaginal or vulvar erythema, burning, pruritus, urticaria, rash. Rarely similar symptoms in sexual partner.

* From 2005 Drug Topics Red Book, Medical Economics Data and Hospital Formulary Pricing Guide. **Price is average wholesale price (AWP).** See page 2 for abbreviations. All dosage recommendations are for adults (unless otherwise indicated) and assume normal renal function.

TABLE 11B (3)

DRUG NAME, GENERIC (TRADE)/ USUAL DOSAGE/COST*	ADVERSE EFFECTS/COMMENTS
Itraconazole (Sporanox) 100 mg cap $10 _____ 10 mg per mL oral solution (fasting state) (150 mL: $141) (AAC 42:1862, 1998) _____ IV usual dose 200 mg bid times 4 doses followed by 200 mg q24h for a maximum of 14 days ($213/250 mg)	**Itraconazole tablet and solution forms are not interchangeable, solution preferred.** Many authorities recommend measuring drug serum concentration after 2 wks to ensure satisfactory absorption. To obtain the highest plasma concentration, the tablet is given with food and acidic drinks (e.g., cola) while the solution is taken in the fasted state; under these conditions, the peak conc. of the capsule is approx. 3 mcg per mL and of the solution 5.4 mcg per mL. Peak levels are reached faster (2.2 vs 5 hrs) with the solution. Protein-binding for both preparations is over 99%, which explains the virtual absence of penetration into the CSF (**do not use to treat meningitis**). Most common adverse effects are dose-related nausea 10%, diarrhea 8%, vomiting 6%, and abdominal discomfort 5.7%. Allergic rash 8.6%, ↑ bilirubin 6%, edema 3.5%, and hepatitis 2.7% reported. ↑ doses may produce hypokalemia 8% and ↑ blood pressure 3.2%. Delirium & peripheral neuropathy reported (Psychosomatics 44:260, 2003; Diabetes Care 28:225, 2005). **Reported to produce impairment in cardiac function** (see footnote 2 page 80). Severe liver failure requiring transplant in pts receiving pulse rx or chronic rx/onychomycosis: FDA reports 24 cases with 11 deaths out of 50 million people who received the drug prior to 2001 (Eur J Acad Derm & Venereol 19:205, 2005). Other concern, as with fluconazole and ketoconazole, is **drug-drug interactions; see Table 22.** Some interactions can be life-threatening. **Peak plasma concentrations after IV injection (200 mg) compared to oral capsule (200 mg): 2.8 mcg per mL (on day 7 of rx) vs 2 mcg per mL (on day 36 of rx).**
Ketoconazole (Nizoral) 200 mg tab $2.25	Gastric acid required for absorption—cimetidine, omeprazole, antacids block absorption. In achlorhydria, dissolve tablet in 4 mL 0.2N HCl, drink with a straw. Coca-Cola ↑ absorption by 65% (AAC 39:1671, 1995). CSF levels "none". **Drug-drug interactions important, see Table 22. Some interactions can be life-threatening. Dose-dependent nausea and vomiting.** At doses of ≥800 mg per day serum testosterone and plasma cortisol levels fall. With high doses, adrenal (Addisonian) crisis reported. Liver toxicity of hepatocellular type reported in about ↑:10,000 exposed pts—usually after several days to weeks of exposure.
Miconazole (Monistat IV) 200 mg—not available in U.S.	IV miconazole indicated in patient critically ill with Scedosporium (Pseudallescheria boydii) infection. Very toxic due to vehicle needed to get drug into solution.
Nystatin (Mycostatin) 30 gm cream NB $28, G $2.30 500,000 units oral tab $0.70	Topical: virtually no adverse effects. Less effective than imidazoles and triazoles. PO: large doses give occasional GI distress and diarrhea.
Posaconazole (FDA approval pending) 200 mg po q6h or 400 mg po bid with food. No cost data available. (See Drugs 65:1552, 2005)	An oral triazole with activity against a wide range of fungi refractory to other antifungal rx including: aspergillosis, zygomycosis, fusariosis, Scedosporium (Pseudallescheria), phaeohyphomycosis, histoplasmosis, refractory candidiasis, refractory cryptococcosis, & refractory chromoblastomycosis. Clinical response in 75% of 176 AIDS pts with azole-refractory oral/esophageal candidiasis. Posaconazole has similar toxicities as other triazoles: nausea 9%, vomiting 6%, abd. pain 5%, headache 5%, diarrhea, ↑ ALT, AST, & rash (3% each). In pts rx for >6 mos. serious side-effects reported in 12/112 pts included adrenal insufficiency, nephrotoxicity, & QTc interval prolongation. Significant drug-drug interactions, inhibits CYP3A4 (see Table 22).
Terbinafine (Lamisil) 250 mg tab $10.50	In pts receiving terbinafine for onychomycosis, rare cases (8) of idiosyncratic & symptomatic hepatic injury and more rarely liver failure leading to death or liver transplantation. The drug is **not recommended** for pts with **chronic or active liver disease;** hepatotoxicity may occur in pts with or without pre-existing disease. Pretreatment serum transaminases (ALT & AST) advised & alternate rx used for those with abnormal levels. Pts started on terbinafine should be warned about symptoms suggesting liver dysfunction (persistent nausea, anorexia, fatigue, vomiting, RUQ pain, jaundice, dark urine or pale stools). If symptoms develop, drug should be discontinued & liver function immediately evaluated. AEs: usually mild, transient and rarely caused discontinuation of rx with AE, terbinafine vs placebo: nausea/diarrhea 2.6–5.6 vs 2.9; rash 5.6 vs 2.2: taste abnormality 2.8 vs 0.7. Inhibits CYP2D6 enzymes (see Table 22). Major drug-drug interaction is 100% ↑ in rate of clearance by rifampin. An acute generalized exanthematous pustulosis has been reported in 13 cases (Brit J Derm 152:780, 2005) & 5 cases of subacute cutaneous lupus erythematosus (Acta Derm Venerol 84:472, 2004).
Voriconazole (Vfend) IV: **Loading dose 6 mg per kg q12h times 1 day, then 4 mg per kg q12h** IV for invasive aspergillus & serious mold infections; **3 mg per kg IV q12h** for serious candida infections. Oral: **≥40 kg body weight: 400 mg po q12h times 1 day, then** 200 mg po q12h **<40 kg body weight:** 200 mg po q12h times 1 day, then 100 mg po q12h **Take oral dose 1 hour before or 1 hour after eating.** Oral suspension (40 mg per mL) $36 49/200 mg dose. Oral suspension dosing: Same as for oral tabs. Reduce to ½ maintenance dose for moderate hepatic insufficiency	A triazole with activity against Aspergillus sp., **including Ampho resistant strains of A. terreus** (J Clin Micro 37:2343, 1999). Active vs Candida sp. (including krusei), Fusarium sp., & various molds. Steady state serum levels reach 2.5–4 mcg per mL. Toxicity similar to other azoles/triazoles including uncommon serious hepatic toxicity (hepatitis, cholestasis & fulminant hepatic failure. Liver function tests should be monitored during rx & drug dc'd if abnormalities develop. Rash reported in up to 20%, occ. photosensitivity & rare Stevens-Johnson, hallucinations [including musical hallucinations (Infection 32:293, 2004)] & anaphylactoid infusion reactions with fever and hypertension (Clin Exp Dermato 26:648, 2001). 1 case of QT prolongation with ventricular tachycardia in a 15 y/o pt with ALL reported (CID 39:884, 2004). Approx. 21% experience a transient visual disturbance following IV or po (↑ altered/enhanced visual perception/" blurred or colored visual change or photophobia) within 30–60 minutes. Visual changes resolve within 30–60 min. after administration & are attenuated with repeated doses (**do not drive at night for outpatient rx**). No persistence of effect reported. Cause unknown. In patients with ClCr <50 mL per min., the drug should be given orally, not IV, since the intravenous vehicle (SBECD-sulfobutylether-B cyclodextrin) may accumulate. Hallucinations, hypoglycemia, electrolyte disturbance & pneumonitis attributed to ↑ drug concentrations (CID 39:1241, 2004). Potential for drug-drug interactions high—see Table 22 (CID 36:630, 1087, 1122, 2003). **NOTE:** Not in urine in active form. **Cost:** 50 mg tab $9: 200 mg tab $35: 200 mg IV $109

* From 2005 Drug Topics Red Book, Medical Economics Data and Hospital Formulary Pricing Guide. **Price is average wholesale price (AWP).**
See page 2 for abbreviations. All dosage recommendations are for adults (unless otherwise indicated) and assume normal renal function

TABLE 12A: TREATMENT OF MYCOBACTERIAL INFECTIONS*

Tuberculin skin test (TST). Same as PPD [MMWR 52(RR-2):15, 2003]:
Criteria for positive TST after 5 tuberculin units (intermediate PPD) read at 48–72 hours:
≥5 mm induration: + HIV, immunosuppressed, ≥15 mg prednisone per day, healed TBc on chest x-ray, recent close contact
≥10 mm induration: foreign-born, countries with high prevalence; IVDUsers; low income; NH residents; chronic illness; silicosis
≥15 mm induration: otherwise healthy
Two-stage to detect sluggish positivity: If 1st PPD pos. but <10 mm, repeat intermediate PPD in 1 week. Response to 2nd PPD can also happen if pt received BCG in childhood.
BCG vaccine as child: if ≥10 mm induration, & from country with TBc, should be attributed to M. tuberculosis. In areas of low TB prevalence, TST reactions of ≤18 mm more likely from BCG than TB [CID 40:211, 2005]. Prior BCG may result in booster effect in 2-stage TST [AnIM 161:1760, 2001; Clin Micro Inf 10:980, 2005].
Routine anergy testing no longer recommended in HIV+ or HIV-negative patients [JAMA 283:2003, 2000].
Whole blood interferon-gamma release assay (QuantiFERON-TB [QFT]) approved by U.S. FDA as diagnostic test for TB [JAMA 286:1740, 2001; CID 34:1449 & 1457, 2002]. CDC recommends TST for TB suspects & pts at ↑ risk for progression to active TB & suggests either TST or QFT for individuals at ↑ risk for latent TB [MMWR 52(RR-2):15, 2003]. A more sensitive assay based on M. tbc-specific antigens (QuantiFERON-TB GOLD) and an enzyme-linked immunospot method (ELISpot) using antigens specific for MTB (do not cross-react with BCG) are under evaluation & look promising [Thorax 58:916, 2003; Ln 361:1168, 2003; AnIM 140:709, 2004; LnID 4:761, 2005; CID 40:246, 2005; JAMA 293:2756, 2005].

CAUSATIVE AGENT/DISEASE	MODIFYING CIRCUMSTANCES	SUGGESTED REGIMENS	
		INITIAL THERAPY	**CONTINUATION PHASE OF THERAPY**
I. Mycobacterium tuberculosis TST negative (household members & other close contacts of potentially infectious cases)	Neonate—Rx essential	INH (10 mg per kg per day for 3 months)	Repeat tuberculin skin test (TST) in 3 mos. If mother's smear negative & infant's TST negative & chest x-ray (CXR) normal, stop INH. In UK, BCG is then given [Ln 2:1479, 1990], unless mother HIV+. If infant's repeat TST positive &/or CXR abnormal (hilar adenopathy &/or infiltrate), INH + RIF (10–20 mg per kg per day) (or SM). Total rx 6 months. If mother is being rx, separation of infant from mother not indicated.
	Children <5 years of age—Rx indicated	As for neonate for 1st 3 months.	If repeat TST at 3 months is negative, stop. If repeat TST positive, continue INH for total of 9 months. If INH not given initially, repeat TST at 3 mos. If positive rx with INH x9 mos. (see Category II below).
	Older children & adults— Risk 2–4% 1st year	No rx	

CAUSATIVE AGENT/DISEASE	MODIFYING CIRCUMSTANCES			
II. Treatment of latent infection with M. tuberculosis (formerly known as "prophylaxis) [NEJM 347:1860, 2002; NEJM 350:2060, 2004; JAMA 293:2776, 2005]

A. INH indicated due to high-risk
Assumes INH susceptibility likely. INH 54–88% effective in preventing active TB for ≥20 years. | (1) + tuberculin reactor (risk of active disease 10% per yr, AIDS 170 times ↑, HIV+ 113 times ↑)*. Development of active TBc in HIV+ pts after INH usually due to reinfection, not INH failure [CID 34:386, 2002]. (2) Newly infected persons (TST conversion in past 2 yrs— risk 3.3% 1st yr) (3) Past tuberculosis, not rx with adequate chemotherapy (INH, RIF, or alternatives) (4) + tuberculin reactors with CXR consistent with non-progressive tuberculous disease (risk 0.5–5.0% per yr) (5) + tuberculin reactors with specific predisposing conditions: illicit injection drug use [MMWR 38:236, 1989], silicosis, diabetes mellitus, prolonged adrenocorticoid rx (≥15 mg prednisone per day), immunosuppressive rx, hematologic diseases (Hodgkin's, leukemia), endstage renal disease, clinical condition with substantial rapid weight loss or chronic under-nutrition, previous gastrectomy [ARRD 134:355, 1986]

* **NOTE: For HIV, see SANFORD GUIDE TO HIV/AIDS THERAPY and/or MMWR 48:RR-10, 1999** | | | |

CAUSATIVE AGENT/DISEASE	MODIFYING CIRCUMSTANCES	SUGGESTED REGIMENS		
		INITIAL THERAPY	**ALTERNATIVE**	
		INH (5 mg per kg per day, maximum 300 mg per day for adults; 10 mg per kg per day not to exceed 300 mg per day for children). May use twice-weekly INH with DOT [MMWR 52:735, 2003]

Optimal duration 9 mos. (includes children, HIV–, HIV+, old fibrotic lesions on chest x-ray). In some cases, 6 mos. may be given for cost-effectiveness [AJRCCM 161:S221, 2000]. Do not use 6 mo. regimen in HIV+ persons <18 yrs old, or those with fibrotic lesions on chest film [NEJM 345:189, 2001]. | If compliance problem: **INH** by DOT† 15 mg per kg 2 times per wk times 9 mos.

2-month **RIF + PZA** regimen effective in HIV– and HIV+ [AJRCCM 161:S221, 2000; JAMA 283:1445, 2000]. **However, there are recent descriptions of severe & fatal hepatitis in immunocompetent pts on RIF + PZA** [MMWR 50:289, 2001]. Therefore, this regimen is no longer recommended for LTBI [MMWR 52:735, 2003; CID 39:488, 2004]. The risk appears lower in HIV+ pts [CID 39:561, 2004].

RIF 600 mg per day po for 4 mos. (HIV– and HIV+). Meta-analysis suggests 3 months of INH + RIF may be equivalent to "standard" (6–12 mos.) INH therapy [CID 40:670, 2005]. | |

CAUSATIVE AGENT/DISEASE	MODIFYING CIRCUMSTANCES	SUGGESTED REGIMENS		
		INITIAL THERAPY	**ALTERNATIVE**	COMMENTS
B. TST positive (organisms likely to be INH-susceptible)	Age no longer considered modifying factor (see Comments)	**INH** (5 mg per kg per day, max. 300 mg per day for adults; 10 mg per kg per day not to exceed 300 mg per day for children) with 6 mos. rx not quite as effective as 12 mos. (65% vs 75% reduction in disease). 9 mos. is current recommendation. See IIA above for details and alternate rx.		Reanalysis of earlier studies favors **INH** prophylaxis (if INH related, hepatitis case fatality rate <1% and TB case fatality rate ≥6.7%, which appears to be the case) [AnIM 127:1051, 1997]. Recent data warrant INH prophylaxis has positive risk-benefit ratio in pts ≥35 if monitored for hepatotoxicity [AnIM 127:1014, 1999].
	Pregnancy—Any risk factors (II.A above)	Treat with **INH** as above. For women at risk for progression of latent to active disease, esp. those who are HIV+ and those who have been recently infected, rx should not be delayed even during the first trimester.		Overall risk of hepatotoxicity 0.1–0.15% [JAMA 281:1014, 1999]. Risk of INH hepatitis may be ↑ [Ln 346:199, 1995].

See page 2 for abbreviations, page 90 for footnotes   * Dosages are for adults (unless otherwise indicated) and assume normal renal/renal function   † **DOT** = directly observed therapy

II. Treatment of latent infection with M. tuberculosis ("prophylaxis")/TST positive (organisms likely to be INH-susceptible) (continued)

CAUSATIVE AGENT/DISEASE	MODIFYING CIRCUMSTANCES	SUGGESTED REGIMENS — INITIAL THERAPY	SUGGESTED REGIMENS — ALTERNATIVE	COMMENTS
C. TST positive & drug resistance likely (For data on worldwide prevalence of drug resistance, see NEJM 344:1294, 2001; JID 185:1197, 2002)	Pregnancy—No risk factors	No initial rx (see Comment)	Delay rx until after delivery (AJRCCM 149:1359, 1994)	
	INH-resistant (or adverse reaction to INH), RIF-sensitive organisms likely	RIF 600 mg per day po for 4 mos. (HIV+ or HIV–)		IDSA guideline lists rifabutin in 600 mg per day dose as another alternative; however, current recommended max. dose of rifabutin is 300 mg per day. Estimate RIF alone has protective effect of 56%; 26% of pts reported adverse effects (only 2/157 did not complete 6 mos. rx) (AJRCCM 155:1735, 1997).
	INH- and RIF-resistant organisms likely	Efficacy of all regimens unproven. (HIV+ or HIV–) [(PZA 25-30 mg per kg per day to max. of 2 gm per day) + ETB 15-25 mg per kg per day po] times 6-12 mos.	[(PZA 25-30 mg per kg per day to max. of 2 gm per day) + (levoflox 500 mg per day or oflox 400 mg per day po)], all po. times 6-12 mos.	PZA + oflox has been associated with asymptomatic hepatitis (CID 24:1264, 1997).

SUGGESTED REGIMENS FOR DOSAGE AND DIRECTLY OBSERVED THERAPY (DOT) REGIMENS

CAUSATIVE AGENT/DISEASE	MODIFYING CIRCUMSTANCES	INITIAL PHASE[8] — Regimen: in order of preference	INITIAL PHASE[8] — Drugs	INITIAL PHASE[8] — Interval/Doses[1] (min. duration)	CONTINUATION PHASE OF THERAPY[7] (in vitro susceptibility known) — Regimen	— Drugs	— Interval/Doses[1,2] (min. duration)	— Range of Total Doses (min. duration)
III. Mycobacterium tuberculosis **A. Pulmonary TB** [General reference on rx in adults & children: Ln 362: 887, 2003; MMWR 52(RR-11):1, 2003; CID 40(Suppl):S1, 2005]	Rate of INH resistance known to be <4% (drug-susceptible organisms) [Modified from MMWR 52 (RR-11):1, 2003]	1 (See Fig. 1, page 89)	INH RIF PZA ETB	7 days per wk times 56 doses (8 wk) or 5 days per wk times 40 doses (8 wk)[3]	1a	INH/RIF	7 days per wk times 126 doses (18 wk) or 5 days per wk times 90 doses (18 wk)[3]	182-130 (26 wk)
					1b	INH/RIF	2 times per wk times 36 doses (18 wk)	92-76 (26 wk)[4]
					1c[5]	INH/RFP	1 time per wk times 18 doses (18 wk)	74-58 (26 wk)
	Isolation essential! Pts with active TB should be isolated in single rooms, not cohorted. Older observations on infectivity of susceptible & resistant M. tbc before and after rx (ARRD 85:5111, 1962) may not be applicable to MDR M. tbc or to the HIV+ individual. Extended isolation may be appropriate.	2 (See Fig. 1, page 89)	INH RIF PZA ETB	7 days per wk times 14 doses (2 wk), then 2 times per wk times 12 doses (6 wk) or 5 days per wk times 10 doses (2 wk)[3] then 2 times per wk times 12 doses (6 wk)	2a	INH/RIF	2 times per wk times 36 doses (18 wk)	62-58 (26 wk)[4]
					2b[5]	INH/RFP	1 time per wk times 18 doses (18 wk)	44-40 (26 wk)
	See footnotes, page 90 USE DOT REGIMENS IF POSSIBLE (continued on next page)	3 (See Fig. 1, page 89)	INH RIF PZA ETB	3 times per wk times 24 doses (8 wk)	3a	INH/RIF	3 times per wk times 54 doses (18 wk)	78 (26 wk)
		4 (See Fig. 1, page 89)	INH RIF ETB	7 days per wk times 56 doses (8 wk) or 5 days per wk times 40 doses (8 wk)[3]	4a	INH/RIF[6]	7 days per wk times 217 doses (31 wk) or 5 days per wk times 155 doses (31 wk)[3]	273-195 (39 wk)
					4b	INH/RIF[6]	2 times per wk times 62 doses (31 wk)	118-102 (39 wk)

COMMENTS

† DOT = directly observed therapy

Regimen*	Dose in mg per kg (max. q24h dose)					
	INH	RIF	PZA	ETB	SM	RFB
q24h:						
Child	10-20 (300)	10-20 (600)	15-30 (2000)	15-25	20-40 (1000)	10-20 (300)
Adult	5 (300)	10 (600)	15-30 (2000)	15-25	15 (1000)	5 (300)
2 times per wk						
Child	20-40 (900)	10-20 (600)	50-70 (4000)	50	25-30 (1500)	10-20 (300)
Adult	15 (900)	10 (600)	50-70 (4000)	50	25-30 (1500)	5 (300)
3 times per wk						
Child	20-40 (900)	10-20 (600)	50-70 (3000)	25-30	25-30 (1500)	NA
Adult	15 (900)	10 (600)	50-70 (3000)	25-30	25-30 (1500)	NA

Second-line anti-TB agents can be dosed as follows to facilitate DOT: Cycloserine 500-750 mg po q24h (5 times per wk) Ethionamide 500-750 mg po q24h (5 times per wk) Kanamycin or capreomycin 15 mg per kg IM/IV q24h (3-5 times per wk) Ciprofloxacin 750 mg po q24h (5 times per wk) Ofloxacin 600-800 mg po q24h (5 times per wk) Levofloxacin 750 mg po q24h (5 times per wk) CID 21:1245, 1995

Risk factors for drug-resistant TB: Recent immigration from Latin America or Asia or living in area of ↑ resistance (≥4%) or previous rx without RIF; exposure to known MDR TB. Incidence of MDR TB in U.S. appears to have stabilized and may be slightly decreasing in early 1990s (JAMA 278:833, 1997). Incidence of primary drug resistance is particularly high (>25%) in parts of China, Thailand, Russia, Estonia & Latvia (NEJM 344:1294, 2001; NEJM 347:1850, 2002) (continued on next page)

* Dosages are for adults (unless otherwise indicated) and assume normal renal function

See page 2 for abbreviations, page 90 for footnotes

TABLE 12A (3)

CAUSATIVE AGENT/DISEASE	MODIFYING CIRCUM-STANCES	SUGGESTED REGIMEN[8]	DURATION OF TREATMENT (mo.)[8]	SPECIFIC COMMENTS[8]	COMMENTS
III. Mycobacterium tuberculosis A. Pulmonary TB (continued from previous page) REFERENCE: CID 22:683, 1996	INH (± SM) resistance	RIF, PZA, ETB (an FQ may strengthen the regimen for pts with extensive disease). Emergence of FQ resistance a concern (LnID 3:432, 2003)	6	(continued from previous page) In British Medical Research Council trials, 6-mo. regimens yielded ≥95% success rates despite resistance to INH if 4 drugs were used in the initial phase & RIF + SM was used throughout (ARRD 133: 423, 1986). Additional studies suggested that results were best if PZA was also used throughout the 6 mos (ARRD 136:1339, 1987). FQs were not employed in BMRC studies, but may strengthen the regimen for pts with more extensive disease. INH should be stopped in cases of INH resistance [see MMWR 52(RR-11):1, 2003 for additional discussion].	(continued from previous page) For MDR TB, consider rifabutin (~30% RIF-resistant strains are rifabutin-susceptible). Note that CIP not as effective as PZA + ETB in multidrug regimen for susceptible TB (CID 22:287, 1996). Moxifloxacin, gatifloxacin and levofloxacin have enhanced activity compared with CIP against M. tuberculosis (AAC 46: 1022, 2002; AAC 47:2442, 2003, AAC 47:3117, 2003; JAC 53:441, 2004; AAC 48:780, 2004). FQ resistance may be seen in pts previously treated with FQ (CID 37:1448, 2003). Linezolid has excellent in vitro activity, including MDR strains (AAC 47: 416, 2003). Mortality reviewed: Ln 349:71, 1997. Rapid (24-hr) diagnostic tests for M. tuberculosis: (1) the Amplified Mycobacterium tuberculosis Direct Test amplifies and detects M. tuberculosis ribosomal RNA; (2) the AMPLICOR Mycobacterium tuberculosis Test amplifies and detects M. tuberculosis DNA. Both tests have sensitivities & specificities >95% in sputum samples that are AFB-positive. In negative smears, specificity remains >95% but sensitivity is 40-77% (AJRCCM 155:1497, 1997). Note that MTB may grow out on standard blood agar plates in 1-2 wks (J Clin Micro 41: 1710,2003).
Multidrug-Resistant Tuberculosis (MDR TB): Defined as resistant to at least 2 drugs. Pt clusters with high mortality (AnIM 118:17, 1993; EJCMID 23: 174, 2004).	Resistance to INH & RIF (± SM)	FQ, PZA, ETB, IA, ± alternative agent[7]	18-24	In such cases, extended rx is needed to ↓ the risk of relapse. In cases with extensive disease, the use of an additional agent (alternative agents) may be prudent to ↓ the risk of failure & additional acquired drug resistance. Resectional surgery may be appropriate.	
	Resistance to INH, RIF (± SM), & PZA	FQ (ETB or PZA if active), IA, & 2 alternative agents[7]	24	Use the first-line agents to which there is susceptibility. Add 2 or more alternative agents in case of extensive disease. Surgery should be considered. Survival ↑ in pts receiving active FQ & surgical intervention (AJRCCM 169:1103, 2004).	
See footnotes, page 90 Reviews of therapy for MDR TB: JAC 54:593, 2004; Med Lett 2:83, 2004	Resistance to RIF	INH, ETB FQ supplemented with PZA for the first 2 mos. (an IA may be included for the first 2-3 mos in pts with extensive disease)	12-18	Q24h & 3 times per wk regimens of INH, PZA, & SM given for 9 mos. were effective in a BMRC trial (ARRD 115:727, 1977). However, extended use of an IA may not be feasible. It is not known if ETB would be as effective as SM in these regimens. An all-oral regimen times 12-18 mos. should be effective. But for more extensive disease &/or to shorten duration (e.g., to 12 mos.), an IA may be added in the initial 2 mos. of rx.	

SUGGESTED REGIMENS

CAUSATIVE AGENT/DISEASE; MODIFYING CIRCUMSTANCES	INITIAL THERAPY	CONTINUATION PHASE OF THERAPY (in vitro susceptibility known)	COMMENTS
B. Extrapulmonary TB	INH + RIF (or RFB) + PZA q24h times 2 months. Authors add pyridoxine 25-50 mg po q24h to regimens that include INH.	INH + RIF (or RFB)	6-month regimens probably effective. Most experience with 9-12 mo. regimens. Am Acad Ped (1994) recommends 6 mos. rx for isolated cervical adenitis, renal and 12 mos. for meningitis, miliary, bone/joint. DOT useful here as well as for pulmonary tuberculosis. IDSA recommends 6 mos. for lymph node, pleural, pericarditis, disseminated disease, genitourinary & peritoneal TBc; 6-9 mos. for bone & joint; 9-12 mos. for CNS (including meningeal) TBc. Corticosteroids "strongly recommended" only for pericarditis & meningeal TBc [MMWR 52(RR-11):1, 2003].
C. Tuberculous meningitis For critical appraisal of adjunctive steroids: CID 25:872, 1997	INH + RIF + PZA + ETB	May omit ETB when susceptibility to INH and RIF established. See Table 9, page 62, for CSF drug penetration.	3 drugs often recommended for initial rx; we prefer 4. May substitute ethionamide for ETB. Infection with MDR TB ↑ mortality & morbidity (CID 38:851, 2004; JID 192:79, 2005). Dexamethasone (for 1st month) has been shown to ↓ complications (Pediatrics 99:226, 1997) & ↑ survival in pts >14 yrs old (NEJM 351:1741, 2004). PCR of CSF markedly increases diagnostic sensitivity and provides rapid dx (Neurol 45:2228, 1995; ArNeurol 53:771, 1996) but considerable variability in sensitivity depending on method used (LnID 3:633, 2003).
D. Tuberculosis during pregnancy	INH + RIF + ETB for 9 months	Directly observed therapy (DOT). Check susceptibilities. (See section III.A, page 87 & 88 above)	PZA not recommended: teratogenic data inadequate. Because of potential ototoxicity to fetus throughout gestation (16%), SM should not be used unless other drugs contraindicated. Add pyridoxine 25 mg per kg per day for pregnant women on INH. Breast-feeding should not be discouraged in pts on first-line rx [MMWR 52(RR-11):1, 2003].
E. Treatment failure or relapse: Usually due to poor compliance or resistant organisms (AJM 102:164, 1997)		Pts whose sputum has not converted after 4-6 mos. = treatment failures. Failures may be due to non-compliance or resistant organisms. Check susceptibilities of original isolates and obtain susceptibility on current isolates. Non-compliance common, therefore institute DOT. If isolates show resistance, modify regimen to include at least 2 effective agents, preferably ones which pt has not received. Surgery may be necessary. In HIV+ patients, reinfection is a possible explanation for "failure".	

See page 2 for abbreviations, page 90 for footnotes. * Dosages are for adults...

89

FIGURE 1: TREATMENT ALGORITHM FOR TUBERCULOSIS [Modified from MMWR 52(RR-11):1, 2003]

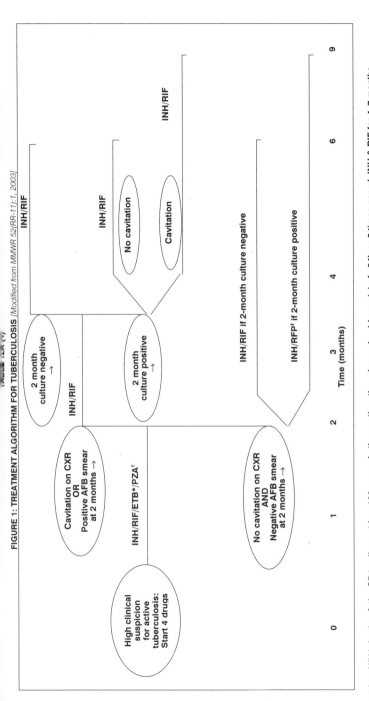

If the pt has HIV infection & the CD4 cell count is <100 per mcL, the continuation phase should consist of q24h or 3 times per wk INH & RIF for 4–7 months.
* ETB may be discontinued in <2 months if drug susceptibility testing indicate no drug resistance. † PZA may be discontinued after 2 months (56 doses). ‡ RFP should not be used in HIV patients with tuberculosis or in patients with extrapulmonary tuberculosis.

See page 2 for abbreviations

TABLE 12A (5)

CAUSATIVE AGENT/DISEASE	MODIFYING CIRCUMSTANCES	SUGGESTED REGIMENS PRIMARY/ALTERNATIVE	COMMENTS
III. Mycobacterium tuberculosis *(continued)*			
F. HIV infection or AIDS— pulmonary or extrapulmonary	INH + RIF (or RFB) q24h times 2 months.	**INH + RIF (or RFB) + PZA** q24h times 2 months. May treat up to 9 mos.) with delayed response.	1. Because of the possibility of developing resistance to RIF in pts with low CD4 cell counts who receive weekly or biweekly therapy during q24x or (or minimally 3 times weekly) doses of RFB for initiation & continuation phase of rx *(MMWR 51:214, 2002)*.
		(Authors add **pyridoxine** *25–50 mg po q24h to regimens that include INH.)*	2. Clinical and microbiologic response same as in HIV-negative patient although there is considerable variability in outcomes among currently available studies *(CID 32:623, 2001)*.
			3. Post-treatment suppression not necessary for drug-susceptible strains.
			4. Rate of INH resistance known to be <4% (for ↑ rates of resistance, see *Section III.A*).
			5. For more information, see *MMWR 47(RR-20):1, 1998; CID 28:139, 1999; MMWR 52(RR-11):1, 2003*
			6. May use partially intermittent therapy: 1 dose per day for 2 weeks followed by 2–3 doses per week for 24 weeks *[MMWR 47(RR-20), 1998]*.
Concomitant protease inhibitor (PI) therapy *(Modified from MMWR 49:185, 2000; AJRCCM 162:7, 2001)*	**Initial & cont. therapy:** INH 300 mg + RFB *(see below for dose)* + PZA 25 mg per kg + ETB 15 mg per kg q24h times 2 mos. : then INH + RFB times 4 mos. (up to 7 mos.)	**Alternative regimen:** INH + SM + PZA + ETB times 2 mos., then INH + SM + PZA 2–3 times per wk for 7 mos. May be prolonged up to 12 mos. in pts with delayed response.	**Comments:** Rifamycins induce cytochrome CYP450 enzymes (RIF > RFP > RFB) & reduce serum levels of concomitantly administered PIs. Conversely, PIs (ritonavir > amprenavir > indinavir = nelfinavir > saquinavir) inhibit CYP450 & cause ↑ serum levels of RIF, RFP & RFB. If dose of RFB is not reduced, toxicity ↑. RFB/PI combinations are therapeutically effective *(CID 30:779, 2000)*. RFB has no effect on nelfinavir levels at dose of 1250 mg bid *(Can JID 10:21B, 1999)*.
	PI Regimen	**RFB Dose**	**Although RFB is preferred, RIF can be used for rx of active TB in pts on regimens containing efavirenz or ritonavir. RIF should not be administered to pts on ritonavir + saquinavir because drug-induced hepatitis with marked transaminase elevations has been seen in healthy volunteers receiving this regimen (Roche; www.fda.gov).**
	Nelfinavir 1200 mg q12h or indinavir 1000 mg q8h or amprenavir 1200 mg q12h	150 mg q24h or 300 mg intermittently	
	Lopinavir/ritonavir—standard dose	150 mg 2 times per wk	

FOOTNOTES: ¹ When DOT is used, drugs may be given 5 days per wk & the necessary number of doses adjusted accordingly. Although if there are no studies that compare 5 with 7 q24h doses, extensive experience indicates this would be an effective practice. ² Patients with cavitation on initial chest x-ray & positive cultures at completion of 2 months of rx should receive a 7-month (31 wk; either 217 doses [q24h] or 62 doses [2 times per wk] continuation phase. ³ 5-day a wk administration is always given by DOT. ⁴ Not recommended for HIV-infected pts with CD4 cell counts <100 cells per mcL. ⁵ Options 1c & 2b should be used only in pts who have neg. sputum smears at the time of completion of 2 months of rx & who do not have cavitation on initial chest x-ray. For pts started on this regimen & found to have a pos. culture from the 2-month specimen, rx should be extended an extra 3 months. ⁶ Options 4a & 4b should be considered only when options 1–3 cannot be given. ⁷ Alternative agents = ethionamide, cycloserine, p-aminosalicylic acid, clarithromycin, AM-CL, linezolid. ⁸ Modified from *MMWR 52(RR-11):1, 2003. See also TB 11:329, 2002.*

CAUSATIVE AGENT/DISEASE	MODIFYING CIRCUMSTANCES	SUGGESTED REGIMENS PRIMARY/ALTERNATIVE	COMMENTS
IV. Other Mycobacterial Disease ("Atypical") *(See ATS Consensus, AJRCCM 152:51, 1997; IDC No. Amer, March 2002; CMR 15:716, 2002)*			
A. M. bovis		INH + RIF + ETB	The M. tuberculosis complex includes M. bovis. All isolates resistant to PZA. 9–12 months of rx used by some authorities. Isolation not required.
B. Bacillus Calmette-Guerin (BCG) (derived from M. bovis)	Only fever (>38.5°C) for 12–24 hrs. Systemic illness or sepsis	INH 300 mg q24h times 3 months (INH 300 mg) + (RIF 600 mg) + (ETB 1200 mg) po q24h times 6 mos.	Intravesical BCG effective in superficial bladder tumors and carcinoma in situ. Adverse effects: fever 2.9%, granulomatosis, pneumonitis, hepatitis 0.7%, sepsis 0.4% (*J Urol 147:596, 1992*). With sepsis, consider initial adjunctive prednisolone. Resistant to PZA. BCG may cause regional adenitis or pulmonary disease in HIV-infected children *(CID 37:1226, 2003)*.
C. M. avium-intracellulare complex (MAC, MAI, or Battey bacillus) ATS Consensus: *AJRCCM 156:51, 1997. Clin Chest Med 23:633, 2002*	**Immunocompetent patients** with chronic pulmonary, disseminated disease (subcutaneous, bone)	**Clarithro** 500 mg po bid (or **azithro** 600 mg po q24h) + **ETB** 25 mg per kg po times 2 mos., then 15 mg per kg po + **RIF** 600 mg po q24h (or **RFB** 300 mg po q24h). May also add **SM** or **AMK** 15 mg per kg 3 times per wk for 2–6 mos. for severe disease. May also add **CLO** 100–200 mg po q24h (until "tan"; then 50 mg po q24h or 100 mg po 3 times per week). Rx until culture neg. times 1 yr. Alternative: **Clarithro** 500 mg po bid + **ETB** 15–25 mg per kg q24h + **RFB** 300 mg po q24h for up to 24 mos. *(Curr Inf Dis Repts 2:193, 2000; CID 32:1547, 2001)*. Regimens dosing azithro 600 mg 3 times per week also effective *(CID 32:1547, 2001)*.	**"Classic" pulmonary MAC:** Men 50–75, smokers, COPD. May be associated with hot tub use *(Clin Chest Med 23:675, 2002)*. **"New" pulmonary MAC:** Women 30–70, scoliosis, mitral valve prolapse, (bronchiectasis), pectus excavatum ("Lady Windermere syndrome"). May also be associated with interferon gamma deficiency *(AJM 113:756, 2002)*. Susceptibility testing of MAC not recommended except clarithro testing of isolates from pts who have failed prior clarithro rx. 3 times per wk azithro (600 mg po), RFB (600 mg per kg po), & initial 2 times per wk SM may be effective in immunocompetent patients *(JID 178:121, 1998; CID 30:288, 2000)*. Late "relapses" (following completion of therapy) after treatment with clarithro or azithro in pts with nodular bronchiectasis usually represent reinfection, not failure of rx *(JID 186:266, 2002)*.

TABLE 12A (6)

CAUSATIVE AGENT/DISEASE; MODIFYING CIRCUMSTANCES	SUGGESTED REGIMENS		COMMENTS
	PRIMARY	**ALTERNATIVE**	
IV. Other Mycobacterial Disease ("Atypical") (continued)			
C. M. avium-intra-cellulare complex (continued)			
Immunocompromised pts: Primary prophylaxis—Pts CD4 count <50–100 per mm³. Discontinue when CD4 count >100 per mm³ in response to HAART (NEJM 342:1085, 2000; CID 34: 662, 2002) Guideline: AnIM 137:435, 2002	**Azithro** 1200 mg po weekly OR **RFB** 300 mg po q24h OR **Clarithro** 500 mg po bid	**RFB** 300 mg po q24h OR **Azithro** 1200 mg po weekly + **RIF** 300 mg po q24h	RFB reduces MAC infection rate by 55% (30% survival benefit); clarithro by 68% (no survival benefit); azithro by 68% (30% survival benefit). Azithro + RFB more effective than either alone but not as well tolerated (NEJM 335:392, 1996). **Many drug-drug interactions, see Table 22, pages 148, 150.** Drug-resistant MAI disease seen in 29–58% of pts in whom disease develops while taking clarithro prophylaxis & in 11% of those on azithro but has not been observed with RFB prophylaxis (J Inf 38:6, 1999). Clarithro resistance more likely in pts with extremely low CD4 counts at initiation (CID 27:807, 1998). Need to be sure no active M. tbc; RFB used for prophylaxis may promote selection of rifamycin-resistant M. tbc (NEJM 335:384 & 428, 1996).
Treatment Either presumptive dx or after positive culture of blood, bone marrow, or other usually sterile body fluids, e.g., liver	**(Clarithro** 500 mg po bid **or azithro** 600 mg po q24h) + **ETB** 15–25 mg per kg per day + **RFB** 300 mg po q24h *Higher doses of clari (1000 mg po bid) may be associated with ↑ mortality (CID 29:125, 1999)	**Clarithro or azithro** + **ETB** + **RFB** + one or more of: **CIP** 750 mg po bid or **Oflox** 400 mg po bid or **Amikacin** 7.5–15 mg per kg IV q24h In pts receiving protease inhibitors can use [**clarithro** 500 mg bid (or **azithro** 600 mg q24h) + **ETB** 15–25 mg per kg per day] if the pt has not had previous prophylaxis with a neomacrolide (Johns Hopkins AIDS Report 9:2, 1997)	Median time to neg. blood culture: clarithro + ETB + azithro + ETB >16 wks. At 16 wks, clearance of bacteremia seen in 37.5% of azithro- & 85.7% of clarithro-treated pts (CID 27:1278, 1998). More recent study suggests similar clearance rates for azithro (46%) vs clarithro (56%) at 24 wks when combined with ETB (CID 31:1245, 2000). Azithro 250 mg po q24h not effective, but azithro 600 mg po q24h as effective as 1200 mg q24h & yields fewer adverse effects (AAC 43: 2869, 1999). Addition of RFB to clarithro + ETB ↓ emergence of resistance to clari, ↓ relapse rate & improves survival (CID 37:1234, 2003). Data on clofazimine difficult to assess. Earlier study suggested adding CLO of no value (CID 25:621, 1997). More recent study suggests it may be as effective as RFB in 3 drug regimens containing clari & ETB (CID 29:125, 1999) although it may not be as effective as RFB in preventing clari resistance (CID 28:136, 1999). Thus, pending more data, we still do not recommend CLO for MAI in HIV+ pts. Drug toxicity: With clarithro, 23% pts had to stop drug 2° to dose-limiting adverse reaction (AnIM 121: 905, 1994). Combination of clarithro, ETB and RFB led to uveitis and pseudojaundice (NEJM 330:438, 1994); result is reduction in max. dose of RFB to 300 mg. Treatment failure rate is high. Reasons: drug toxicity, development of drug resistance, & inadequate serum levels of clarithro ↓ in pts also given RIF or RFB (JID 171:747, 1995). If pt not responding to initial regimen after 2–4 weeks, add one or more drugs. Several anecdotal reports of pts not responding to usual primary regimen who gained weight and became afebrile with dexamethasone 2–4 mg per day po (AAC 38:2275, 1994; CID 26:682, 1998).
Chronic post-treatment suppression—secondary prophylaxis	**Always necessary.** [Clarithro or azithro] + **ETB** (lower dose to 15 mg per day) (dosage above)	**Clarithro or azithro or RFB** (dosage above)	Recurrences almost universal without chronic suppression. However, in patients on HAART with robust CD4 cell response, it may be possible to discontinue chronic suppression (JID 178:1446, 1998; NEJM 340:1301, 1999).
D. Mycobacterium celatum	Treatment; optimal regimen not defined	May be susceptible to **clarithro, FQ** (Clin Micro Inf 3:582, 1997). Suggest rx "like MAI" but often resistant to RIF (J Inf 38:157, 1999). Most reported cases received 3 or 4 drugs, usually clarithro + ETB + CIP ± RFB (EID 9:399, 2003).	Isolated from pulmonary lesions and blood in AIDS patients (CID 24:144, 1997). Easily confused with M. xenopi (and MAC). Susceptibilities similar to MAC, but highly resistant to RIF (CID 24:140, 1997).
E. Mycobacterium chelonae ssp. abscessus Mycobacterium chelonae ssp. chelonae	Treatment; Surgical excision may facilitate clarithro rx in subcutaneous abscess and is important adjunct to rx (CID 24:1147, 1997)	**Clarithro** 500 mg po bid times 6 mos. (AnIM 119:482, 1993; CID 24:1147, 1997; E/CMID 19: 43, 2000). Azithro may also be effective. For serious disseminated infections add tobramycin + IMP for 1st 2–6 wks (Clin Micro Rev 15:716, 2002).	M. abscessus susceptible to AMK (70%), clarithro (95%), cefoxitin (70%), CLO, cefmetazole. Single isolates of M. abscessus often not associated with disease. Clarithro-resistant strains now described (J Clin Micro 39: 2745, 2001). M. chelonae susceptible to AMK (80%), clarithro, azithro, tobramycin (100%), IMP (60%), gatifloxacin (90%), moxifloxacin (AAC 46:3283, 2002). Resistant to cefoxitin, FQ (CID 24:1147, 1997; AJRCCM 156:S1, 1997).
F. Mycobacterium fortuitum	Treatment; optimal regimen not defined. Surgical excision of infected areas.	**AMK + cefoxitin + probenecid** 2–6 wks, then **TMP- SMX,** or **doxycycline** 2–6 mos. Usually responds to 6–12 mos. of oral rx with 2 drugs to which it is susceptible (AAC 46: 3283, 2002; Clin Micro Rev 15: 716, 2002). Nail salon-acquired infections respond to 4–6 mos. of minocycline or doxy or CIP (CID 38:38, 2004).	**Resistant to all standard anti-Tbc drugs.** Sensitive in vitro to doxycycline, minocycline, cefoxitin, IMP, AMK, TMP-SMX, CIP, oflox, azithro, clarithro, gatifloxacin (80%) (AAC 46: 3283, 2002), linezolid (Clin Micro Rev 15:716, 2002). May be resistant to azithromycin, rifabutin (JAC 39:567, 1997).

See page 2 for abbreviations.   * Dosages are for adults (unless otherwise indicated) and assume normal renal function   † **DOT** = directly observed therapy

92

TABLE 12A (7)

CAUSATIVE AGENT/DISEASE; MODIFYING CIRCUMSTANCES	SUGGESTED REGIMENS		COMMENTS
	PRIMARY	ALTERNATIVE	
IV. Other Mycobacterial Disease ("Atypical") (continued)			
G. Mycobacterium haemophilum	Regimen(s) not defined. In animal model, **clarithro + rifabutin** (AAC 39:2316, 1995). Combination of **CIP + RFB + clarithro** reported effective but clinical experience limited (Clin Micro Rev 9:435, 1996). Surgical debridement may be necessary (CID 26:505, 1998).		Clinical: Ulcerating skin lesions, synovitis, osteomyelitis. Lab: Requires supplemented media to isolate. Sensitive in vitro to: CIP, cycloserine, rifabutin. Over ½ resistant to: INH, RIF, ETB, PZA (AnIM 120:118, 1994).
H. Mycobacterium genavense	Regimens used include ≥2 drugs: **ETB, RIF, RFB, CLO, clarithro.** In animal model, **clarithro & RFB** (& to lesser extent amikacin & **ETB**) shown effective in reducing bacterial counts; CIP not effective (JAC 42:483, 1998).		Clinical: CD4 <50. Symptoms of fever, weight loss, diarrhea. Lab: Growth in BACTEC vials slow (mean 42 days). Subcultures grow only on Middlebrook 7H11 agar containing 2 mcg per ml mycobactin J—growth still insufficient for in vitro sensitivity testing (Ln 340:76, 1992; AnIM 117:586, 1992. Survival ↑ from 81 to 263 days in pts rx for at least 1 month with ≥2 drugs (AnIM 155:400, 1995).
I. Mycobacterium gordonae	Regimen(s) not defined, but consider **RIF + ETB + KM or CIP** (J Inf 38:157, 1999).		In vitro: sensitive to ETB, RIF, AMK, CIP, clarithro, linezolid (AAC 47:1736, 2003).. Resistant to INH (CID 14:1229, 1992). Surgical excision.
J. Mycobacterium kansasii	Q24h po: INH (300 mg) + **RIF** (600 mg) + **ETB** (25 mg per kg times 2 mos., then 15 mg per kg). Rx for 18 mos. with culture-neg. sputum times 12 mos. if HIV+ pt.) (See Comment)	If RIF-resistant, po q24h: [INH (900 mg) + **pyridoxine** (50 mg) + **ETB** (25 mg per kg)] + **sulfamethoxazole** (1.0 gm tid). Rx until pt culture-neg. times 12–15 mos. (See Comment) **Clari + ETB + RIF** also effective in small study (CID 37:1178, 2003).	**All isolates are resistant to PZA.** Rifapentine, azithro, ETB effective alone or in combination in athymic mice (JAC 42:417, 2001). Highly susceptible to linezolid in vitro (AAC 47:1736, 2003). RIF, substitute either clarithro (500 mg bid) or RFB (150 mg per day) for RIF (AJRCCM 156:S1, 1997). Because of variable susceptibility to INH, some substitute clarithro 500–750 mg q24h for INH. Resistance to clarithro reported (DMID 31:369, 1998), but most strains susceptible to clarithro as well as moxifloxacin (JAC 55:950, 2005) & levofloxacin (AAC 48:4562, 2004). Prognosis related to level of immunosuppression (CID 37:584, 2003).
K. Mycobacterium marinum	(**Clarithro** 500 mg bid) or (**minocycline** 100–200 mg q24h) or (**doxycycline** 100–200 mg q24h), or (**TMP-SMX** 160/800 mg po bid), or (**RIF + ETB**) for 3 mos. (AJRCCM 156:S1, 1997). Surgical excision.		Resistant to INH & PZA (AJRCCM 156:S1, 1997). Also susceptible in vitro to linezolid (AAC 47: 1736, 2003). CIP, gatifloxacin, moxifloxacin also show moderate in vitro activity (AAC 46:1114, 2002).
L. Mycobacterium scrofulaceum	Surgical excision. Chemotherapy seldom indicated. Although regimens not defined, **clarithro** + **CLO** with or without **ETB**, **INH**, **RIF**, **strep** + **cycloserine** have also been used.		In vitro resistant to INH, RIF, ETB, PZA, AMK, CIP (CID 20: 549, 1995). Susceptible to clarithro, strep, erythromycin.
M. Mycobacterium simiae	Regimen(s) not defined. Start 4 drugs as for disseminated MAI.		Most isolates resistant to all 1st-line anti-tbc drugs. Isolates often not clinically significant (CID 26: 625, 1998).
N. Mycobacterium ulcerans (Buruli ulcer)	[**RIF + AMK** (7.5 mg per kg IM bid)] or [**ETB + TMP-SMX** (160/800 mg po tid)] for 4–6 weeks. Surgical excision.		Susceptible in vitro to RIF, strep, CLO, clarithro, CIP, oflox, amikacin (AAC 42:2070, 1998; JAC 45: 231, 2000; AAC 46:3193, 2002). Monotherapy with RIF selects resistant mutants in mice (AAC 47:1228, 2003). RIF + strep effective in small study (AAC 49:3182, 2005). Treatment generally disappointing—see review, Ln 354:1013, 1999. RIF + dapsone only slightly better (82% improved) than placebo (75% in small study (Intl J Inf Dis 6:60, 2002).
O. Mycobacterium xenopi	Regimen(s) not defined (CID 24:226 & 233, 1997). Some recommend a **macrolide + (RIF or rifabutin) + ETB ± SM** (AJRCCM 156:S1, 1997) or **RIF + INH ± ETB** (Resp Med 97:439, 2003) but recent study suggests no need to treat in most pts with HIV (CID 37:1250, 2003).		In vitro: sensitive to clarithro (AAC 36:2841, 1992) and rifabutin (JAC 39:567, 1997) and many standard antimycobacterial drugs. Clarithro-containing regimens more effective than RIF/INH/ETB regimens in mice (AAC 45:3229, 2001). FQs, linezolid also active in vitro.
Mycobacterium leprae (leprosy) - Paucibacillary (tuberculoid or indeterminate) - Multibacillary (lepromatous or borderline) **See Comment for erythema nodosum leprosum** Rev. Lancet 363:1209, 2004	**Dapsone** 100 mg q24h unsupervised + **RIF** 600 mg po once per month supervised for 6 months [**Dapsone** 100 mg q24h + **CLO** 50 mg q24h unsupervised] + [**RIF** 600 mg + **CLO** 300 mg q24h 1 time per month supervised] for 24 months (WHO Tech Rpt 874:1, 1998). Recent data suggest 12 mos. rx effective (Ln 353:655, 1999)	[**mg** + oflox 400 mg + minocycline 100 mg] (Ln 353:655, 1999). For erythema nodosum leprosum: prednisone 60–80 mg per day q24h) or **prothionamide** (375 mg q24h) may be substituted for CLO	Side-effects overall 0.4%. Single lesion paucibacillary disease may be treated with single-dose rx (RIF 600 mg + oflox 400 mg + minocycline 100 mg) (Ln 353:655, 1999). Side-effects overall 5.1%. CLO available from Ciba-Geigy ((908) 277-3572]. Oflox 400 mg po q24h, bactericidal and effective clinically with 4 log ↓ in organisms in small trials (AAC 38:662, 1994; AAC 38:61, 1994). Clarithro also rapidly bactericidal (AAC 38:515, 1994). (Good reference: Ln 345:4, 1995.) 1 recent study suggests dapsone monotherapy as effective as combination rx for multibacillary leprosy (AAC 38:2249, 1994). Regimens incorporating clarithro, minocycline, RIF, moxifloxacin, and/or oflox also show promise (AAC 44:2919, 2000). High relapse rate in pts treated with q24h RIF + oflox for 4 wks (AAC 41:1953, 1997). Resistance to dapsone, RIF & oflox reported (Ln 349:103, 1997). Dapsone (or acedapsone^NUS) effective for prophylaxis (J Inf 41:137, 2000).

See page 2 for abbreviations.   * Dosages are for adults (unless otherwise indicated) and assume normal renal function   † **DOT** = directly observed therapy

TABLE 12B: DOSAGE, PRICE AND SELECTED ADVERSE EFFECTS OF ANTIMYCOBACTERIAL DRUGS[1]

AGENT (TRADE NAME)	USUAL DOSAGE*	ROUTE/1° DRUG RESISTANCE (RES) US[2]/COST**	SIDE-EFFECTS, TOXICITY AND PRECAUTIONS	SURVEILLANCE
FIRST LINE DRUGS				
Ethambutol (Myambutol)	25 mg per kg per day for 2 months & then 15 mg per kg per day q24h as 1 dose [Bacteriostatic to both extracellular & intracellular organisms]	po RES: 0.3% (0–0.7%) 400 mg tab $1.80	**Optic neuritis** with decreased visual acuity, central scotomata, and loss of green and red perception; peripheral neuropathy and headache (~1%), rashes (rare), arthralgia (rare), hyperuricemia (rare). Anaphylactoid reaction (rare). *Comment:* Primarily used to inhibit resistance. Disrupts outer cell membrane in M. avium with ↑ activity to other drugs.	Monthly visual acuity & red/green with dose >15 mg per kg per day; ≥10% loss considered significant. Usually reversible if drug discontinued
Isoniazid (INH) (Nydrazid, Laniazid, †Teebaconin)	Q24h dose: 5–10 mg per kg per day up to 300 mg per day as 1 dose. Twice weekly dose: 15 mg per kg (900 mg maximum dose) (< 10% protein binding) [Bactericidal to both extracellular and intracellular organisms] Add pyridoxine in alcoholic, pregnant, or malnourished pts.	po RES: 4.1% (2.6–8.5%) 300 mg tab $0.02 IM (IV route not FDA-approved but has been used, esp. in AIDS) 100 mg per ml in 10 ml vials (IM) $16.64	Overall ~1%. Liver: **Hepatitis** (children 10% mild ↑ SGOT, normalizes with continued rx, age <20 yrs rare, 20–34 yrs 1.2%; ≥50 yrs 2.3%) [also ↑ with q24h alcohol & previous exposure to Hepatitis C (usually asymptomatic—*CID 36:293, 2003*). May be fatal. With prodromal sx, dark urine do LFTs; discontinue if SGOT >3–5 times normal. **Peripheral neuropathy** (17% on 6 mg kg per day, less on 300 mg, incidence ↑ in slow acetylators); **pyridoxine 10 mg q24h will ↓ incidence.** other neurologic sequelae, convulsions; optic neuritis, toxic encephalopathy, psychosis, muscle twitching, dizziness, coma (all rare); allergic skin rashes, fever, minor disulfiram-like reaction, flushing after Swiss cheese; blood dyscrasias (rare); + antinuclear (20%). **Drug-drug interactions** common, see *Table 22.*	Pre-rx liver functions. Repeat if symptoms (fatigue, weakness, malaise, anorexia, nausea or vomiting) >3 days *(AJRCCM 152: 1705, 1995)*. Some recommend SGOT at 2, 4, 6 months esp. if age >50 years. Clinical evaluation every month.
Pyrazinamide	25 mg per kg per day (maximum 2.5 gm per day) q24h as 1 dose [Bactericidal for intracellular organisms]	po 500 mg tab $1.09	**Arthralgia; hyperuricemia** (with or without symptoms); hepatitis (not over 2% if recommended dose not exceeded); gastric irritation; photosensitivity (rare).	Pre-rx liver functions. Monthly SGOT, uric acid. Measure serum uric acid if symptomatic gouty attack occurs.
Rifamate®—combination tablet	2 tablets single dose q24h	po (1 hr before meal) 1 tab $2.65	1 tablet contains 150 mg INH, 300 mg RIF	As with individual drugs
Rifampin (Rifadin, Rimactane, †Rifocin)	10.0 mg per kg per day up to 600 mg per day q24h as 1 dose (60–90% protein binding) [Bactericidal to all populations of organisms]	po RES: 0.2% (0–0.3%) 300 mg cap $1.90 (IV available, Merrell-Dow. Cost 600 mg $90.28)	INH/RIF dc'd in ~3% for toxicity; gastrointestinal irritation, antibiotic-associated colitis, drug fever (1%), pruritus with or without skin rash (1%), anaphylactoid reactions in HIV+ pts, mental confusion, thrombocytopenia (1%), leukopenia (1%), hemolytic anemia, transient **abnormalities in liver function. "Flu syndrome"** (fever, chills, headache, bone pain, shortness of breath) seen if RIF taken irregularly or if q24h dose restarted after an interval of no rx. **Discolors urine, tears, sweat, contact lens an orange-brownish color.** May cause drug-induced lupus erythematosus *(Ln 349:1521, 1977)*.	Pre-rx liver function. Repeat if symptoms. **Multiple significant drug-drug interactions, see Table 22.**
Rifater®—combination tablet (See Side-Effects)	Wt ≥55 kg. 6 tablets single dose q24h	po (1 hr before meal) 1 tab $1.96	1 tablet contains 50 mg INH, 120 mg RIF, 300 mg PZA. Used in 1st 2 months of rx. (PZA 25 mg per kg). Purpose is convenience in dosing, ↑compliance *(AnIM 122: 951, 1995)* but cost 1.58 more. Side-effects = individual drugs.	As with individual drugs. PZA 25 mg per kg
Streptomycin	15 mg per kg IM q24h, 0.75–1.0 gm per day initially for 60–90 days, then ↑ 1.0 gm 2–3 times per week (15 mg per kg per day) q24h as 1 dose	IM (or IV) RES: 3.9% (2.7–7.6%) 1.0 gm $9.10	Overall 8%. **Ototoxicity**, vestibular dysfunction (vertigo); paresthesias; dizziness & nausea (all less in pts receiving 2–3 doses per week); tinnitus and high frequency loss (1%); nephrotoxicity (rare); peripheral neuropathy (rare); allergic skin rashes (4–5%); drug fever. Available from X-Gen Pharmaceuticals, 607-732-4411. Ref. re: IV—*CID 19:1150, 1994.* Toxicity similar with qd vs tid dosing *(CID 38:1538, 2004).*	Monthly audiogram. In older pts, serum creatinine or BUN at start of rx and weekly if pt stable

* Adult dosage only; §Mean (range) (higher in Hispanics, Asians, and patients <10 years old).

---

[1] Note: Malabsorption of antimycobacterial drugs may occur in patients with AIDS enteropathy. For review of adverse effects, see *AJRCCM 167:1472, 2003.*
[2] **RES** = % resistance of M. tuberculosis

* Average wholesale price according to 2005 Drug Topics RED Book, Medical Economics

* Adult dosage only; §Mean (range) (higher in Hispanics, Asians, and patients <10 years old)

Dosages are for adults (unless otherwise indicated) and assume normal renal function † **DOT** = directly observed therapy

See page 2 for abbreviations

TABLE 12B (2)

AGENT (TRADE NAME)	USUAL DOSAGE*	ROUTE/¹° DRUG RESISTANCE (RES) US¹⁹/COST**	SIDE-EFFECTS, TOXICITY AND PRECAUTIONS	SURVEILLANCE
SECOND LINE DRUGS (more difficult to use and/or less effective than first line drugs)				
Amikacin (Amikin)	7.5–10.0 mg per kg q24h [Bactericidal for extracellular organisms]	IV or IM RES: (est. 0.1%) 500 mg $7.80	See Table 10, pages 64 & 74. Toxicity similar with qd vs tid dosing (CID 38:1538, 2004).	Monthly audiogram. Serum creatinine or BUN weekly if pt stable
Capreomycin sulfate (Capastat sulfate)	1 gm per day (15 mg per kg per day) q24h as 1 dose	IM or IV RES: 0.1% (0–0.9%) 1 gm $25.54	Nephrotoxicity (36%), ototoxicity (auditory 11%), eosinophilia, leukopenia, skin rash, fever, hypokalemia, neuromuscular blockade.	Monthly audiogram, biweekly serum creatinine or BUN
Ciprofloxacin (Cipro)	750 mg bid	po, IV 750 mg (po) $5.33	TB not an FDA-approved indication for CIP. Desired CIP serum levels 4–6 mcg per mL, requires median dose 800 mg (AJRCCM 151:2006, 1995). Discontinuation rates 6–7%. CIP well tolerated (AJRCCM 151:2006, 1995). FQ-resistant M. Tb identified in New York (Ln 345:1148, 1995). See Table 10, pages 66 & 71 for adverse effects.	None
Clofazimine (Lamprene)	50 mg per day (unsupervised) + 300 mg 1 time per month supervised or 100 mg per day	po (with meals) 50 mg $0.20	Skin: **pigmentation (pink-brownish black)** 75–100% dryness 20%, pruritus 5%. GI: abdominal pain 50% (rarely severe leading to exploratory laparoscopy), splenic infarction (VR), bowel obstruction (VR), GI bleeding (VR). Eye: conjunctival irritation, retinal crystal deposits.	None
Cycloserine (Seromycin)	750–1000 mg per day (15 mg per kg per day) 2–4 doses per day [Bacteriostatic for both extracellular & intracellular organisms]	po RES: 0.1% (0–0.3%) 250 mg cap $3.50	Convulsions, **psychoses** (5–10% of those receiving 1.0 gm per day); headache; somnolence; hyperreflexia; increased CSF protein and pressure, **peripheral neuropathy**. 100 mg pyridoxine (or more) q24h should be given concomitantly. Contraindicated in epileptics.	None
Dapsone	100 mg per day	po 100 mg $0.20	Blood: ↓ hemoglobin (1–2 gm) & ↑ retics (2–12%), in most pts. Hemolysis in G6PD deficiency. **Methemoglobinemia.** CNS: peripheral neuropathy (rare). GI: nausea, vomiting. Renal: albuminuria, nephrotic syndrome. Erythema nodosum leprosum in pts rx for leprosy (2 pts 1st year).	None
Ethionamide (Trecator-SC)	500–1000 mg per day (15–20 mg per kg per day) 1–3 doses per day [Bacteriostatic for extracellular organisms only]	po RES: 0.8% (0–1.5%) 250 mg tab $3.09	**Gastrointestinal irritation** (up to 50% on large dose); goiter; peripheral neuropathy (rare); convulsions (rare); changes in affect (rare); difficulty in diabetes control; rashes; hepatitis; purpura, stomatitis, gynecomastia, menstrual irregularity. Give drug with meals or antacids; 50–100 mg pyridoxine per day concomitantly; SGOT monthly. Possibly teratogenic.	
Ofloxacin (Floxin)	400 mg bid	po, IV 400 mg (po) $4.2	Not FDA-approved indication. Overall adverse effects 11%, 4% discontinued due to side-effects. GI: nausea 3%, diarrhea 1%. **CNS:** insomnia 3%, headache 1%, dizziness 1%.	None
Para-aminosalicylic acid (PAS, Paser) (Na⁺ or K⁺ salt)	4–6 gm bid (200 mg per kg per day) [Bacteriostatic for extracellular organisms only]	po RES: 0.8% (0–1.5%) 450 mg tab $0.08 (see Comment)	**Gastrointestinal irritation** (10–15%); goitrogenic action (rare); depressed prothrombin activity (rare); G6PD-mediated hemolytic anemia (rare), drug fever, rashes, hepatitis, myalgia, arthralgia. Retards hepatic enzyme induction, may ↓ INH hepatotoxicity. Available from CDC, (404) 639-3670, Jacobus Pharm. Co. (609) 921-7447.	None
Rifabutin (Mycobutin)	300 mg per day (prophylaxis or treatment)	po 150 mg $7.19	Polymyalgia, polyarthralgia, leukopenia, granulocytopenia. Anterior uveitis when given with concomitant clarithromycin; avoid 600 mg dose (NEJM 330:438, 1994). Uveitis reported with 300 mg per day (AnIM 12:510, 1994). Reddish urine, orange skin (pseudojaundice).	None
Rifapentine (Priftin)	600 mg twice weekly for 1st 2 mos., then 600 mg q week	po 150 mg $3.00	Similar to other rifabutins. (See RIF, RFB). Hyperuricemia seen in 21%. Causes red-orange discoloration of body fluids. Note ↑ prevalence of RIF resistance in pts on weekly rx (Ln 353:1843, 1999).	None
Thalidomide (Thalomid)	100–300 mg po q24h (may use up to 400 mg po q24h for severe erythema nodosum leprosum)	po 50 mg $42.36	**Contraindicated in pregnancy. Causes severe life-threatening birth defects. Both male and female patients must use barrier contraceptive methods (Pregnancy Category X). Frequently causes drowsiness or somnolence. May cause peripheral neuropathy.** (AJM 108:487, 2000) For review, see Ln 363:1803, 2004	Available only through pharmacists participating in System for Thalidomide Education and Prescribing Safety (S.T.E.P.S.)

* Adult dosage only; ⁵Mean (range) (higher in Hispanics, Asians, and patients <10 years old); ** Average wholesale price according to 2005 Drug Topics Red Book, Medical Economics

† **RES** = % resistance of M. tuberculosis

See page 2 for abbreviations * Dosages are for adults (unless otherwise indicated) and assume normal renal function   † **DOT** = directly observed therapy

TABLE 13A: TREATMENT OF PARASITIC INFECTIONS

Many of the drugs suggested are not licensed in the United States. The following are helpful resources available through the Center for Disease Control and Prevention (CDC) in Atlanta. Website is www.cdc.gov. General advice for parasitic diseases other than malaria: (770) 488-7760 or (770) 488-7775.

For CDC Drug Service[1] 8:00 a.m.–4:30 p.m. EST: (404) 639-3670 (or -2888); emergency after hours: (404) 639-2888; fax: (404) 639-3717.
For malaria: Prophylaxis advice (770) 488-3228 or (877) 394-8747; treatment (770) 488-7788; website: www.cdc.gov/travel; fax (888) 232-3299

NOTE: All dosage regimens are for adults with normal renal function unless otherwise stated.
For licensed drugs, suggest checking package inserts to verify dosage and side-effects. Occasionally, post-licensure data may alter dosage as compared to package inserts.
For abbreviations of journal titles, *see page 3*. **Reference with pediatric dosages:** *Medical Letter on-line version:* **www.medletter.com** *(August 2004)*

INFECTING ORGANISM	SUGGESTED REGIMENS		COMMENTS
	PRIMARY	ALTERNATIVE	
PROTOZOA—INTESTINAL (non-pathogenic: E. hartmanni, E. dispar, E. coli, Iodamoeba butschlii, Endolimax nana, Chilomastix mesnili)			
Balantidium coli	**Tetracycline** 500 mg po qid times 10 days	**Metronidazole** 750 mg po tid times 5 days	*See Table 10C for side-effects.*
Blastocystis hominis: Role as pathogen controversial	**Nitazoxanide:** Adults 500 mg tabs (children 200 mg oral suspension)—both po q12h times 3 days (*TRSM 91:701, 1997*).	**Metronidazole** 500 mg po tid times 5 days. Based on 1 placebo-controlled trial (*J Travel Med 10:128, 2003*). **Alternatives: iodoquinol** 650 mg po tid times 20 days or **TMP-SMX-DS**, one bid times 7 days	**Nitazoxanide:** Approved in liquid formulation for rx of children & 500 mg tabs for adults. Ref.: *CID 40:1173, 2005.*
Cryptosporidium parvum and hominis Treatment is unsatisfactory Ref.: *CID 39:504, 2004*	**Immunocompetent—No HIV: Nitazoxanide** 500 mg po bid times 3 days	**HIV with immunodeficiency:** (1) Effective anti-retroviral therapy best therapy. (2) **Nitazoxanide** 500 mg po bid times 14 days in adults (60% response). No response in HIV+ children.	**C. hominis** assoc. with ↑ in post-infection eye & joint pain, recurrent headache, & dizzy spells (*CID 39:504, 2004*).
Cyclospora cayetanensis	Immunocompetent pts: **TMP-SMX-DS** tab 1 po bid times 7–10 days	AIDS pts: **TMP-SMX-DS** tab 1 po qid times 10 days; then tab 1 po 3 times per week	If sulfa-allergic: **CIP** 500 mg po bid times 7 days & then 1 tab po 3 times per wk times 2 wks.
Dientamoeba fragilis	**iodoquinol** 650 mg po tid times 20 days	**Tetracycline** 500 mg po qid times 10 days OR **Metronidazole** 500–750 mg po tid times 7 days	Other alternatives: doxy 100 mg po bid times 10 days; paromomycin 500 mg po tid times 7 days
Entamoeba histolytica; amebiasis Reviews: *Ln 361:1025, 2003; NEJM 348:1563, 2003.*			
Asymptomatic cyst passer	**Paromomycin** (aminosidine in U.K.) 500 mg po tid times 7 days OR **iodoquinol** 650 mg po tid times 20 days	**Diloxanide furoate**[NUS] (Furamide) 500 mg po tid times 10 days (Source: Panorama Compound. Pharm., 800-247-9767)	Metronidazole not effective vs cysts.
Patient with diarrhea/dysentery; mild/moderate disease. Oral rx possible	**Metronidazole** 500–750 mg po tid times 10 days or **tinidazole** 2 gm once daily times 3 days, followed by: Either [**paromomycin** 500 mg po tid times 7 days] or [**iodoquinol** 650 mg po tid times 20 days]	(**Tinidazole** 1 gm po q12h times 3 days) or **ornidazole**[NUS] 500 mg po q12h times 5 days) followed by: Either [**paromomycin** 500 mg po tid times 7 days] or [**iodoquinol** (was diiodohydroxyquin) 650 mg po tid times 20 days]	Drug side-effects in Table 10C. Colitis can mimic ulcerative colitis; ameboma can mimic adenocarcinoma of colon. **Dx:** antigen detection & PCR better than O&P (*Clin Micro Rev 16:713, 2003*). Watch out for non-pathogenic E. dispar (*Ln 351:1672, 1998*).
Severe or extraintestinal infection, e.g., hepatic abscess	[**Metronidazole** 750 mg **IV to PO** tid times 10 days or **tinidazole** 2 gm once daily times 5 days] followed by **paromomycin** 500 mg po times 7 days		**Serology positive (antibody present) with extraintestinal disease.**
Giardia lamblia; giardiasis	(**Tinidazole** 2 gm po times 1) OR (**nitazoxanide** 500 mg po bid times 3 days)	**Metronidazole** 500–750 mg po tid times 5 days (high frequency of GI side-effects). *See Comment.* Rx if pregnant: **Paromomycin** 500 mg po 4 times per day times 7 days	**Refractory pts: (metro 750 mg po + quinacrine**[2] **100 mg po)** —both 3 times per day times 3 wks. Ref: *CID 33:22, 2001.* **Nitazoxanide** ref.: *CID 40:1173, 2005.*
Isospora belli	**TMP-SMX-DS** tab 1 po bid times 10 days; if AIDS pt.: TMP-SMX-DS qid times 10 days & then bid times 3 wks.	(**Pyrimethamine** 75 mg per day po + **folinic acid** 10 mg per day po) times 14 days **CIP** 500 mg po bid times 7 days— 87% response (*AnIM 132:885, 2000*).	Chronic suppression in AIDS pts; either 1 TMP-SMX-DS tab 3 times per wk OR (pyrimethamine 25 mg per day po + folinic acid 5 mg per day po)

[1] **Drugs available from CDC Drug Service: 404-639-2888 or -3670 or www.cdc.gov/ncidod/srp/drugs/formulary.html:** Bithionol, dehydroemetine, diethylcarbamazine (DEC), melarsoprol, nifurtimox, stibogluconate (Pentostam), suramin.
[2] Quinacrine available from Panorama Compounding Pharmacy, (800) 247-9767; (818) 988-7979.
* *See page 2 for abbreviations. All doses are for adults(unless otherwise indicated) and assume normal renal function.*

TABLE 13A (2)

INFECTING ORGANISM	SUGGESTED REGIMENS		COMMENTS
	PRIMARY	**ALTERNATIVE**	
PROTOZOA—INTESTINAL (continued)			
Microsporidiosis			
Ocular: Encephalitozoon hellum or cuniculi, Vittaforma (Nosema) corneae, Nosema ocularum	For HIV pts: antiretroviral therapy key. **Albendazole** 400 mg po bid times 3 weeks	In HIV+ pts, reports of response of E. hellum to **fumagillin** eyedrops (see Comment). For V. corneae, may need keratoplasty.	To obtain fumagillin: 800-292-6773 or www.leiterx.com. Neutropenia & thrombocytopenia serious adverse events. Dx: Most labs use modified trichrome stain. Need electron micrographs for species identification. FA and PCR methods in development. Peds dose ref.: PIDJ 23:915, 2004
Intestinal (diarrhea): Enterocytozoon bieneusi, Encephalitozoon (Septata) intestinalis	**Albendazole** 400 mg po bid times 3 weeks; peds dose: 15 mg per kg per day div. into 2 daily doses times 7 days	Oral **fumagillin 20 mg po tid** reported effective for E. bieneusi (NEJM 346:1963, 2002)—see Comment	
Disseminated: E. hellum, cuniculi or intestinalis; Pleistophora sp., others in Comment	**Albendazole** 400 mg po bid times 3 weeks	No established rx for Pleistophora sp.	For Trachipleistophora sp., try itraconazole + albendazole (NEJM 351:42, 2004). Other pathogens: Brachiola vesicularum & algerae (NEJM 351:42, 2004).
PROTOZOA—EXTRAINTESTINAL			
Amebic meningoencephalitis			
Acanthamoeba sp.— no proven rx Rev.: Clin Micro Rev 16:273, 2003	Success with IV **pentamidine**, topical **chlorhexidine** & 2% **ketoconazole** cream & then po rx: **TMP-SMX** + **rifampin** + **keto** (PIDJ 20:623, 2001).		For treatment of keratitis, see Table 1, page 11
Balamuthia mandrillaris	**Pentamidine + clarithro + flucon + sulfadiazine + flucytosine** (CID 37:1304, 2003; Arch Path Lab Med 128:466, 2004).		
Naegleria fowleri: >95% mortality	A cause of chronic granulomatous meningitis **Ampho B** 1.5 mg per kg per day in 2 div. doses & then 1 mg per kg per day IV times 6 days		Case report: Ampho, miconazole, & RIF (NEJM 306:346, 1982).
Sappinia diploidea	**Azithro + pentamidine + itra + flucytosine** (JAMA 285:2450, 2001)		
Babesia microti; babesiosis (CID 22:1117, 2001)	**Atovaquone** 750 mg times 7–10 days + **azithromy** 600 mg daily times 7–10 days (NEJM 343:1454, 2000).	(**Clindamycin** 600 mg po tid) + (**quinine** 650 mg po tid) times 7–10 days For adults, can give **clinda** IV as 1.2 gm bid.	Can cause overwhelming infection in asplenic patients. Reported in Washington State (EID 10:622, 2004).
Ehrlichiosis—See Table 1, page 42			
Leishmaniasis. NOTE: Responses of various species differ—see references. U.S. military experience: CID 39:1674, 2004			
Visceral—Kala-azar L. donovani: India/Africa L. infantum: Mediterranean L. chagasi: New World **WARNING: Avoid combined antimony & ampho B** (Ln 351:1928, 1998)	**Miltefosine**[NUS] drug of choice—see Comment. **Adults:** 2.5 mg per kg per days po either as once or twice daily times 28 days **Children** (<12 yrs old): 2.5 mg per kg per day in 3 div. doses after meals times 28 days Refs.: NEJM 347:1737, 1739, & 1794, 2002; PIDJ 22:434, 2003	**Lipid formulations of ampho B** effective in short-course regimens but impractical due to expense: **Children:** Liposomal ampho B → >98% success (CID 36:560, 2003) in dose of 10 mg per kg per day times 2 days. **Adults:** Liposomal Ampho B 2 mg per kg per day times 5 days (CID 38:377, 2004).	**Antimony** (**stibogluconate** or **meglumine antimonate**) 20 mg per kg per day of antimony (Sb) (in 2 div. doses) IM or IV times 28 days. Not marketed in U.S. Contact CDC Drug Service: (404) 639-3670. **Miltefosine:** Available from Zentaris, Frankfurt, Germany: impavido@zentaris.de.
Mucosal—L. brazilliensis	**Antimony**, as for Visceral	**Ampho B**[1] mg per kg IV every other day times 20–30 doses	Approx. cure rates: antimony 60%, AmB >75%
Cutaneous: ***Most resolve spontaneously; Rx goal:*** ↓ time to cure & prevention of mucocutaneous spread New World: Multiple species Old World: L. tropica & L. major	**Fluconazole** 200 mg po once daily times 6 wks. Effective vs L. major (NEJM 346:891, 2002). New World vs L.v. panamensis: **Miltefosine**[NUS] 2.5 mg per kg po 1 time per day times 28 days 91% success (CID 38:1266, 2004).	Other options all IV: **Antimony**: as for visceral, or **Pentamidine** 2–4 mg per kg per day or q2 days IV times 15 doses	For **miltefosine**, contact Zentaris: impavido@zentaris.de. Treatment is species-specific. Good review (does not include miltefosine): JAC 53:158, 2004. **Other reported options:** (1) Physical destruction by heat (CID 40:1148 & 1156, 2005 (2) Parenteral antimony + topical imiquimod (CID 40:1395, 2005), (3) Parenteral antimony + topical GM-CSF (JID 190:1793, 2004).

INFECTING ORGANISM	SUGGESTED REGIMENS — PRIMARY	SUGGESTED REGIMENS — ALTERNATIVE	COMMENTS
PROTOZOA—EXTRAINTESTINAL *(continued)*			
Malaria (Plasmodia species)—NOTE: CDC Malaria info—prophylaxis (877) 394-8747; treatment (770) 488-7788. After hours: 770-488-7100. Websites: www.cdc.gov/ncidod/dpd/parasites/malaria/default.htm; www.who.int/health-topics/malaria.htm.			
Prophylaxis—Drugs plus personal protection: screens, nets, 30–35% DEET skin repellent (avoid 95% products in children), permethrin spray on clothing and nets *(AnIM 128:931, 1998)*			
For areas **free** of chloroquine (CQ)-resistant P. falciparum: Haiti, Dominican Republic, Central America west and north of the Panama Canal, and parts of the Middle East	**CQ** 500 mg (300 mg base) po per week starting 1–2 wks before travel, during travel, & 4 wks post-travel **or AP** 1 adult tab per day (1 day prior to, during, & 7 days post-travel). Note: May exacerbate psoriasis.	**CQ Peds dose:** 8.3 mg per kg (5 mg per kg of base) po 1 time per wk up to 300 mg (base) max. dose **or** **AP** by weight (peds tabs): 11–20 kg, 1 tab; 21–30 kg, 2 tabs; 31–40 kg, 3 tabs; >40 kg, 1 adult tab per day.	CQ safe during pregnancy. **The areas free of CQ-resistant falciparum malaria continue to shrink:** Central America west of Panama Canal, Haiti, and parts of Middle East. CQ-resistant falciparum malaria reported from Saudi Arabia, Yemen, Oman, & Iran.
For areas with **CQ-resistant P. falciparum** CDC voice info on prophylaxis at (888) 232-3228 or website: www.cdc.gov	**Atovaquone** 250 mg—**proguanil** 100 mg (**Malarone**) comb. tablet, 1 per day with food 1–2 days prior to, during, & 7 days post-travel. Peds dose in footnote[1]. Cost per 2 wks: $125. Another option for adults: **primaquine (PQ)** 30 mg base po daily in non-pregnant G6PD-neg. travelers 88% protective vs P. falciparum & >92% vs P. vivax *(CID 33:1990, 2001)*.	**Doxycycline** 100 mg po daily for adults & children >8 years of age[1]. Cost per 2 wks: $30 **OR** **Mefloquine (MQ)**[1] 250 mg (228 mg base) po per week, 1 wk before, during, and for 4 wks after travel. Cost per 2 wks: $80 Peds dose in footnote[1]	**Pregnancy: MQ current best option**. Insufficient data with **Malarone**. **Avoid doxycycline and primaquine.** **Primaquine**: Used only if prolonged exposure to endemic area (e.g., Peace Corps). **Can cause hemolytic anemia if G6PD deficiency present.** **MQ not recommended** if cardiac conduction abnormalities, seizures, or psychiatric disorders, e.g., depression, psychosis. MQ outside U.S.: 275 mg tab, contains 250 mg of base. Do not use halofantrine due to cardiac adverse events.

Treatment—Based on CDC Guidelines (8/05) for drugs currently available in U.S. **Artesunate drugs of major import in SE Asia & Africa but presently not available in U.S.** CDC Hotline: 770-488-7788.

Clinical Severity/ Plasmodia sp.	Region Acquired	Suggested Treatment Regimens (Drug): Primary—Adults	Suggested Treatment Regimens (Drug): Alternative & Peds	Comments
Uncomplicated/ P. falciparum (or not identified)	Central America, west of Panama Canal; Haiti, Dominican Republic, & most of Middle East—**CQ-sensitive**	**CQ** 1 gm salt (600 mg base) po, then 0.5 gm in 6 hrs, then 0.5 gm daily times 2 days. Total: 2500 mg salt	**Peds**: **CQ** 10 mg per kg of base po; then 5 mg per kg of base at 6, 24, & 48 hrs. Total: 25 mg per kg base	**Peds dose should never exceed adult dose.**
	CQ-resistant or unknown resistance	(**QS** 650 mg po tid) + [(**Doxy** 100 mg po bid) or (**tetra** 250 mg po qid)] times 7 days **OR** **AP** 1 gm–400 mg (4 adult tabs) po once daily times 3 days with food	**MQ** 750 mg po, then 500 mg po in 12 hrs. **Peds**: (**QS** 10 mg per kg po tid) + (**clinda** 20 mg per kg per day div. tid)—both times 7 days	Can substitute clinda for doxy/tetra: 20 mg per kg per day po div. tid times 7 days. MQ alternative due to neuropsych. reactions. Avoid if malaria acquired in SE Asia due to resistance.
Uncomplicated/ P. malariae	All regions	**CQ** as above: adults & peds		
Uncomplicated/ P. vivax or P. ovale	All except Papua, New Guinea & Indonesia (CQ-resistant)	**CQ** as above + **PQ** base: 30 mg po once daily times 14 days	**Peds**: **CQ** as above + **PQ** base 0.5 mg po once daily times 14 days	PQ added to eradicate latent parasites in liver. Screen for G6PD def. before starting PQ; if G6PD positive, dose PQ as 45 mg po once weekly times 8 weeks. Avoid PQ in pregnancy.
Uncomplicated/ P. vivax	CQ-resistant: Papua, New Guinea & Indonesia	[**QS** + (**doxy** or **tetra**) + **PQ**] as above	**MQ** + **PQ** as above. **Peds** (<8 yrs old): **QS** alone times 7 days or **MQ** alone. If latter fail, add **doxy** or **tetra**	

[1] **Peds prophylaxis dosages** (Ref.: *CID 34:493, 2002*)**: Mefloquine** weekly dose by **weight** in kg: <15 = 5 mg/kg; 15–19: ¼ adult dose; 20–30 = ½ adult dose; 31–45 = ¾ adult dose; >45 = adult dose. **Atovaquone/proguanil** by **weight** in kg, single daily dose using peds tab (62.5 mg atovaquone & 25 mg proguanil): <11 kg—do not use; 11–20 kg, 1 tab; 21–30 kg, 2 tabs; 31-40 kg, 3 tabs; ≥41 kg, one adult tab. **Doxycycline**, ages >8–12 yrs: 2 mg per kg per day up to 100 mg/day

* *See page 2 for abbreviations. All dosage recommendations are for adults (unless otherwise indicated) and assume normal renal function.*

TABLE 13A (4)

PROTOZOA—EXTRAINTESTINAL/Malaria/Treatment (continued)

Clinical Severity/ Plasmodia sp.	Region Acquired	Suggested Treatment Regimens (Drug)		Comments
		Primary—Adults	**Alternative & Peds**	
Uncomplicated/ Pregnancy	CQ-sensitive areas	**CQ** as above		Doxy or tetra used if benefits outweigh risks. No controlled studies of AP in pregnancy. Possible association of MQ & increased number of stillbirths. If P. vivax or P. ovale, after pregnancy check for G6PD & give PQ 30 mg po daily times 14 days.
	CQ-resistant P. falciparum	**QS + clinda** as above	If failing or intolerant, **QS + doxy**	
	CQ-resistant P. vivax	**QS** 650 mg po tid times 7 days		
Severe malaria, i.e., impaired consciousness, severe anemia, renal failure, pulmonary edema, ARDS, DIC, jaundice, acidosis, seizures, parasitemia >5%. One or more of latter. Almost always P. falciparum	All regions	**Quinidine gluconate** in normal saline: 10 mg per kg (salt) IV over 1 hr & then 0.02 mg per kg per min. by constant infusion OR 24 mg per kg IV over 4 hrs & then 12 mg per kg over 4 hrs q8h. Continue until parasite density <1% & can take po QS. **QS** as above times 7 days (SE Asia) or 3 days elsewhere **PLUS** (**Doxy** 100 mg IV q12h times 7 days) OR (**clinda** 10 mg per kg IV load & then 5 mg per kg IV q8h times 7 days)	**Peds: Quinidine gluconate** IV—same mg per kg dose as for adults **PLUS** (**Doxy**: if <45 kg, 4 mg per kg IV q12h; if ≥45 kg, dose as for adults) OR **Clinda**, same mg per kg dose as for adults	During quinidine IV: monitor BP, EKG (prolongation of QTc), & blood glucose (hypoglycemia). Consider exchange transfusion if parasitemia >10%. Switch to oral QS, doxy, & clinda when patient able. Steroids not recommended for cerebral malaria. **Outside U.S., the artemisinins (artemether, artesunate) are widely used in combination because of their efficacy vs resistant plasmodia, modest cost, & relative safety,** e.g., artesunate 2 mg per kg po + clinda (CID 40:1777, 2005). For more info: NEJM 352:1565, 2005 & WHO website: www.rbm.WHO.int. Not available to date in U.S.

INFECTING ORGANISM	SUGGESTED REGIMENS		COMMENTS
	PRIMARY	**ALTERNATIVE**	
Malaria—self-initiated treatment: Only for emergency situation where medical care not available	Atovaquone-proguanil (**AP**) 4 adult tabs (1 gm per 400 mg) po daily times 3 days	**Peds:** Using adult **AP** tabs for 3 consecutive days: 11–20 kg, 1 tab; 21–30 kg, 2 tabs; 31–40 kg, 3 tabs; ≥41 kg, 4 tabs.	Do not use for renal insufficiency pts. Do not use if weight <11 kg, pregnant, or breast-feeding.

Microsporidia—systemic—see page 96, Intestinal Protozoa

Pneumocystis carinii Pneumonia (PCP). New name is **Pneumocystis jiroveci** (yee-row-vek-ee). Refs.: NEJM 350:2487, 2004; CID 40(Suppl.3):S131, 2005			
Not acutely ill, able to take po meds. PaO₂ >70 mmHg	(**TMP-SMX-DS**, 2 tabs po q8h times 21 days) OR (**Dapsone** 100 mg po q24h + **trimethoprim** 5 mg per kg po tid times 21 days) **NOTE:** Concomitant use of corticosteroids usually reserved for sicker pts with PaO₂ <70 (see below)	[**Clindamycin** 300–450 mg po q6h + **primaquine** 15 mg base po q24h] times 21 days OR Atovaquone suspension 750 mg po bid with food times 21 days.	Mutations in the gene of the enzyme target (dihydropteroate synthetase) of sulfamethoxazole identified. Unclear whether mutations result in resistance to TMP-SMX or dapsone + TMP (EID 10:1721, 2004). Dapsone ref.: CID 27:191, 1998. **After 21 days, chronic suppression in AIDS pts (see below).**
Acutely ill, po rx not possible. PaO₂ <70 mmHg	[**Prednisone** (15–30 min. before TMP-SMX): 40 mg po bid times 5 days, then 40 mg q24h times 5 days, then 20 mg po q24h times 11 days] + **TMP-SMX** (15 mg of TMP component per kg per day) IV div. q6-8h times 21 days] Can substitute IV prednisolone (reduce dose 25%) for po prednisone	**Prednisone** as in primary rx PLUS [(**Clinda** 600 mg IV q8h) + (**primaquine** 30 mg base po q24h)] times 21 days OR **Pentamidine** 4 mg per kg per day IV times 21 days (**Pentamidine** 300 mg IV in 6 mL sterile water by aerosol q4 wks) OR (**dapsone** 200 mg po + **pyrimethamine** 75 mg po + **folinic acid** 25 mg po—all once a week) or **atovaquone** 1500 mg po q24h with food.	**After 21 days, chronic suppression in AIDS pts (see below).** **PCP can occur in absence of HIV infection and steroids (CID 25:215 & 219, 1997).** Wait at least 4–8 days before declaring treatment failure & switching to clinda + primaquine or pentamidine. See above regarding gene mutations.
Primary prophylaxis and post-treatment suppression	(**TMP-SMX-DS** or **-SS,** 1 tab po q24h or 1 DS 3 times per wk) OR (**dapsone** 100 mg po q24h). DC when CD4 >200 times 3 mos. (NEJM 344:159, 2001).		**TMP-SMX-DS** regimen provides cross-protection vs toxo and other bacterial infections. Dapsone + pyrimethamine protects vs toxo. Atovaquone suspension 1500 mg daily as effective as daily dapsone (NEJM 339:1889, 1998) or inhaled pentamidine (JID 180:369, 1999)

* See page 2 for abbreviations. All dosage recommendations are for adults (unless otherwise indicated) and assume normal renal function.

TABLE 13A (6)

INFECTING ORGANISM	SUGGESTED REGIMENS		COMMENTS
	PRIMARY	ALTERNATIVE	
PROTOZOA—EXTRAINTESTINAL/Trypanosomiasis/East African sleeping sickness (continued)			
Late: Encephalitis	**Melarsoprol**[1] 2–3.6 mg per kg per day IV times 3 days; repeat after 7 days & for 3rd time 7 days after 2nd course	**Prednisone** may prevent/attenuate encephalopathy	
T. cruzi—**Chagas disease** or acute American trypanosomiasis Ref.: Ln 357:797, 2001	**Nifurtimox**[1] 8–10 mg per kg per day po div. 4 times per day after meals times 120 days Ages 11–16 yrs: 12.5–15 mg per kg per day div. qid po times 90 days Children <11 yrs: 15–20 mg per kg per day div. qid po times 90 days	**Benznidazole**[NUS] 5–7 mg per kg per day po div. 2 times per day times 30–90 days (AJTMH 63:111, 2000). NOTE: Avoid tetracycline and steroids.	Treatment of no benefit in chronic late disease. Nifurtimox reported 70–95% effective. Immunosuppression for heart transplant can reactivate chronic Chagas disease.
NEMATODES—INTESTINAL (Roundworms)			
Ascaris lumbricoides (**ascariasis**)	**Albendazole** 400 mg po times 1 dose or **mebendazole** 100 mg po bid times 3 days or 500 mg po times 1 dose	**Ivermectin** 150–200 mcg per kg po times 1 dose or **mebendazole** 100 mg po bid times 3 days; **Nitazoxanide: Adults**—500 mg po bid times 3 days; **children 4–11**—200 mg oral susp. po q12h	For significance of eosinophilia, see CID 34:407, 2002 Can present with intestinal obstruction.
Capillaria philippinensis (**capillariasis**)	**Mebendazole** 200 mg po bid times 20 days	**Albendazole** 200 mg po bid times 10 days	Side-effects in Table 13B, pages 103, 105
Enterobius vermicularis (**pinworm**)	**Albendazole** 400 mg po times 1, repeat in 2 wks OR **mebendazole** 100 mg po times 1, repeat in 2 wks	**Pyrantel pamoate** 11 mg per kg (to max. dose of 1 gm) po times 1 dose; repeat every 2 wks times 2.	
Hookworm (Necator americanus and Ancylostoma duodenale)	**Albendazole** 400 mg po times 1 dose or **mebendazole** 500 mg po times 1 dose	**Pyrantel pamoate** 11 mg per kg (to max. dose of 1 gm) po daily times 3 days	NOTE: Ivermectin not effective. Eosinophilia may be absent but eggs in stool (NEJM 351:799, 2004).
Strongyloides stercoralis (**strongyloidiasis**)	**Ivermectin** 200 mcg per kg per day po times 2 days	**Albendazole** 400 mg po bid times 2 days (7–10 days for hyperinfection syndrome)	Case report of ivermectin failure in pt with hypogamma-globulinemia (Am J Med Sci 311:178, 1996).
Trichostrongylus orientalis	**Albendazole** 400 mg po times 1 dose	**Pyrantel pamoate** 11 mg per kg (max. 1 gm) po times 1	**Mebendazole** 100 mg po bid times 3 days
Trichuris trichiura (**whipworm**)	**Albendazole** 400 mg po once daily times 3 days	**Mebendazole** 100 mg po bid times 3 days or 500 mg once	**Ivermectin** 200 mcg per kg daily po times 3 days
NEMATODES—EXTRAINTESTINAL (Roundworms)			
Angiostrongylus cantonensis—a cause of eosinophilic meningitis	Supportive care. Serial LPs to ↓ intracranial pressure	Anthelminth therapy may worsen meningitis (NEJM 346:668, 2002). Prednisone may help.	Mortality rate <1%. Ref.: AJM 114:217, 2003)
Anisakis simplex (**anisakiasis**)	Physical removal: endoscope or surgery	Questionable response to albendazole (Ln 360:54, 2002)	Anisakiasis acquired by eating raw fish: herring, salmon, mackerel, cod, squid. Similar illness due to Pseudoterranova species acquired from cod, halibut, red snapper.
Ancylostoma braziliense & caninum: causes **cutaneous larva migrans**	**Ivermectin** 200 mcg per kg po times 1 dose per day times 1–2 days	**Albendazole** 200 mg po bid times 3 days	Also called "creeping eruption," dog and cat hookworm. Ivermectin cure rate 77% (1 dose) to 97% (2–3 doses) (CID 31:493, 2000).
Baylisascariasis (Raccoon ascaris)	No drug proven efficacious. Try po **albendazole**.	Peds: 25–50 mg per kg per day; Adults: 400 mg bid. Both times 10 days	Some add steroids (CID 39:1484, 2004).
Dracunculus medinensis: **Guinea worm**	Slow extraction of pre-emergent worm	**Metronidazole** 250 mg po tid times 10 days used to ↓ inflammatory response and facilitate removal. Immersion in warm water promotes worm emergence. Mebendazole 400–800 mg per day times 6 days may kill worm.	
Filariasis. Wolbachia bacteria needed for filarial development. Rx with doxy 100–200 mg per day times 4–6 wks ↓ number of wolbachia & number of microfilaria (BMJ 326:207, 2003) Lymphatic (**Elephantiasis**): Wuchereria bancrofti or Brugia malayi or B. timori	Prospective random DB trial shows efficacy of **doxy** vs both adult worms & microfilaria: 200 mg po per day times 8 wks (Ln 365: 2067 & 2116, 2005).	**Diethylcarbamazine**[1][2] (DEC) po over 14 days: Day 1, 50 mg; day 2, 50 mg tid; day 3, 100 mg tid; days 4–14, 2 mg per kg tid.	**Diethylcarbamazine**[1][2] (DEC) 6 mg per kg po once—similar effect as multiple doses

---

[1] Available from CDC Drug Service; see footnote 1 page 95

[2] May need antihistamine or corticosteroid for allergic reaction from disintegrating organisms

* See page 2 for abbreviations. All dosage recommendations are for adults (unless otherwise indicated) and assume normal/renal function.

INFECTING ORGANISM	SUGGESTED REGIMENS		COMMENTS
	PRIMARY	ALTERNATIVE	
NEMATODES—Extraintestinal (Roundworms)/Filariasis *(continued)*			
Cutaneous			
Loiasis: **Loa loa**, eyeworm disease	Diethylcarbamazine (DEC)[1,2]—6 mg per kg po times 1 dose		DEC: 300 mg per wk. po effective prophylaxis.
Onchocerca volvulus (**onchocerciasis**)—river blindness (*Ln 360:203, 2002*)	**Ivermectin** 150 mcg per kg po times 1 dose; repeat q6 months to suppress dermal and ocular microfilariae. If eye involved, start **prednisone** 1 mg per kg po several days before ivermectin. NOTE: Worm survival requires symbiotic bacteria Wolbachia (*Science 296:1365, 2002*)		Ivermectin ↓ number of microfilariae in skin and impairs female worm fertility; does not kill adult worms (nothing does). Ivermectin OK in pregnancy.
Body cavity			
Mansonella perstans (dipetalonemiasis)	**Mebendazole**[1] 100 mg po bid times 30 days or **albendazole** 400 mg po bid times 10 days	Usually no or vague allergic symptoms + eosinophilia. Ivermectin has no activity against this species.	
Mansonella streptocerca	**Diethylcarbamazine**[1,2] as above for Wuchereria OR **ivermectin** 150 mcg per kg times 1	Chronic pruritic hypopigmented lesions that may be confused with leprosy. Can be asymptomatic.	
Mansonella ozzardi	**Ivermectin** 200 mcg per kg times 1 dose may be effective	Usually asymptomatic. Articular pain, pruritus, lymphadenopathy reported. May have allergic reaction from dying organisms.	
Dirofilariasis: **Heartworms**			
D. immitis, dog heartworm	No effective drugs; surgical removal only option		Can lodge in pulmonary artery → coin lesion. Eosinophilia rare.
D. tenius (raccoon), D. ursi (bear), D. repens (dogs, cats)	No effective drugs		Worms migrate to conjunctivae, subcutaneous tissue, scrotum, breasts, extremities
Gnathostoma spinigerum: eosinophilic myeloencephalitis	**Albendazole** 400 mg po q24h or bid times 21 days	**Ivermectin** 200 mcg per kg per day times 2 days	
Toxocariasis: *Clin Micro Rev 16:265, 2003*	**Rx directed at relief of symptoms as infection self-limited, e.g., steroids & antihistamines; use of anthelminthics controversial.**		
Visceral larval migrans	**Albendazole** 400 mg po bid times 5 days	**Mebendazole** 100–200 mg po bid times 5 days	Severe lung, heart or CNS disease may warrant steroids. Differential dx of larval migrans syndromes: Toxocara canis and catis, Ancylostoma spp., Gnathostoma spp., Spirometra spp.
Ocular larval migrans	First 4 wks of illness: (Oral **prednisone** 30–60 mg po q24h) + subtenon **triamcinolone** 40 mg weekly) times 2 weeks		No added benefit of antihelminthic drugs. Rx of little effect after 4 wks.
Trichinella spiralis (**trichinosis**)—muscle infection	**Albendazole** 400 mg po bid times 8–14 days	**Mebendazole** 200–400 mg po tid times 3 days, then 400–500 mg po tid times 10 days	Use albendazole/mebendazole with caution during pregnancy.
	Concomitant **prednisone** 40–60 mg po q24h		
TREMATODES (Flukes)			
Clonorchis sinensis (liver fluke)	**Praziquantel** 25 mg per kg po tid times 1 day or **albendazole** 10 mg per kg per day po times 7 days		Same dose in children
Fasciola buski (intestinal fluke)	**Praziquantel** 25 mg per kg po tid times 1 day		Same dose in children
Fasciola hepatica (sheep liver fluke)	**Triclabendazole**[NUS] (Fasinex; Novartis Agribusiness) 10 mg per kg po times 1 dose. Ref.: *CID 32:1, 2001*		**Bithionol**[1] Adults and children: 30–50 mg per kg (max. dose 2 gm per day) every other times 10–15 doses
Heterophyes heterophyes (intestinal fluke); Metagonimus yokogawai (intestinal fluke); Opisthorchis viverrini (liver fluke)	**Praziquantel** 25 mg per kg po tid times 1 day		Same dose in children. Same regimen for **Metorchis conjunctus (North American liver fluke)**. **Nanophyetus salmincola:** Praziquantel 20 mg per kg po tid times 1 day
Paragonimus westermani (lung fluke)	**Praziquantel** 25 mg per kg po tid times 2 days or **bithionol**[1] 30–50 mg per kg po times 1 every other day times 10 days		Same dose in children

[1] Available from CDC Drug Service; see footnote 1 page 95

[2] May need antihistamine or corticosteroid for allergic reaction from disintegrating organisms

* See page 2 for abbreviations. All dosage recommendations are for adults (unless otherwise indicated) and assume normal renal function.

TABLE 13A (8)

INFECTING ORGANISM	SUGGESTED REGIMENS		COMMENTS
	PRIMARY	ALTERNATIVE	
TREMATODES (Flukes) *(continued)*			
Schistosoma haematobium; GU bilharziasis. (NEJM 346:1212, 2002)	**Praziquantel** 20 mg per kg po bid times 1 day (2 doses)		Same dose in children. Alternative: metrifonate 10 mg per kg per dose po q2 wks for 3 doses.
Schistosoma intercalatum.	**Praziquantel** 20 mg per kg po bid times 1 day (2 doses)		Same dose in children.
Schistosoma japonicum; Oriental schisto. (NEJM 346:1212, 2002)	**Praziquantel** 20 mg per kg po **tid** times 1 day (**3 doses**)		Same dose in children. Cures 60–90% pts.
Schistosoma mansoni (intestinal bilharziasis) Possible **praziquantel resistance** (JID 176:304, 1997) (NEJM 346:1212, 2002)	**Praziquantel** 20 mg per kg po bid times 1 day (2 doses)	**Oxamniquine**[NUS] single dose of 15 mg per kg po once; in North and East Africa 20 mg per kg po daily times 3 days Do not use during pregnancy.	Same dose for children. Cures 60–90% pts. Report of success treating myeloradiculopathy with single po dose of praziquantel, 50 mg per kg, + prednisone for 6 months (CID 39:1618, 2004).
Schistosoma mekongi	**Praziquantel** 20 mg per kg po **tid** times 1 day (**3 doses**)		Same dose for children
Toxemic schisto; Katayama fever	**Praziquantel** 25 mg per kg po q4h with food times 3 doses		Massive infection with either S. japonicum or S. mansoni
CESTODES (Tapeworms)			
Echinococcus granulosus (hydatid disease) (CID 37:1073, 2003; Ln 362:1295, 2003)	Meta-analysis supports percutaneous aspiration-injection-reaspiration (PAIR) + albendazole. Before **and** after drainage: **albendazole** ≥60 kg, 400 mg po bid or <60 kg, 15 mg per kg per day div, with meals. Then: Puncture (P) & needle aspirate (A) cyst content. Instill (I) hypertonic saline (15–30%) or absolute alcohol & wait 20–30 min., then re-aspirate (R) with final irrigation. **Continue albendazole times 28 days** Cure in 96% as compared to 90% pts with surgical resection.		
Echinococcus multilocularis (alveolar cyst disease) (COID 16:437, 2003)	**Albendazole** efficacy not clearly demonstrated, can try in dosages used for hydatid disease. Wide surgical resection only reliable rx; technique evolving (Radiology 198:259, 1996).		
Intestinal tapeworms Diphyllobothrium latum (fish), Dipylidium caninum (dog), Taenia saginata (beef), and Taenia solium (pork)	**Praziquantel** 5–10 mg per kg po times 1 dose for children and adults. **Alternative: Niclosamide** 2 gm po times 1. **NOTE:** Niclosamide preferred for Taenia solium because it is not absorbed; hence, avoid risk of CNS symptoms if pt has neurocysticercosis.		
Hymenolepis diminuta (rats) and H. nana (humans)	**Praziquantel** 25 mg per kg po times 1 dose for children and adults. **Alternative: Niclosamide** 500 mg po q24h times 3 days		
Neurocysticercosis (NCC): Larval form of T. solium Ref.: AJTMH 72:3, 2005 **Parenchymal NCC**	**NOTE: Treat T. solium intestinal tapeworms,** if present, with **niclosamide**		
"Viable" cysts by CT/MRI	[**Albendazole** ≥60 kg: 400 mg bid with meals or <60 kg, 15 mg per kg per day in 2 div. doses (max. 800 mg per day) + **Dexamethasone** 0.1 mg per kg per day ± Anti-seizure medication) — all times 8 days.	(**Praziquantel** 50–100 mg per kg per day in 3 div. doses) + **Dexamethasone** 0.1 mg per kg per day ± Anti-seizure medication) — all times 15 days	Albendazole assoc. with 46% ↓ in seizures (NEJM 350:249, 2004). Praziquantel less cysticidal activity. Steroids decrease serum levels of praziquantel.
Degenerating cysts	**Albendazole + dexamethasone** as above		Treatment improves prognosis of associated seizures.
Dead calcified cysts	No treatment indicated		
Subarachnoid NCC	**Albendazole + steroids** as above) + shunting for hydrocephalus. Without shunt, 50% died within 9 yrs (J Neurosurg 66:686, 1987).		
Intraventricular NCC	**Albendazole + dexamethasone** + neuroendoscopic removal (if available)		
Sparganosis (Spirometra mansonoides) Larval cysts; source—frogs/snakes	Surgical resection or ethanol injection of subcutaneous masses (NEJM 330:1887, 1994).		

* See page 2 for abbreviations. All dosage recommendations are for adults (unless otherwise indicated) and assume normal renal & ...

TABLE 13A (9)

DISEASE	INFECTING ORGANISM	SUGGESTED REGIMENS		COMMENTS
		PRIMARY	ALTERNATIVE	
ECTOPARASITES Ref.: *CID* 36:1355, 2003; *Ln* 363:889, 2004. **NOTE: Due to potential neurotoxicity, lindane not recommended.**				
Head lice *Med Lett* 47:68, 2005	Pediculus humanus, var. capitis	**Permethrin** 1% generic lotion or cream rinse (Nix): Apply to shampooed dried hair for 10 min.; repeat in 1 wk. **OR** **Malathion** 0.5% (Ovide): Apply to dry hair for 8–14 hrs, then shampoo	**Ivermectin** 200–400 mcg per kg po once; repeat in 7–10 days	**Permethrin:** success in 78%. Extra combing of no benefit. Resistance increasing. No advantage to 5% permethrin. **Malathion:** Report that 1–2 20-min. applications 98% effective *Ped Derm* 21:670, 2004). In alcohol—potentially flammable.
Pubic lice (crabs)	Phthirus pubis	**Pubic hair: Permethrin** OR **malathion** as for head lice	**Eyelids: Petroleum jelly** applied qid times 10 days OR **yellow oxide of mercury** 1% qid times 14 days	Costs: Permethrin 1% lotion/cream $8–9 Malathion 0.5% lotion $119 Ivermectin $20
Body lice	Pediculus humanus, var. corporis	No drugs for pt; treat the clothing. Organism lives in & deposits eggs in seams of clothing. Discard clothing; if not possible, treat clothing with 1% malathion powder or 10% DDT powder.		
Scabies Immunocompetent patients	Sarcoptes scabiei	**Primary: Permethrin** 5% cream (ELIMITE). Apply entire skin from chin to toes. Leave on 8–10 hrs. Repeat in 1 week. Safe for children >2 mos. old. **Alternative: Ivermectin** 200 mcg per kg po times 1 (*NEJM* 333:26, 1995) **or** 10% crotamiton topically 1 time per day times 2 days		Trim fingernails. Reapply to hands after handwashing. Pruritus may persist times 2 wks after mites gone.
AIDS patients, CD4 <150 per mm³ (Norwegian scabies—see *Comments*)		For Norwegian scabies: **Permethrin** 5% as above on day 1, then 6% sulfur in petrolatum daily on days 2–7, then repeat times several weeks. **Ivermectin** 200 mcg per kg po times 1 reported effective.		Norwegian scabies in AIDS pts: Extensive, crusted. Can mimic psoriasis. Not pruritic. ELIMITE: 60 gm $18.60; ivermectin $19.62 Highly contagious—isolate!
Myiasis Due to larvae of flies		Usually cutaneous/subcutaneous nodule with central punctum. Treatment: Occlude punctum to prevent gas exchange with petrolatum, fingernail polish, makeup cream or bacon. When larva migrates, manually remove.		

TABLE 13B: DOSAGE, PRICE, AND SELECTED ADVERSE EFFECTS OF ANTIPARASITIC DRUGS

NOTE: Drugs available from CDC Drug Service indicated by "CDC": Call (404) 639-3670 (or -2888).
Doses vary with indication. For convenience, drugs divided by type of parasite; some drugs used for multiple types of parasites, e.g., albendazole.
COMMENT: Cost data represent average wholesale prices as listed in 2005 Drug Topics Red Book, Medical Economics.

CLASS, AGENT, GENERIC NAME (TRADE NAME)	USUAL ADULT DOSAGE (Cost)	ADVERSE REACTIONS/COMMENTS
Antiprotozoan Drugs		
Intestinal Parasites		
Albendazole (Albenza)	Doses vary with indication, 200–400 mg bid po 200 mg tab $1.58	Teratogenic. Pregnancy Cat. C; give after negative pregnancy test. Abdominal pain, nausea/vomiting, alopecia. ↑ serum transaminase. Rare leukopenia.
Dehydroemetine *(CDC)**	1.5 mg per kg per day to max. of 90 mg IM	Local pain, ECG changes, cardiac arrhythmias, precordial pain, paresthesias, weakness, peripheral neuropathy. GI: nausea/vomiting, diarrhea. Avoid strenuous exercise for 4 wks after rx.
Iodoquinol (Yodoxin) (650 mg $0.47)	Adults: 650 mg po tid; children: 40 mg per kg per day div. tid	Rarely causes nausea, abdominal cramps, rash, acne. Contraindicated if iodine intolerance.
Metronidazole/Ornidazole[NUS] (Tiberal) Paromomycin (Humatin) Aminosidine in U.K.	See *metronidazole in Table 10A, page 66, & 10C, page 73*. Up to 750 mg qid. 250 mg tab $3.37	Side-effects similar for all. See *metronidazole in Table 10A, page 66 & 10C, page 73*. Drug is aminoglycoside similar to neomycin; if absorbed due to concomitant inflammatory bowel disease can result in oto/nephrotoxicity. Doses >3 gm assoc. with nausea, abdominal cramps, diarrhea.
Quinacrine[NUS] (Atabrine, Mepacrine)	100 mg tid. No longer available in U.S.; 2 pharmacies will prepare as a service: (1) Connecticut 203-785-6818; (2) California 800-247-9767	Contraindicated for pts with history of psychosis or psoriasis. Yellow staining of skin. Dizziness, headache, vomiting, toxic psychosis (1.5%), hemolytic anemia, leukopenia, thrombocytopenia, urticaria, rash, fever, minor disulfiram-like reactions.

* See page 2 for abbreviations. *All dosage recommendations are for adults (unless otherwise indicated) and assume normal renal function.*

104

TABLE 13B (2)

CLASS, AGENT, GENERIC NAME (TRADE NAME)	USUAL ADULT DOSAGE (Cost)	ADVERSE REACTIONS/COMMENTS
Antiprotozoan Drugs **Tinidazole (Tindamax)**	500 mg tabs, with food. Regimen varies with indication. Cost: 500 mg tab $4.56	Chemical structure similar to metronidazole but better tolerated. Seizures/peripheral neuropathy reported. **Adverse effects:** Metallic taste 4–6%, nausea 3–5%, anorexia 2–3%.
Extraintestinal Parasites **Antimony compounds**[NUS] Stibogluconate sodium (Pentostam, Tricostam) *(CDC)* Meglumine antimonate (Glucaratine, Glucontim—French tradenames)	Solution containing 30–34% pentavalent antimony	Cough/vomiting if IV infusion too fast. Arthralgia 50%. Others: myalgia, bradycardia, cramps/diarrhea, pruritus/rash, renal toxicity,↑ amylase. **NOTE: EKG abnormalities occur. Combination rx with, or sequential rx with, ampho B may trigger fatal arrhythmias (Ln 351:1928, 1998).**
Atovaquone (Mepron) Ref.: *AAC 46:1163, 2002*	Suspension: 1 tsp (750 mg) po bid 750 mg per 5 mL. Cost: 210 mL $744.00	No. pts stopping rx due to side-effects was 9%; rash 22%, GI 20%, headache 16%, insomnia 10%, fever 14%
Atovaquone and proguanil (Malarone) For prophylaxis of P. falciparum; little data on P. vivax	**Prophylaxis:** 1 tab po (250 mg + 100 mg) q24h with food **Treatment:** 4 tabs po (1000 mg + 400 mg) once daily with food times 3 days Adult tab: 250/100 mg; Peds tab 62.5/25 mg. Peds dosage: *footnote 1 page 97.* Cost: 250/100 mg tab $5.04	Adverse effects in rx trials: Adults—abd. pain 17%; N/V 12%. Children—cough, headache, anorexia, vomiting, abd. pain. Rx stopped in 1%. Asymptomatic mild ↑ in ALT/AST. Children—cough, headache, anorexia, vomiting, abd. pain. *See drug interactions, Table 22.* Safe in G6PD-deficient pts. Can crush tabs for children and give with milk or other liquid nutrients. Renal insufficiency: contraindicated if CrCl <30 mL per min.
Benznidazole[NUS] **(Rochagan,** Roche, Brazil)	7.5 mg per kg per day po	Photosensitivity in 50% of pts. GI: abdominal pain, nausea/vomiting/anorexia. CNS: disorientation, insomnia, twitching/seizures, paresthesias, polyneuritis
Chloroquine phosphate (Aralen)	Dose varies—see *Malaria prophylaxis and rx, pages 97–98.* 500 mg tabs $6.04	Minor: anorexia/nausea/vomiting, headache, dizziness, blurred vision, pruritus in dark-skinned pts. Major: protracted rx in rheumatoid arthritis can lead to retinopathy. Can exacerbate psoriasis. Can block response to rabies vaccine. Contraindicated in pts with epilepsy.
Dapsone Ref.: *CID 27:191, 1998*	100 mg po q24h 100 mg tabs $0.20	Usually tolerated by pts with rash after TMP-SMX. Adverse effects: nausea/vomiting, rash, oral lesions *(CID 18:630, 1994).* Methemoglobinemia (usually asymptomatic); if >10–15%, stop drug. Hemolytic anemia if G6PD deficient. Sulfone syndrome: fever, rash, hemolytic anemia, atypical lymphocytes, and liver injury *(West J Med 156:303, 1992).*
Eflornithine[NUS] **(Ornidyl)**	Approved in U.S. for trypanosome infections but not marketed. Contact Hoechst Marion Roussel. (800) 552-3656.	Diarrhea in ½ pts, vomiting, abdominal pain, anemia/leukopenia in ½ pts, seizures, alopecia, jaundice, ↓ hearing
Fumagillin	Eyedrops + po. 20 mg po tid. Call 800-547-1392.	Adverse events: Neutropenia & thrombocytopenia
Mefloquine (Lariam)	One 250 mg tab per week for malaria prophylaxis; for rx, 1250 mg times 1 or 750 mg plus then 500 mg in 6–8 hrs. 250 mg tab $12.93. In U.S.: 250 mg tab = 228 mg base; outside U.S. 275 mg tab = 250 mg base	Side-effects in roughly 3%: Minor: headache, irritability, insomnia, weakness, diarrhea. Toxic psychosis, seizures can occur. Teratogenic—do not use in pregnancy. Do not use with quinine, quinidine, or halofantrine. Rare: Prolonged QT interval and toxic epidermal necrolysis *(Ln 349:101, 1997).* Not used for self-rx due to neuropsychiatric side-effects.
Melarsoprol *(CDC)* **(Mel B, Arsobal)** (Manufactured in France)	See Trypanosomiasis for adult dose. Peds dose: 0.36 mg per kg IV, then gradual ↑ to 3.6 mg per kg q1–5 days for total of 9–10 doses.	Post-rx encephalopathy (10%) with 50% mortality overall; risk of death 2° to rx 4–8%. Prednisolone 1 mg per kg per day po may ↓ encephalopathy. Other: Heart damage, albuminuria, abdominal pain, vomiting, peripheral neuropathy. Herxheimer-like reaction, pruritus.
Miltefosine[NUS] **(Zentaris, Impavido)**	100–150 mg (approx. 2.25 mg per kg per day) po times 28 days Cutaneous leishmaniasis 2.25 mg per kg po q24h times 6 wks	**Pregnancy—No;** teratogenic. Side-effects vary; kala-azar pts. vomiting in up to 40%, diarrhea in 17%; mild to moderate in severity—may resolve in <1 day. Contact Astra Medica, Ger.
Nifurtimox (Lampit) *(CDC)* (Manufactured in Germany by Bayer)	8–10 mg per kg per day po. 4 times per day	Side-effects in 40–70% of pts. GI: abdominal pain, nausea/vomiting. CNS: polyneuritis (1/3), disorientation, insomnia, twitching, seizures. Skin rash. Hemolysis with G6PD deficiency.
Nitazoxanide (Alinia)	Adults: 500 mg po q12h. Children 4–11: 200 mg susp. po q12h.Take with food. 500 mg tabs $13.02.	Abdominal pain 7.8%, diarrhea 2.1%. Rev.: *CID 40:1173, 2005*
Pentamidine (NebuPent)	300 mg via aerosol q month. Also used IM. 300 mg $98.75 + admin. costs	Hypotension, hypocalcemia, hypoglycemia followed by hyperglycemia, pancreatitis. Neutropenia (15%), thrombocytopenia. Nephrotoxicity. Others: nausea/vomiting, ↑ liver tests, rash.
Primaquine phosphate	26.3 mg (=15 mg base) $0.77	In G6PD def. pts, can cause hemolytic anemia with hemoglobinuria, esp. African, Asian peoples. Methemoglobinemia. Nausea/abdominal pain if pt. fasting. *(CID 39:1336, 2004)*

* See page 2 for abbreviations. All dosage recommendations are for adults (unless otherwise indicated) and assume normal renal function.

TABLE 13B (3)

CLASS, AGENT, GENERIC NAME (TRADE NAME)	USUAL ADULT DOSAGE (Cost)	ADVERSE REACTIONS/COMMENTS
Antiprotozoan Drugs/Extraintestinal Parasites *(continued)*		
Pyrimethamine (Daraprim, Malocide) Also combined with sulfadoxine as Fansidar (25–500 mg) $4.13	100 mg po, then 25 mg per day. 25 mg/day $0.43. Cost of folinic acid (leucovorin) 5 mg $2.36	Major problem is hematologic: megaloblastic anemia, ↓ WBC, ↓ platelets. Can give 5 mg folinic acid per day to ↓ bone marrow depression and not interfere with antitoxoplasmosis effect. If high-dose pyrimethamine, ↑ folinic acid to 10–50 mg per day. Pyrimethamine + sulfadiazine can cause mental changes due to carnitine deficiency (*AJM 95:112*, 1993). Other: Rash, vomiting, diarrhea, xerostomia
Quinacrine[NUS]	For giardiasis: 100 mg po tid times 5 days Peds dose: 2 mg per kg po tid (max. 300 mg per day) times 5 days	Compounded by Med. Center Pharm., New Haven, CT: (203) 688-6816 or Panorama Compound. Pharm., Van Nuys, CA: (800) 247-9767
Quinidine gluconate	Loading dose of 10 mg (equivalent to 6.2 mg of quinidine base) per kg IV over 1–2 hrs, and then constant infusion of 0.02 mg of quinidine gluconate per kg per minute. 80 mg IV $21.56	Adverse reactions of quinidine/quinine similar: (1) IV bolus injection can cause fatal hypotension, (2) hyperinsulinemic hypoglycemia, esp. in pregnancy, (3) ↓ rate of infusion of IV quinidine if QT interval ↑ >25% of baseline, (4) reduce dose 30–50% after day 3 due to ↓ renal clearance and ↓ vol. of distribution.
Quinine sulfate (300 mg salt = 250 mg base)	325 and 650 mg tabs. No IV prep. in U.S. Oral rx of chloroquine-resistant falciparum malaria: 650 mg po tid times 3 days, then tetracycline 250 mg po qid times 7 days 325 mg $0.16	Cinchonism: tinnitus, headache, nausea, abdominal pain, blurred vision. Rarely: blood dyscrasias, drug fever, asthma, hypoglycemia. Transient blindness in <1% of 500 pts (*AnIM 136:339, 2002*). Contraindicated if G6PD deficiency.
Spiramycin (Rovamycine) /*JAC 42:572, 1998*/	Up to 3–4 gm per day	GI and allergic reactions have occurred. Not available in U.S.
Sulfadiazine	1–1.5 gm po q6h. 500 mg $0.34	See *Table 10C, page 73*, for sulfonamide side-effects
Sulfadoxine and pyrimethamine combination (Fansidar)	Contains 500 mg of sulfadoxine and 25 mg of pyrimethamine One tab $4.13	Very long mean half-life of both drugs: Sulfadoxine 169 hrs, pyrimethamine 111 hrs allows weekly dosage. Do not use in pregnancy. Fatalities reported due to Stevens-Johnson syndrome and toxic epidermal necrolysis. Renal excretion—use with caution in pts with renal impairment.
DRUGS USED TO TREAT NEMATODES, TREMATODES, AND CESTODES		
Bithionol *(CDC)*	Adults & children: 30–40 mg per kg (to max. of 2 gm per day) po every other day times 10–15 doses	Photosensitivity, skin reactions, urticaria, GI upset
Diethylcarbamazine (Hetrazan) *(CDC)*	Used to treat filariasis. Licensed (Lederle) but not available in U.S.	Headache, dizziness, nausea, fever. Host may experience inflammatory reaction to death of adult worms: fever, urticaria, asthma, GI upset (Mazzotti reaction).
Ivermectin (Stromectol, Mectizan)	Strongyloidiasis dose: 200 mcg per kg times 1 dose po Onchocerciasis: 150 mcg per kg times 1 po Scabies: 200 mcg per kg po times 1 3 mg tabs $4.35	Mild side-effects: fever, pruritus, rash. In rx of onchocerciasis, can see tender lymphadenopathy, headache, bone/joint pain. Can cause Mazzotti reaction (see above).
Mebendazole (Vermox)	Doses vary with indication. 100 mg tab $5.91	Rarely causes abdominal pain, nausea, diarrhea. Contraindicated in pregnancy and children <2 yrs old.
Oxamniquine (Vansil)[NUS]	For S. mansoni. Some experts suggest 40–60 mg per kg over 2–3 days in all of Africa.	Rarely: dizziness, drowsiness, neuropsychiatric symptoms, GI upset. EKG/EEG changes. Orange/red urine.
Praziquantel (Biltricide)	Doses vary with parasite; see *Table 13A*. 600 mg $11.90	Mild: dizziness/drowsiness, N/V, rash, fever. Only contraindication is ocular cysticercosis. Metab.-induced by anticonvulsants and steroids; can negate effect with cimetidine 400 mg po tid.
Pyrantel pamoate (over-the-counter as Reese's Pinworm Medicine)	Oral suspension. Dose for all ages: 11 mg per kg (to max. of 1 gm) times 1 dose	Rare GI upset, headache, dizziness, rash
Suramin (Germanin) *(CDC)*	For early trypanosomiasis. Drug powder mixed to 10% solution with 5 mL water and used within 30 minutes.	Does not cross blood-brain barrier; no effect on CNS infection. Side-effects: vomiting, pruritus, urticaria, fever, paresthesias, albuminuria (discontinue drug if casts appear). Do not use if renal/liver disease present. Deaths from vascular collapse reported.
Thiabendazole (Mintezol)	Take after meals. Dose varies with parasite; see *Table 12A*. 500 mg $1.25	Nausea/vomiting, headache, dizziness. Rarely: liver damage, ↓ BP, angioneurotic edema, Stevens-Johnson syndrome. May ↓ mental alertness.

* *See page 2 for abbreviations. All dosage recommendations are for adults (unless otherwise indicated) and assume normal renal function.*

TABLE 14A: ANTIVIRAL THERAPY (Non-HIV)*

VIRUS/DISEASE	DRUG/DOSAGE	SIDE EFFECTS/COMMENTS
Adenovirus: Cause of RTIs including fatal pneumonia in children & young adults. **Findings include:** fever, ↑ liver enzymes, leukopenia, thrombocytopenia, diarrhea, pneumonia, or hemorrhagic cystitis.	**No proven rx. Cidofovir** 5 mg per kg q wk times 2 wks, then q2 wks + **probenecid** 1.25 gm per M given 3 hrs before adult's and 3 & 9 hrs after each infusion (CID 38:45, 2004) successful in 3/8 immunosuppressed children. Intravesical cidofovir (5 mg per kg in 100 mL saline instilled into bladder) successful rx of adenovirus hemorrhagic cystitis (CID 40:199, 2005).	↓ in virus load predicted response to cidofovir (CID 38:45, 2004). Value of rx controversial (CID 40:1244, 2005).
Coronavirus—SARS-CoV (Severe Acute Respiratory Distress Syn.) (see CID 36:1420, 2004) A new coronavirus, isolated in spring 2003 (NEJM 348:1953 & 1967, 2003) emerged from China & spread from Hong Kong to 32 countries. Effective infection control guidelines likely responsible for controlling the epidemic. Only 4 mini-outbreaks in 2004, 3/4 from research labs testing live virus (Science 304:1097, 2004); none reported so far in 2005 (7/05).	**Therapy remains predominantly supportive care.** (see Comments): **Ribavirin**—ineffective. Interferon alfa ± steroids—small case series. Pegylated interferon alfa effective in monkeys. Value of corticosteroids alone unclear. Inhaled nitric oxide improved oxygenation & improved chest x-ray (CID 39:1531, 2004).	Therapy tried or under evaluation Other coronaviruses (HCOV-229E, OC43, NL63, etc.) implicated as cause of croup, asthma exacerbations, & other RTIs in children (CID 40:1721, 2005; JID 191:492, 2005) may be associated with Kawasaki disease (JID 191:489, 2005).
Enterovirus—Meningitis: most common cause of aseptic meningitis. PCR on CSF valuable for early dx (Scand J Inf Dis 34:359, 2002) but ↓ sensitivity > 2 days of symptoms. PCR on feces pos. in 12/13 specimens, 5–16 days after clinical onset (CID 40:982, 2005).	**No rx currently recommended;** however, **pleconaril** (VP 63843) still under investigation. [For compassionate use call Viropharma (610) 458-7300; ext. 6297 [Donna Kolbush, RN]	No clinical benefit demonstrated in double-blind placebo-controlled study in 21 infants with enteroviral aseptic meningitis (PIDJ 22:335, 2003).

Hemorrhagic Fever Virus Infections: For excellent reviews, see Med Lab Observer, May 2005, p. 16, www.mlo-online.com and LnID 4:487, 2004

VIRUS/DISEASE	DRUG/DOSAGE	SIDE EFFECTS/COMMENTS
Congo-Crimean Hemorrhagic Fever (HF) (CID 39:284, 2004) Tickborne; symptoms include N/V, fever, headache, myalgias, & stupor (1/3). Signs: conjunctival injection, hepatomegaly, petechiae (1/3). Lab: ↓ platelets, ↓ WBC, ↑ ALT, AST, LDH & CPK (100%).	Oral **ribavirin. 30 mg per kg** as initial loading dose & 15 mg per kg q6h times 4 days & then 7.5 mg per kg times 6 days (WHO recommendation) (see Comment)	3/3 healthcare workers in Pakistan had complete recovery (Ln 346:472, 1995) & 61/69 (89%) with confirmed CCHF rx with ribavirin survived in Iran (CID 36:1613, 2003).
Ebola/Marburg HF (Central Africa) Severe outbreak in Angola, 308 cases with 277 deaths by 5/3/05 (NEJM 352:2155, 2005; LnID 5:331, 2005).	**No effective antiviral rx** (J Virol 77:9733, 2003).	An intense inflammatory response within 4 days after infection may control viral proliferation & result in asymptomatic infection (Ln 355:2210, 2000). Can infect gorillas & chimps that come in contact with other dead animal carcasses (Science 303:387, 2004). Bats also suspected (LnID 5:331, 2005).
With pulmonary syndrome: Hantavirus pulmonary syndrome, "sin nombre virus"	**No benefit from ribavirin has been demonstrated** (CID 39:1307, 2004).	Acute onset of fever, headache, myalgias, non-productive cough, thrombocytopenia and non-cardiogenic pulmonary edema with respiratory insufficiency following exposure to rodents.
With renal syndrome: Lassa, Venezuelan, Korean, HF, Sabia, Argentinian HF, Bolivian HF, Junin, Machupo	**Ribavirin** IV 2 gm loading dose, then 1 gm q6h times 4 days, then 0.5 gm q8h times 6 days (See Comment: Congo-Crimean HF)	Toxicity (mild, hemolysis reported but recovery when treatment stopped. No significant changes in WBC, platelets, hepatic or renal function. Effective in Lassa and in 2 cases of Bolivian HF (CID 24:718, 1997). No data on others. See CID 36:1254, 2003; for management of contacts.
Dengue and dengue hemorrhagic fever (DHF) (see AnIM 104:545, 2004) www.cdc.gov/ncidod/dvbid/dengue/dengue-hcp.htm Think dengue in traveler to tropics or subtropics (incubation period usually 4-7 days) with fever, bleeding, thrombocytopenia, and hemoconcentration with shock. Dx by viral isolation or serology serum to CDC. (telephone 787-706-2399).	**No data on antiviral rx.** Fluid replacement with careful hemodynamic monitoring critical. For **DHF** with colloids may be more effective than crystalloids in pts with low pulse pressures (J Ped 140: 629, 2002).	Of 77 cases dx at CDC (2001-2004), recent (2-wk) travel to Caribbean island 39%, Asia 17%, Central America 15%, S. America 15% (MMWR 54:556, June 10, 2005). 5 pts with severe **DHF** rx with dengue antibody neg. gamma globulin 500 mg per kg q24h IV for 3-5 days; rapid ↑ in platelet count (Transpl Inf Dis 4:160, 2003).
West Nile virus (see AnIM 104:545, 2004) A flavivirus transmitted by mosquitoes, blood transfusions, transplanted organs (NEJM 348: 2196, 2003; CID 38:1257, 2004), & breast-feeding (MMWR 51:877, 2002). Birds (>200 species) are main host in man & horses incidental hosts. Usually nonspecific febrile disease but 1/150 cases develops meningo-encephalitis, aseptic meningitis or polio-like paralysis (AnIM 104:545, 2004; JCI 113: 1102, 2004). Longterm sequelae (neuromuscular weakness & psychiatric) common (IDCP 13:101, 2005).	**No proven rx to date.** 2 clinical trials in progress: (1) Interferon alfa-N3 (CID 40:764, 2005). See www.nyha.org/posting/rahal.html (2) IVIG from Israel with high titer antibody West Nile (JID 188:5, 2003; Transpl Inf Dis 4:160, 2003). Contact NIH, 301-496-7453; see www.clinicaltrials.gov/show/NCT00068055.	Dx by ↑ IgM in serum & CSF or CSF PCR (contact State Health Dept./ CDC). Blood supply now tested in U.S. ↑ serum lipase in 11/17 cases (NEJM 352:420, 2005).
Yellow fever		Reemergence in Africa & South America. Vaccination effective. (JAMA 276:1157,1996)
Hepatitis Viral Infections		
Hepatitis A (Ln 351:1643, 1998)	No therapy recommended. If within 2 wks of exposure, IVIG 0.02 mL per kg IM times 1 protective.	Vaccine recommendations in Table 20. Coverage of only 50% in states that recommend Hep A vaccination (MMWR 54:1141, 2005). 40% of pts with chronic Hep C who developed superinfection with Hep A developed fulminant hepatic failure (NEJM 338:286, 1998).

* See page 2 for abbreviations. NOTE: All dosage recommendations are for adults (unless otherwise indicated) and assume normal renal function.
Costs from 2005 DRUG TOPICS RED BOOK, Medical Economics. Price is average wholesale price (AWP).

VIRUS/DISEASE	DRUG/DOSAGE	SIDE EFFECTS/COMMENTS
Hepatitis Viral Infections (continued)		
Hepatitis B		
Acute	No therapy recommended	Most common cause of death from acute hepatitis in Italy (Dig Liver Dis 35:404, 2003). Screen for HIV.
Chronic	Data on treatment changing rapidly. 4 approved options now approved & available—no	**Goal of rx:** ↓ liver inflammation; stop progression of cirrhosis & prevent hepato-
HBeAg+:	consensus on initial rx, but guidelines consider all equivalent.	cellular carcinoma. For all drugs listed, ideal response:
Consider rx if:	• **Lamivudine** (LAV) 100 mg po q24h until HBsAg seroconversion. If hepatitis flare or persistent viral load elevation (NEJM 351:1521, 2004),	↓ plasma HB DNA to <20,000 copies/ml;
(1) Persistent ↑ ALT/AST	switch to ENT or ADF. Don't use for first-line rx in cirrhotics: ↑ clinical breakthrough	Normal ALT/AST;
(2) HBsAg positive	with resistance & hepatitis flares.	HBsAg to anti-HBs;
(3) HBV DNA plasma "viral	• **Entecavir** (ENT) 0.5 mg po fasting q24h. If previous LAV treatment or known	HBeAg to anti-HBe.
load" >10⁵ copies/mL; if	YMDD mutation, use 1 mg q24h. Treat 1 year or min. 6 mos. after seroconversion.	**Combination rx:** e.g. PEG alfa-2a + LAV disappointing (NEJM 352:26, 2005;
>10⁴–<10⁵ copies/mL, no rx	• **Adefovir** (ADF) 10 mg po q24h. For HBeAg(+), treat 1 year or min. 6 mos. & recheck HBeAg;	AnIM 142:240, 2005).
unless active inflammation/	for HBeAg(−), treat ≥1 year. 6 mos. after seroconversion or indefinitely.	**Specific drug comments** (side-effects & cost in Table 14B):
fibrosis on biopsy. <10⁴, no	• Another option: (**Tenofovir** 300 mg + **emtricitabine** 200 mg) as Truvada^[NFDA] 1	**LAV:** Non-toxic. YMDD mutants less virulent than wild type. Sustained viral
rx.	tab po q24h looks promising, but don't use alone in HIV co-infected patients.	response (SVR) if initial ALT >2x normal is 65% at 3 yrs (J Viral Hep 9:208, 2002).
HBeAg−: Rx indefinitely;	• **PEG IFN alfa-2a** 180 mcg subcut. OR **PEG IFN alfa-2b** 1.5 mcg per kg once	**ENT.** Min. toxicity. Active vs YMDD mutants & ADV-resistant strains.
consult specialist!	weekly times at least 1 year OR	**ADV.** Effective vs YMDD mutant strains.
Refs: NEJM 350:1118, 2004;	**Interferon alfa-2b** 10 million units 3 times per week or 5 million units q24h subcut.	**Interferon:** PEG IFN 2 times more effective than standard IFN (J Viral Hep
Clin Gastro & Hep 2:87, 2004	for 16–24 weeks. Don't use IFNs in cirrhosis or decompensated liver dis-	10:298, 2003) & more effective than LAV for HBeAg(−) pts (NEJM 351:1206,
	eases—hepatitis flares common & associated with further decompensation.	2004). Genotypes A & B respond better (40–50%) than C & D (25–30%).
"Prevention of re-infection after	**Lamivudine** 100 mg q24h from 4 wks pre-transplant to 12 wks post-transplant.	Based on uncontrolled studies: Hpt 30:2224, 1999; J Hpt 34:888 & 895, 2001.
liver transplant for Hepatitis B		Some add HBIG (Hpt 28:585, 1998).
Hepatitis C (up to 3% of world infected. 4 million in U.S., 36,000 new cases annually). Co-infection with HIV common—see Sanford Guide to HIV/AIDS Therapy. See AnIM 136:747, 2002; www.va.gov/hepatitis; www.hepnet.com/hepc.html		
Acute	Follow plasma HCV viral load by PCR:	Sustained viral response with IFN alfa-2b therapy 32% vs 4% with placebo. P
Usually asymptomatic (>75%). Can detect by	If clear within 3–4 mos., no treatment.	0.00007 (Cochrane Database Sys & Rev CD000369, 2002).
PCR within 13 days; antibody in 36 or more	If persists: PEG IFN ± ribavirin as below, albeit controversial	
days (JID 189:3, 2004; CID 40:951, 2005).	(NEJM 346:1091, 2002).	
Chronic: www.va.gov/hepatitis; Sem Liver Dis 23(Suppl.1):35, 2003; AASLD/IDSA Guidelines: Hpt 39:1147, 2004		
	Treat if: persistent elevated ALT/AST, pos. HCV plasma viral load, fibrosis &/or inflammation on biopsy.	In U.S., 90% due to genotype 1. Sustained viral response
		(SVR) to 48-wk rx of genotype 1 42–51%. SVR to 24-wk rx of
Genotypes 1 & 4		**Pegylated interferon**			**+**		**Ribavirin**		genotype 2 or 3 76–82%.
AnIM 140:346, 2004	PEG IFN: Either alfa-2a (Pegasys) 180 mcg subcut. once			HIV accelerates HCV disease.
	weekly OR					**Weight**	**Ribavirin Dose**	Avoid alcohol—accelerates HCV disease
	Alfa-2b (PEG-INTRON) 1.5 mcg per kg subcut. once weekly				<75 Kg	400 mg a.m. & 600 mg p.m.	See Table 14B for drug adverse effects & cost. Interferon alfa
					>75 Kg	600 mg a.m. & 600 mg p.m.	can cause serious depression.
	Monitor response by quantification:						Ribavirin is teratogenic & has dose-related hematologic
		HCV RNA		**Result**			**Action**	toxicity.
	After 4 wks rx:	<1 log ↓					Discontinue therapy	For drugs in development, see Hepatol Res, July 12, 2005.
		<2 log ↓					Discontinue therapy	For genotypes 2 & 3, some use standard IFN; results similar &
	After 12 wks rx:	>2 log ↓ or undetectable					Treat 48 wks	↓ cost.
Genotype 2 or 3	PEG IFN alfa-2a or 2b—**dose as for types 1 & 4 above** + **Ribavirin 400** mg po bid						
		Quant. HCV RNA		**Result**			**Action**	
	After 4 wks rx:	Undetectable					Treat 12 wks (NEJM 352:2609, 2005)	
		>1 log ↓					Treat 24 wks	
For prevention of acute and chronic infection, see Table 15D, page 128		

* See page 2 for abbreviations. NOTE: All dosage recommendations are for adults (unless otherwise indicated) and assume normal renal function.
Costs from 2005 Drug Topics Red Book, Medical Economics. Price is average wholesale price (AWP).

TABLE 14A (3)

VIRUS/DISEASE	DRUG/DOSAGE	SIDE EFFECTS/COMMENTS
Herpesvirus Infections (see review: CID 26:541, 1998)		
Cytomegalovirus (CMV)		
Normal host	No rx for acute mononucleosis-like syndrome and not established for congenital CMV (Sem Ped Inf Dis 16:50, 2005). Colitis reported in 44 immunocompetent pts with ↑ mortality in elderly (Dig Dis Sci 50:609, 2005).	
Immunocompromised host	**Treatment of AIDS patients with highly active antiretroviral therapy (HAART) is effective in reducing mortality in pts with CMV infection by 81%** (CID 37: 1365, 2003) **and in suppressing CMV viremia** (AIDS 13:1203, 1999). Monitoring CMV DNA of value in organ transplant pts; CMV DNA level >13 ng per mL correlated with active infection (JID 166:829, 2002). Pos. CMV DNA by PCR independent predictor of death in AIDS pts even in HAART era (JAIDS 38:538, 2005).	
Colitis/esophagitis Consider in transplant & AIDS pts with dysphagia & retrosternal pain (Dig Dis Sci 50:609, 2005).	**Ganciclovir** as with retinitis except induction period extended for 3–6 wks. No agreement on use of maintenance (ArIM 158:957, 1998). Responses less predictable than for retinitis (AJM 98:109, 1995). **Foscarnet** 90 mg per kg q12h effective in 9/10 pts (AAC 41:1226, 1997). **Valganciclovir also likely effective.** Switch to oral valganciclovir when po tolerated.	
CMV of the nervous system: Encephalitis & ventriculitis. Treatment not defined, but disease develops while taking ganciclovir as suppressive therapy.		
Lumbosacral poly-radiculopathy	**Ganciclovir,** as with retinitis. Consider combination of ganciclovir and foscarnet if prior CMV rx used. Switch to valganciclovir when possible.	About 50% will respond (CID 20:747, 1995); survival ↑ (5.4 wks to 14.6 wks) (CID 27:345, 1998).
Mononeuritis multiplex	Not defined	Due to vasculitis and may not be responsive to antiviral rx (AnNeurol 29:139, 1991).
CMV pneumonia—predominantly transplants, rare in HIV	**Ganciclovir** 5 mg per kg IV q12h times 3 wks followed by maintenance valganciclovir 900 mg po q24h or ganciclovir 5 mg per kg IV q24h	In BMT recipients, serial measure of CMV interstitial pneumonia; good results if GCV initiated within 6 days of antigen positivity (Bone Marrow Transplant 26:413, 2000). For preventive therapy, see Table 15E, page 131.
Retinitis (most common in AIDS) Differential dx: HIV retinopathy, herpes simplex retinitis, varicella-zoster retinitis (rare, hard to diagnose) (Ophthal 111:1326, 2004). Marked reduction in CMV associated mortality with HAART plus anti-CMV therapy (CID 37: 1365, 2003; Ophthalmology 112:771, 2005). 33–63% with inactive CMV retinitis who responded to HAART (↑ of ≥60 CD4 cells per mL) devel. immune recovery vitritis (vision ↓ & floaters — with posterior segment inflammation—vitreitis, papillitis & macular changes) an avg. of 43 wks after rx started (JID 179:697, 1999; JID CID 14: 1163, 2000; CID 36:1063, 2003). Continued ophthalmologic follow-up needed. Corticosteroid rx ↓ inflammatory reaction of immune recovery vitritis without reactivation of CMV retinitis (5th CRV, Abst.751).	**Induction therapy, primary. Valganciclovir** (GCV) 5 mg per kg IV q12h times 21 days **OR ganciclovir** (GCV) 5 mg per kg IV q12h (adjust for renal function) times 14–21 days **OR foscarnet** (FOS) 90 mg per kg IV q12h (adjust for renal function) at constant rate (requires infusion pump) over minimum of 1 hr times 14–21 days **OR** combination of **intraocular ganciclovir (GCV) implant** (delivers 1–2 mcg per hr times 6–7 mos.) + (either concomitant **IV GCV** 5 mg per kg IV q24h or **oral valganciclovir** 900 mg q24h with food). **Induction therapy, alternative: Cidofovir** 5 mg per kg IV q week times 2 wks with **probenecid** (2 gm po 3 hrs before cidofovir dose, 1 gm 2 hrs immediately after dose, and 1 gm 8 hrs after dose) and 1 liter of normal saline IV 1 hr before cidofovir infusion (J AIDS & HR 17:339, 1998; Blood 97:388, 2001) **OR** for pts who fail monotherapy with GCV or FOS, consider combination rx with both: (1) **GCV** 5 mg per kg q12h or q24h IV and (2) **FOS** 90 mg per kg q12h up to total of 125 mg per kg q24h IV. **Suppression** (maintenance therapy): See CID 28:534, 1999. With immune reconstitution from response to HAART. USPHS/IDSA guidelines recommend suppressive rx may be dc if **CD4 >100 per mm³ after 6 mos of HAART**(see www.aidsinfo.nih.gov for guidelines) and retinitis inactive.	**Alternative:** Combination of **GCV intraocular implant of 6 mos. + valganciclovir** 900 mg q24h **OR cidofovir** 5 mg per kg IV q2 wks + probenecid & hydration (as above under induction rx)

Cannot use GCV ocular implant as approx. 50% risk of CMV retinitis in other eye at 6 mos. & 31% risk visceral disease. Risk ↓ with systemic rx (NEJM 337:83, 1997). Similarly, intraocular injections of fomivirsen will not prevent contralateral eye or systemic/visceral disease (Am J Ophth 133:467, 475, 484, 552, 2002). **Concurrent systemic rx recommended!** Intravitreal foscarnet used in Thailand in 193 AIDS pts with 66% either improved or stabilized but 35% developed vitreitis in the other eye (J Med Assoc Thai 88:103, 2005).

Watch for retinal detachments; 50–60% within 1 yr of dx of retinitis.
Equal efficacy of IV GCV & FOS. GCV avoids nephrotoxicity of FOS; FOS avoids bone marrow suppression of GCV. **Oral valganciclovir should replace both.** Emergence of resistance to GCV & valganciclovir minimal even with prophylactic use (JID 189:1615, 2004; AAC 49:873, 2005).

Reports indicate success of combination rx with GCV at 5 mg per kg q24h & FOS up to 125 mg per kg per day for GCV-resistant isolates in solid organ transplants (CID 34:1337, 2002). Hypomagnesemia common complication. Valganciclovir 900 mg q24h has similar efficacy (17% progressed over 1 year) & toxicity profile as IV ganciclovir but with fewer IV-related events (JAIDS 30:392, 2002). |
| **EBV—Mononucleosis** (Ln ID 3:131, 2003) | **No treatment** Corticosteroids for tonsillar obstruction or CNS complications. | (See JAC 56:277, 2005 for current status of drugs in development.) |

CMV in transplant patients: The prevention and management of CMV infections in transplant pts is beyond the scope of this Guide. Use of valganciclovir to prevent infections in CMV seronegative recipients who receive organs from a seropositive donor & in seropositive receivers has been highly effective (Ln 365:2105, 2005). Others suggest preemptive rx when pt develops CMV antigenemia post-transplant (Transplant 79:85, 2005).

* See page 2 for abbreviations. NOTE: All dosage recommendations are for adults (unless otherwise indicated) and assume normal renal function.

TABLE 14A (4)

VIRUS/DISEASE	DRUG/DOSAGE	SIDE EFFECTS/COMMENTS
Herpesvirus Infections *(continued)*		
HHV-6—Implicated as cause of roseola (exanthem subitum) & other febrile diseases of childhood *(NEJM 352:768, 2005)*. Fever & rash documented in transplant pts *(JID 179:311, 1999)*. Reactivation in 47% of 110 U.S. HSCT pts assoc. with delayed monocytes & platelet engraftment *(CID 40:932, 2005)*. Recognized in assoc. with meningoencephalitis in immunocompetent adults. Dx made by pos. PCR in CSF ↓ viral copies in response to **ganciclovir** rx *(CID 40:890 & 894, 2005)*. Foscarnet rx improved thrombotic microangiopathy *(Am J Hematol 76:156, 2004)*.		
HHV-7—ubiquitous virus (>90% of the population is infected by age 3 yrs). No relationship to human disease. Infects CD4 lymphocytes via CD4 receptor, transmitted via saliva.		
HHV-8—The agent of Kaposi's sarcoma, Castleman's disease, & body cavity lymphoma	**No antiviral treatment.** Effective anti-HIV rx may help.	Localized lesions: radiotherapy, laser surgery or intralesional chemotherapy. Systemic: chemotherapy. Castleman's disease responded to ganciclovir *(Blood 103:1632, 2004)*. Valganciclovir reduced HHV8 replication in saliva by 79% vs placebo *(IDSA 2005, Abst. 0066)*
Herpes simplex virus (HSV Types 1 & 2) *(See Ln 357:1513, 2001 & CID Suppl. 39:S237, 2004 for x HSV in HIV-infected persons)*		
Bell's palsy (May also be caused by H. zoster, Lyme disease. HHV-6) *(CID 30:529, 2000)*	Either **[Acyclovir** (400 mg) po 5 times per day for 10 days] with or without **[prednisone** po (30 mg bid or 1 mg per kg daily dose given bid times 5 days, then taper to 5 mg bid and dc after total of 10 days)] **or rx.**	99 pts with symptoms <3 days had better recovery and less neural degeneration when rx with acyclovir + prednisone compared to prednisone alone *(Ann Oto/Rhino/Laryngol 105:371, 1996)*, but another study was inconclusive. More data needed *(Cochrane Database Syst Rev 2004:CD001869, 2004)*. Surgical decompression within 14 days of symptoms controversial *(NEJM 352:416, 2005)*. If caused by VZV, acyclovir may help *(PID 21:615, 2002)*.
Encephalitis (Excellent reviews: CID 35: 254, 2002) UK experience (EID 9:234, 2003) & Eur J Neurol 12:331, 2005)	**Acyclovir** IV 10 mg per kg IV (infuse over 1 hr) q8h times 14–21 days. Up to 20 mg per kg q8h in children <12 yrs	HSV-1 is most common cause of sporadic encephalitis. Survival & recovery from neurological sequelae are related to mental status at time of initiation of rx. **Early dx and rx imperative**. Mortality rate reduced from >70% to 19% with acyclovir rx. PCR analysis of CSF for HSV-1 DNA is 100% specific & 75–98% sensitive. 8/33 (25%) CSF samples drawn before day 3 were neg. by PCR; neg. PCR assoc. with ↓ protein & <10 WBC per mm³ in CSF *(CID 36:1335, 2003)*. All were + after 3 days. Relapse after successful rx reported in 7/27 (27%) children. Relapse was associated with a lower total dose of initial acyclovir (285 ± 82 mg per kg in relapse group vs. 462 ± 149 mg per kg, p <0.03) *(CID 30:185, 2000; Neuropediatrics 35:371, 2004)*.
Genital, immunocompetent: Emerging problem in adolescents *(Sem in Ped In Dis 16:24, 2005)*. ACOG guidelines for management: *Ob Gyn 104:1111, 2004*. Recommendations from International Herpes Management Forum, *Herpes 12:15, 2005*		
Primary (initial episode) See excellent reviews: *NEJM 350:1970, 2004 & AnIM 137:257, 2002 or CDC 2002 Guidelines*	**Acyclovir** (Zovirax or generic) 400 mg po tid times 7–10 days (FDA-approved dosage is 200 mg po 5 times per day times 10 days). (NB $150 per course). **OR** **Valacyclovir** (Valtrex) 1000 mg po bid times 10 days (~$90 per course) **OR** **Famciclovir** (Famvir) 250 mg po tid times 7–10 days (not FDA-approved for this indication) ($97–139 per course).	↓ by 2 days time to resolution of signs & symptoms, ↓ by 4 days time to healing of lesions, ↓ by 7 days duration of viral shedding. Does not prevent recurrences. For severe cases only: 5 mg per kg IV q8h times 5–7 days. An ester of acyclovir, which is well absorbed, bioavailability 3–5 times greater than acyclovir. Found to be **equal to acyclovir**. *(Sex Trans Dis 24:481, 1997)*. Metabolized to penciclovir, which is active component. Side effects and activity similar to acyclovir. Famciclovir 250 mg po tid found to be **equal to acyclovir** 200 mg 5 times per day.
Episodic recurrences	**Acyclovir** 400 mg po tid **times 5 days** or 800 mg po tid **times 2 days** **or** **famciclovir** 125 mg po bid **times 5 days** or **valacyclovir** 500 mg po bid **times 3 days**	All effective with few differences. Choice can be made on basis of cost & convenience. Trend is to ↓ duration of rx. The 2-day course of acyclovir ↓ duration of episode & lesions from 6 to 4 days vs placebo, & viral shedding from 58 to 25 hrs *(CID 34:944, 2002)*. The 3-day course of valacyclovir was equivalent to 5 days, duration of episode & lesions 4.4 days *(CID 34:958, 2002)*.
Chronic suppression *(JAMA 280:928, 1998; JID 178:603, 1998)* Decision to rx arbitrary, but rx sig. improves quality of life over 1 yr *(Sex Trans Infect 75:398, 1999)*.	**Suppressive rx reduces the frequency of genital herpes recurrences by 70–80% among pts who have frequent recurrences (i.e., >6 recurrences per yr) & many report no symptomatic outbreaks** *(MMWR 51:RR-6, 2002)*. **Acyclovir** 400 mg po bid (cost per yr $2993), **or famciclovir** 250 mg po bid times 7–10 days **or valacyclovir** 1 gm po q24h (if $3268 per yr); for pts with <9 recurrences per yr, use 500 mg po q24h ($1825 per yr). May use 1 gm po q24h if breakthrough at lower dose.	All suppress subclinical HSV-2 shedding between episodes of active disease. Vala = acyclovir in 69 immunocompetent pts & sig. better than placebo in double-blind crossover study *(JID 190:1374, 2004)*. Drug resistance unlikely to develop with ↑ use: 0.2% after 20 yrs of use in immunocompetent pts *(J Clin Virol 32:7, 2005)*. However, in immunocompromised pts (HIV+ & BMT) 6–7% HSV are resistant *(CID 39S:248, 2004)*. Suppressive rx could also ↓ HIV transmission *(JID 191:5107, 2005)*. Since 2/3 of pts demonstrate ↓ in recurrences between yrs 1 & 5, daily suppressive rx should be reassessed periodically, and after 3–5 yrs, episodic rx may become more practical *(AnIM 131:14, 1999)*. Rarely failure of suppression in immunocompetent could indicate resistant virus *(JID 192:156, 2005; CID 41:320, 2005)*.
Gingivostomatitis, primary (children)	**Acyclovir** 15 mg per kg po 5 times per day times 7 days	Efficacy demonstrated in randomized placebo-controlled trial *(BMJ 314:1800, 1997)*.
Kerato-conjunctivitis and recurrent epithelial keratitis	**Trifluridine** (Viroptic), 1 drop 1% solution q2h (max. 9 drops per day) for max. of 21 days *(Ln 363:1772, 2004)*	In controlled trials, response % = idoxuridine. Suppressive rx with acyclovir (400 mg bid) reduced recurrences of ocular HSV from 32% to 19% over 12-month period *(NEJM 339:300, 1998)*
Mollaret's recurrent "aseptic" meningitis (usually HSV-2)	No controlled trials of antiviral rx & resolves spontaneously. In severe cases, IV or po acyclovir or valacyclovir or famciclovir recommended	Pos. PCR for HSV in CSF confirms dx *(EJCMID 23:560, 2004)*. Daily suppression rx might ↓ frequency of recurrence but no clinical trials.

* See page 2 for abbreviations. NOTE: All dosage recommendations are for adults (unless otherwise indicated) and assume normal renal function.
Costs from 2005 DRUG TOPICS RED BOOK, Medical Economics. Price is average wholesale price (AWP).

TABLE 14A (5)

VIRUS/DISEASE	DRUG/DOSAGE	SIDE EFFECTS/COMMENTS

Herpesvirus Infections/Herpes Simplex Virus (HSV Types 1 & 2) *(continued)*

Mucocutaneous

Oral labial, "fever blisters":
Normal host
See AnPharmacotherapy 38:705, 2004; JAC 53:703, 2004

Start rx with prodrome symptoms ((tingling or burning) before lesions appear.

Drug	Dose	Cost	Duration Sx
Oral: Valacyclovir[1]	2 gm po q12h times 1 day	$36	↓ 1 day
Famciclovir[1]	500 mg po bid times 7 days	$123	↓ 2 days
Acyclovir[NFDA]	400 mg po 5 times per day (q4h while awake) times 5 days	$19 (generic)	↓ ½ day

Topical:			
Penciclovir 1% cream	q2h during day times 4 days	$25	↓ 1 day
Docosanol 10% cream	5 times per day until healed	$14	↓ ½ day
Acyclovir 5% cream[2]	6 times per day (q3h) times 7 days	$37 per 2 gm / $86 per 5 gm	↓ ½ day

Penciclovir (*J Derm Treat 13:67, 2002; JAMA 277:1374, 1997; AAC 46: 2848, 2002*). Docosanol (*J Am Acad Derm 45:222, 2001*). Oral acyclovir 5% cream (*AAC 46:2238, 2002*). Oral famciclovir (*JID 179:303, 1999*). Topical fluocinonide (0.05% Lidex gel) q8h times 5 days in combination with famciclovir ↓ lesion size and pain when compared to famciclovir alone (*JID 181:1906, 2000*).

[1] FDA approved only HIV; [2] Approved for immunocompromised
See Table 1, page 21

Oral labial or genital:
Immunocompromised (includes pts with AIDS) and critically ill pts in ICU setting
(See Comment)

Acyclovir 5 mg per kg IV (infused over 1 hr) q8h times 7 days (250 mg per M²) or 400 mg po 5 times per day times 14–21 days (*see Comment if suspect acyclovir-resistant*) **OR Famciclovir:** in HIV infected, 500 mg po bid for 7 days for recurrent episodes of genital herpes **OR Valacyclovir:** in HIV-infected, 500 mg po bid for 5–10 days for recurrent episodes of genital herpes or 500 mg po bid for chronic suppressive rx.

Acyclovir-resistant HSV occurs, esp. in large ulcers. Most will respond to **IV foscarnet**, but recur after drug discontinued [median 6 weeks (*NEJM 325.551, 1991*)]. Suppressive rx with famciclovir (500 mg po bid) reduced viral shedding and clinical recurrences (total days with lesions 18% vs 5%) in HIV-infected pts (*AnIM 128:21, 1998*), similar to findings with acyclovir & valacyclovir 500 mg po bid [at 6 mos. 65% of vala-rx were recurrence-free vs 26% of placebo-rx (*JID 188:1009, 2003*)]. Cidofovir (topical) has been used with moderate success (*JID 176:892, 1997*).

Herpes Whitlow

Perinatal (genital in pregnancy at delivery)

In 25% HSV reactivated in last month of pregnancy. Infant exposure to primary lesion 50% risk, if recurrent lesion 4%. 50% mortality in infected neonates. If visible genital lesion, deliver by **C-section**, regardless of duration of membrane rupture. If no lesions or symptoms, vaginal delivery. Routine HSV cultures no longer recommended. **Acyclovir** useful in dose of 10 mg per kg (20 mg per kg if premature) q8h times 10–21 days IV (*PIDJ 14:827, 1995; NEJM 337:509, 1997*).

Herpes simiae—Monkey bite (Herpes B virus)
CID 35:1191, 2002

Postexposure prophylaxis: Valacyclovir 1 gm po q8h times 14 days or acyclovir 800 mg po 5 times per day times 14 days.
Treatment of disease: (1) CNS symptoms absent: Acyclovir 12.5–15 mg per kg IV q8h or ganciclovir 5 mg per kg IV q12h. (2) CNS symptoms present: Ganciclovir 5 mg per kg IV q12h

Fatal human cases of myelitis and hemorrhagic encephalitis have been reported following bites, scratches, or eye inoculation of saliva from monkeys. Initial sx include fever, headache, myalgias and diffuse adenopathy, incubation period of 2–14 days (*EID 9:246, 2003*)

Herpes Varicella-Zoster Virus (VZV)

Varicella: Vaccination has markedly ↓ incidence of varicella & morbidity (*NEJM 352:450, 2005*). Our understanding of the disease still undeveloped (*COID 18:235, 2005*).

Normal host (chickenpox)
Child (2–12 years)

Rx not recommended by American Academy of Pediatrics. Oral acyclovir recommended for healthy persons at ↑ risk for moderate to severe varicella, i.e., >12 yrs of age; chronic cutaneous or pulmonary diseases; chronic salicylate rx (↑ risk of Reye syndrome), use **acyclovir 20 mg per kg** po qid times 5 days (start within 24 hrs of rash).

Acyclovir slowed development and ↓ number of new lesions; duration of disease ↓ in children receiving acyclovir: 7.6 vs 9.0 days (*PIDJ 21:739, 2002*). Oral dose of acyclovir in children should not exceed 80 mg per kg per day or 3200 mg per day.

Adolescents, young adults

Acyclovir 800 mg po 5 times per day times 5–7 days (start within 24 hrs of rash) or **valacyclovir**[NFDA] 1000 mg po 3 times per day times 5 days). **Famciclovir**[NFDA] 500 mg po 3 times per day also probably effective but data lacking (*AnIM 130:922, 1999*).

↓ duration of fever, time to healing, and symptoms (*AnIM 117:358, 1992*).

Pneumonia or chickenpox in 3rd trimester of pregnancy

Acyclovir 800 mg po 5 times per day or 10 mg per kg IV q8h times 5 days. Risks and benefits to fetus and mother still unknown. Many experts recommend rx, especially in 3rd trimester. Some would add VZIG (varicella-zoster immune globulin).

Varicella pneumonia severe in pregnancy (41% mortality, *Ob Gyn 25:734, 1965*) and acyclovir ↓ incidence and severity (*JID 185:422, 2002*). If varicella-susceptible mother exposed and respiratory symptoms develop within 10 days after exposure, start acyclovir (*CCTID 13:123, 1993*). Acyclovir is pregnancy category B; no evidence of ↑ birth defects (*MMWR 42:806, 1993*). Disseminated 1° varicella infection reported during infliximab rx of rheumatoid arthritis (*J Rheum 31:2517, 2004*).

---

* See page 2 for abbreviations. NOTE: All dosage recommendations are for adults (unless otherwise indicated) and assume normal renal function. Costs from 2005 DRUG TOPICS RED BOOK, Medical Economics. Price is average wholesale price (AWP).

TABLE 14A (b)

VIRUS/DISEASE	DRUG/DOSAGE	SIDE EFFECTS/COMMENTS
Herpesvirus Infections/Herpes Varicella-Zoster Virus (VZV)/Varicella (continued)		
Immunocompromised host	**Acyclovir** 10–12 mg per kg IV (infused over 1 hr) q8h times 7 days (500 mg per M^2)	Continuous infusion of high-dose acyclovir (2 mg per kg per hr) successful in 1 pt with severe hemorrhagic varicella (NEJM 336:732, 1997). Mortality high (43%) in AIDS pts (Int J Inf Dis 6:6, 2002).
Prevention—Post-exposure prophylaxis Varicella was the leading cause of vaccine-preventable deaths in children in the U.S. Now markedly reduced with vaccine, but still deaths in unvaccinated (MMWR 54:272, 2005).	**CDC Recommendations for Prevention:** Since <5% of cases of varicella but >50% of varicella-related deaths occur in adults >20 yrs of age, the CDC recommends a more aggressive approach in this age group: **1st, varicella-zoster immune globulin (VZIG)** (125 units per 10 kg (22 lbs) body weight IM up to a max. of 625 units; minimum dose is 125 units) is recommended for post-exposure prophylaxis in susceptible persons at greater risk for complications (immunocompromised such as HIV, malignancies, pregnancy, and steroid rx) as soon as possible after exposure (<96 hrs). If varicella develops, initiate rx quickly (<24 hrs of rash) with **acyclovir** as below. Some would rx presumptively with acyclovir in high-risk pts. **2nd,** susceptible adults should be vaccinated. Check antibody in adults with negative or uncertain hx of varicella (10–30% will be Ab-neg) and vaccinate those who are Ab-neg. **3rd,** susceptible children should receive vaccination. Recommended routinely before age 12–18 mos. but OK at any age.	
Herpes zoster (shingles) (See NEJM 342:635, 2000 & 347:340, 2002)		
Normal host Effective rx most evident in pts >50 yrs. *(For rx of post-herpetic neuralgia, see CID 36: 877, 2003)* 25-fold ↓ in zoster after immunization (MMWR 48:R-6, 1999) New vaccine ↓ herpes zoster & post-herpetic neuralgia (NEJM 352: 2271, 2005).	[**NOTE: Trials showing benefit of rx: only in pts treated within 3 days of onset of rash**] **Valacyclovir** 1000 mg po tid times 7 days (adjust dose for renal failure). **OR** **Famciclovir** 750 mg po q24h or 500 mg bid or 250 mg 3 times per day times 7 days equal efficacy (J Clin Virol 29:248, 2004). Adjust for renal failure. (see Table 17). **OR** **Acyclovir** 800 mg po 5 times per day times 7–10 days [**Prednisone** 30 mg bid days 1–7, 15 mg bid days 8–14 and 7.5 mg bid days 15–21 also recommended by some authorities in pts >50 yrs of age (NEJM 335:32, 1996)] and especially when pt has large number of lesions (>21) and/or severe pain at presentation (JID 179:9, 1999)	Valacyclovir ↓ post-herpetic neuralgia more rapidly than acyclovir in pts >50 yrs of age: median duration of zoster-associated pain was 38 days with valacyclovir and 51 days on acyclovir (AAC 39:1546, 1995). Toxicity of both drugs similar (Arch Fam Med 9:863, 2000). Famciclovir similar to acyclovir in reduction of duration of PHN with famciclovir 63 days, placebo 163 days. Famciclovir similar to acyclovir in reduction of acute pain and PHN (J Micro Immunol Inf 37:75, 2004). A meta-analysis of 4 placebo-controlled trials (691 pts) demonstrated that acyclovir accelerated by approx. 2-fold pain resolution by all measures employed and reduced post-herpetic neuralgia at 3 & 6 mos (CID 22:347, 1996); med. time to resolution of pain 41 days vs 101 days in those >50 yrs. Prednisone added to acyclovir improved quality of life measurements (↓ acute pain, sleep, and return to normal activity) (AnIM 125:376, 1996). In post-herpetic neuralgia, controlled trials demonstrated effectiveness of gabapentin, the lidocaine patch (5%) & opioid analgesic in controlling pain (Drugs 64:937, 2004; J Clin Virol 29:248, 2004). Nortriptyline & amitriptyline are equally effective but nortriptyline is better tolerated (CID 36:877, 2004). Role of antiviral drugs in rx of PHN unproven (Neurol 64:21, 2005).
Immunocompromised host		
Not severe	**Acyclovir** 800 mg po 5 times per day times 7 days. (**Options: Famciclovir** 750 mg po q24h or 500 mg bid or 250 mg 3 times per day times 7 days **OR valacyclovir** 1000 mg po tid times 7 days, though both are not FDA-approved for this indication)	If progression, switch to IV
Severe: >1 dermatome, trigeminal nerve or disseminated	**Acyclovir** 10–12 mg per kg IV (infusion over 1 hr) q8h times 7–14 days. In older pts, ↓ to 7.5 mg per kg. If nephrotoxicity and pt improving, ↓ to 5 mg per kg q8h.	Acyclovir-resistant VZV occurs in 72 hrs. Acyclovir-resistant VZV occurs in HIV+ pts previously treated with acyclovir. Foscarnet (40 mg per kg q8h for 14–26 days) successful in 4/5 pts but 2 relapsed in 7 and 14 days (AnIM 115:19, 1991).
Influenza (A & B)	**If fever & cough; known community influenza activity; and 1st 48 hrs of illness, consider:**	Pts with COPD or asthma, **potential risk of bronchospasm with zanamivir.** Amantadine & rimantadine equally effective, but rimantadine ↓ side effects (Cochrane Database Sys Rev:CD 001169, 2004). All ↓ duration of symptoms by approx. 50% (1–2 pt days) if given within 30–36 hrs after onset of symptoms. Benefit influenced by duration of sx before rx: initiation of oseltamivir within 1st 12 hrs after fever onset ↓ total median illness duration by 74.6 hrs (JAC 51:123, 2003). ↓ risk of pneumonia (8% vs 2%) with oseltamivir (Curr Med Res Opin 21:761, 2005). **Disturbing report** of oseltamivir-resistant virus detected after 4 days of rx (Ln 364: 733 & 759, 2004). In another study of 298 rx cases of adults & children, no oseltamivir-resistant viruses found (JID 189:440, 2004). ↑ concern about post-influenza complications including community-acquired MRSA pneumonia (CID 40:1693, 2005).
Suspect or proven acute disease Rapid diagnostic tests available. Antiviral rx cost-effective without viral testing in febrile pt with typical symptoms during influenza season. Pathogenic avian influenza (H5N1) in poultry (mainly chickens & ducks) in East & Southeast Asia. As of Aug. 2005, 112 human cases reported with 57 deaths since Jan. 2004 (see www.cdc.gov/flu/avian). Human-to-human transmission reported (NEJM 352:333, 2005); most have had direct contact with poultry (NEJM 350:1179, 2004). Human isolates resistant to amantadine/rimantadine. Oseltamivir recommended if avian H5N1 suspected (MMWR 53:97, 2004). ↑ dose & duration of oseltamivir necessary for maximum effect in mouse model (JID 192:665, 2005; Nature 435:419, 2005). Consider flu in returning travelers from Asia, Africa, Latin America, & esp. India (CID 40:1282, 2005).	**For influenza A & B; also** **Oseltamivir** 75 mg po bid times 5 days (also approved for rx of children age 1–12 yrs, dose 2 mg per kg up to a total of 75 mg po bid times 5 days) or **Zanamivir** 2 inhalations (2 times 5 mg) bid times 5 days **For influenza A only: Rimantadine** or **amantadine**—Age— 1–9 yrs, 5 mg per kg per day to max. of 75 mg po bid; 10–65 yrs, 100 mg po bid; >65 yrs, 100 mg po q24h (adjust for ↓ renal function) for **3–5 days or 1–2 days after the disappearance of symptoms.**	A common manifestation of immune reconstitution following HAART in HIV-infected children (J All Clin Immun 113:742, 2004). Rx must be begun within 72 hrs.

* See page 2 for abbreviations. NOTE: All dosage recommendations are for adults (unless otherwise indicated) and assume normal renal function.
Costs from 2005 DRUG TOPICS RED BOOK, Medical Economics. Price is average wholesale price (AWP).

TABLE 14A (7)

VIRUS/DISEASE	DRUG/DOSAGE	SIDE EFFECTS/COMMENTS
Influenza (A & B) (continued) **Prevention:** See MMWR 54:RR-8:1, 2005	**Prevention of influenza A & B:** give vaccine and if ≥13 yrs age, consider **oseltamivir** 75 mg po q24h for duration of peak influenza in community or outbreak control in high-risk populations (CID 39:459, 2004). (Consider for similar populations as immunization recommendations.)	**Prevention of influenza A:** give vaccine followed by **rimantadine** or **amantadine** (dosages as above) for duration of influenza A activity in community or for outbreak control in high-risk populations (CID 39:459, 2004). (Consider for similar populations as immunization recommendations.)	Immunization contraindicated if hypersensitivity to hen's eggs. Both amantadine and rimantadine are about 60–90% effective against influenza A. Both oseltamivir and zanamivir reported efficacious (82 & 84% respectively) in clinical trials (JAMA 285:748, 2001; JID 186:1582, 2002). In families, rx of index case as well as contact cases was more effective than rx index case alone (p <0.01) (JID 189:440, 2004).
Measles Children	No therapy or **vitamin A** 200,000 units po times 2 days	Vitamin A ↓ severity of measles in one study (NEJM 323:160, 1990), not in others.
Adults	No rx or **ribavirin** IV (i) 20–35 mg per kg per day times 7 days	↓ severity of illness in adults (CID 20:454, 1994).
Metapneumovirus (HMPV) A paramyxovirus isolated from pts of all ages, with mild bronchiolitis/bronchospasm to pneumonia (PIDJ 23:S215, 2004).	**No proven antiviral therapy**	Human metapneumovirus isolated from 6.2% of children with respiratory infections (JID 190:20, 2004), 12% of children with lower respiratory infections (NEJM 350:443, 2004) & 21% of hospitalized children with URI (PIDJ 23:436, 2004; JID 190:27, 2004). Dual infection with RSV assoc. with severe bronchiolitis (JID 191:382, 2005).
Monkey pox (orthopox virus) (see LnID 4:17, 2004) In 2003, 72 pts contracted monkey pox from contact with ill prairie dogs. Source likely imported Gambian giant rats (MMWR 42:642, 2003).	**No proven antiviral therapy.** Cidofovir is active in vitro & in mouse model (AAC 46:1329, 2002; Antiviral Res 57:13, 2003).	Incubation period of 12 days, then fever, headache, cough, adenopathy, & a vesicular papular rash that pustulates, umbilicates, & crusts on the head, trunk, & extremities. Transmission in healthcare setting rare (CID 40:789, 2005).
Norovirus (Norwalk-like virus, or NLV) Caused 93% of outbreaks of non-bacterial gastroenteritis reported to CDC between 1997 & 2000. Transmission is by contaminated food, fecal-oral contact with contaminated surfaces, or fomites.	**No antiviral therapy.** Replete volume.	Sudden onset of nausea, vomiting, & watery diarrhea lasting 12–60 hours. Ethanol-based hand rubs effective against norovirus (J Hosp Inf 60:144, 2005).
Papillomaviruses. 81.7% of 60 adolescent females infected over 2.2 yrs (JID 191:182, 2005). Therapies unsatisfactory with limited efficacy, high recurrence rates & ↑ side-effects (JAC 53:137, 2004).
Anogenital Warts. Condyloma acuminatum (HPV types 6 & 11 most common but types 16 & 18 most likely premalignant) [See CID 28(Suppl.1):S37, 1999] [NOTE: Results of Pap smear should be available prior to rx; **avoid rx in pregnant women**] NOTE: Recurrences common after all treatments	**Podofilox** (Condylox) 2 times daily application with cotton swab for 3 days followed by 4 days without rx; repeat cycle 4–6 times as necessary **OR** [25% **podophyllin** in tincture of benzoin (Podocon-25): apply once weekly for up to 6 wks, wash after 1–4 hrs.] If no regression after 4 weekly applications, use alternate rx.	**Podofilox:** Local reactions—pain, burning, inflammation in 50%. No systemic effects. Efficacy in penile warts 74% vs placebo 8%. Recurrences 55% vs 100% with placebo. (Podocon-25 15 mL $32.40, Condylox 3.5 mL $56.64.) Warts recur in 1/3 with either agent within 1st month after rx.
	interferon alfa-2b (intron A), **alfa-n3** (Alferon N): 1 million units (0.1 mL) into lesion 3 times per week times 3 weeks intralesional injection of skin test antigens (mumps, candida or trichophyton) with or without interferon alfa-2b	**Painful; dilute to 10 million units per 1 mL.** Other concentrations are hypertonic (CID 28:S537, 1999). Use when other rx fails, esp. in AIDS. More effective than placebo in ↓ warts. IFN alfa-2b did not ↑ response rate & given alone, not better than saline placebo in one 235-pt randomized single-blind placebo-controlled trial (ArDerm 141:589, 2005). An in vitro positive monocyte proliferation assay to antigen predicted resolution of wart.
Warts occurred within 36 mos. after infection with HPV-16/18 in 64% (JID 119:731, 2005).	**imiquimod** (5% cream): Apply 3 times per week prior to sleep; remove 6–10 hrs later when awake. Continue until cleared or max. 16 wks.	Clearance rates of 52% vs 14% for controls if applied 3 times per wk overnight for up to 16 wks or until warts completely cured (AAC 42:789, 1998). Less effective in immunosuppressed pts: Benefit in 5/12 pts who completed 24-month course (Brit J Derm 152:122, 2005). Cost of 1–4 wks rx: $108–432.
Skin papillomas	**Topical α-lactalbumin. Oleic acid** (from human milk) applied daily for 3 wks	↓ lesion size & recurrence vs placebo (p <0.001) (NEJM 350:2663, 2004). Further studies warranted.
Parvo B19 Virus (Erythrovirus B19) Uncomplicated or self-limited acute arthritis. May be chronic in children.	See NEJM 350:586, 2004 **No treatment recommended**	Bone marrow shows selective erythrocyte maturation arrest with giant pronormoblasts. IgM antibody for diagnosis. Parvo B19 also associated with respiratory distress syndrome (CID 27:900, 1998) and myocarditis/myocardiopathy (CID 28:1343, 1999). One 14-year-old boy with chronic infection (fatigue, fever, rash) responded to high dose IVIG (PIDJ 24:272, 2005).
Acute profound anemia: in utero, in hemolytic anemia, in HIV	**IVIG** 0.4 gm per kg IV q24h times 5 days in immune def. states with severe anemia has been reported successful.	IVIG contains anti-parvo B19 antibody. Longterm remission reported (Transpl Inf Dis 7:30, 2005) in pts with pre-existing hemolytic anemia, parvo B19-induced bone marrow arrest can result in sudden severe anemia.

* See page 2 for abbreviations. NOTE: All dosage recommendations are for adults (unless otherwise indicated) and assume normal renal function.
Costs from 2005 Drug Topics Red Book, Medical Economics. Price is average wholesale price (AWP).

TABLE 14A (8)

VIRUS/DISEASE	DRUG/DOSAGE	SIDE EFFECTS/COMMENTS
Papovavirus/Polyomavirus		
Progressive multifocal leukoencephalopathy (PML)/JC virus) Pts with advanced HIV disease or organ transplant. Reported in 3 pts receiving natalizumab, a monoclonal antibody against alpha 4 integrins for Crohn's disease (1) & multiple sclerosis. (2) *(NEJM 353:353, 362 & 369, 2005)*	See *SANFORD GUIDE TO HIV/AIDS THERAPY*. **HAART** ↑ survival (545 days vs 60 days, p < 0.001) and either improved (50%) or stabilized (50%) neurological deficits in 12 pts *(AIDS 12: 2467, 1999)*. Others less optimistic *(CID 28: 1152, 1999)*.	Cytarabine of no value in controlled trial *(NEJM 338:1345, 1998)*. Camptothecin, a human topoisomerase I inhibitor, was administered to a single pt with slowing of progression *(Ln 349:1366, 1997)*. Use of cidofovir controversial *(Clin Micro Rev 16:569, 2003; J Child Neurol 19:35, 2004; Transpl Int 17:658, 2005)*. DC immunosuppression in transplant pts resulted in successful outcome *(Am J Transpl 5:1151, 2005)*.
Polyomavirus-associated nephropathy	Due to BK virus, post renal transplant	Possible rx role for **cidofovir** *(LnID 3:611, 2003)*.
Rabies *(see Table 20C, pages 144–145; see Mayo Clin Proc 79:671, 2004; MMWR 54-RR-3:1, 2005)* Rabid dogs account for 50,000 cases per yr worldwide. Most cases in the U.S. are cryptic, i.e., no documented evidence of bite or contact with a rabid animal *(CID 35:738, 2003)*. 70% assoc. with 2 rare bat species *(EID 9:151, 2003)*. An organ donor infected 4 recipients (2 kidneys, liver & artery) who all died of rabies avg. 13 days after transplant *(NEJM 352:1103, 2005)*.	**Mortality 100% with only survivors those who receive rabies vaccine before the onset of illness/symptoms** *(CID 36:61, 2003)*. A 15-year-old female who developed rabies 1 month post-bat bite survived after drug induction of coma (+ other rx) for 7 days; did not receive immunoprophylaxis *(NEJM 352:2508, 2005)*.	Corticosteroids ↑ mortality rate and ↓ incubation time in mice. Therapies that have failed after symptoms develop include rabies vaccine, rabies immunoglobulin, rabies virus neutralizing antibody, ribavirin, alfa interferon, & ketamine.
Respiratory Syncytial Virus Major cause of morbidity in neonates/infants. In adults, RSV accounted for 10.6% of hospitalizations for pneumonia, 11.4% for COPD, 7.2% for asthma & 5.4% for CHF in pts >65 yrs of age *(NEJM 352:1749, 2005)*. RSV caused 11% of clinically important respiratory illnesses in military recruits *(CID 41:311, 2005)*. **Prevention** (1) Children <24 mos. old with bronchopulmonary dysplasia (BPD) requiring supplemental O_2 (2) Perhaps premature infants (<26 wks gestation) and <6 mos. old at start of RSV season	Rapid dx by antigen detection on nasopharyngeal wash. **No rx proven to ↑ survival.** Various combinations of ribavirin, RSV-IVIG & palivizumab have been used; see *Comments (PIDJ 23:707, 2004; Pharmacother 24:932, 2004; Ped Drugs 6:177, 2004)*. **RSV immune globulin intravenous** (RSV-IVIG) 100 mg per kg IV once monthly Nov. through April (for northern hemisphere) 1st year of life for prematures. Perhaps up to 60 months of age for pts with BPD **OR** **Palivizumab** 15 mg per kg IM q month Nov.–April as above *(Scand J Inf Dis 33:323, 2001)*. Cost: $3000–5000/yr.	Ribavirin reported to ↓ fever and other symptoms and signs. However, in controlled studies, **ribavirin had no beneficial effect** *(J Ped 128: 422, 1996; AJRCCM 160:829, 1999)*. Still recommended by some authorities in immunocompromised children *(PIDJ 19:253, 2000)* & still controversial *(PIDJ 22:589, 2003)*. RSV–IVIG very expensive—estimated cost per infusion $1,175. See consensus opinion for details: *Ped Inf Dis J 15:1059, 1996. See Ln 354:847, 1999 for updated review.* Palivizumab reduced hospitalization rates for RSV in 1500 premature infants & children with chronic lung disease from 10.6% to 4.8% *(Pediatrics 102:531, 1998)*. Expense argues against its use, but in 2004 approx. 100,000 infants received drug annually in U.S. *(PIDJ 23:1051, 2004)*.
Rhinovirus (Colds) *See Ln 361:51, 2003* Found in ½ of children with community-acquired pneumonia; role in pathogenesis unclear *(CID 39:681, 2004)*. Antiviral Kleenex may reduce spread *(Med Lett 47:3, 2004)*	No antiviral rx indicated *(Ped Ann 34:53, 2005)*. Symptomatic rx: • ipratropium bromide nasal (2 sprays per nostril tid) • clemastine 1.34 mg 1–2 tab po bid-tid (OTC)	Sx relief: ipratropium nasal spray ↓ rhinorrhea and sneezing vs placebo *(AnIM 125:89, 1996)*. Clemastine (an anti-histamine) ↓ sneezing, rhinorrhea but associated with dry nose, mouth & throat in 6–19% *(CID 22:656, 1996)*. Zinc lozenges were ineffective *(CID 31:1202, 2000)*. Oral **pleconaril** given within 24 hrs of onset reduced duration (1 day) & severity of "cold symptoms" in DBPCT (p < .001) *(CID 36:1523, 2003)*. A combination of intranasal inter-feron alfa-2b, oral chlorpheniramine & ibuprofen ↓ symptom score by 33–73% vs placebo when started 24 hrs after intranasal rhinovirus *(JID 186:147, 2002)*. Echinacea didn't work *(CID 38:1367, 2004 & 40:807, 2005)*—put it to rest!
SARS-CoV. *See page 106*		
Smallpox *(NEJM 346:1300, 2002)* **Contact vaccinia** *(JAMA 288:1901, 2002)*	Smallpox vaccine (if within 4 days of exposure) + cidofovir (dosage uncertain); contact CDC: 770-488-7100) From vaccination: Progressive vaccinia—vaccinia immune globulin may be of benefit. To obtain immune globulin, contact CDC: 770-488-7100. *(CID 39:759, 776 & 819, 2004)*	
West Nile virus. *See page 106*		

---

* See page 2 for abbreviations. NOTE: All dosage recommendations are for adults (unless otherwise indicated) and assume normal/renal function. Costs from 2005 DRUG TOPICS RED BOOK, Medical Economics. Price is average wholesale price (AWP).

TABLE 14B: ANTIVIRAL DRUGS (Other Than Retroviral)

DRUG NAME(S) GENERIC (TRADE)	DOSAGE/ROUTE/COST*	COMMENTS/ADVERSE EFFECTS
CMV (See *SANFORD GUIDE TO HIV/AIDS THERAPY*)		
Cidofovir (Vistide)	5 mg per kg IV q week times 2, then q2 weeks. (375 mg $888). Properly timed IV prehydration with normal saline and oral probenecid **must be used with each cidofovir infusion** (see pkg insert for details). Renal function (serum creatinine and urine protein) must be monitored prior to each dose (see pkg insert for details).	**Adverse effects: Nephrotoxicity;** dose-dependent proximal tubular injury (Fanconi-like syndrome): proteinuria, glycosuria, bicarbonaturia, phosphaturia, polyuria (nephrogenic diabetic insipidus, *Ln 350:413, 1997*), ↑ creatinine. Concomitant saline prehydration, probenecid, extended dosing intervals allowed use. 25% of pts dc IV cidofovir due to nephrotoxicity. Other toxicities: nausea 48%, fever 31%, alopecia 16%, myalgia 16%, neutropenia 29%. No effect on hematocrit, platelets, LFTs. **Comment:** Recommended dosage, frequency or infusion rate must not be exceeded. Dose must be reduced or discontinued if changes in renal function occur during rx. For ↑ of 0.3–0.4 mg per dL in serum creatinine, cidofovir dose must be ↓ from 5 to 3 mg per kg; discontinue cidofovir if ↑ of 0.5 mg per dL above baseline or 3+ proteinuria develops (for 2+ proteinuria, observe pts carefully and consider discontinuation).
Foscarnet (Foscavir)	90 mg per kg IV q12h (induction) 90 mg per kg q24h (maintenance) Dosage adjust. with renal dysfunction (see Table 17) (6 gm $83)	**Adverse effects: Major clinical toxicity is renal impairment (1/3 of patients)**—↑ creatinine, proteinuria, nephrogenic diabetes insipidus, ↓ K+, ↓ Ca++ → ↑ Ca++, ↓ Mg++. Toxicity ↑ with other nephrotoxic drugs [ampho B, aminoglycosides or pentamidine (especially severe ↓ Ca++)]. Adequate hydration may ↓ toxicity. Other: headache, mild (100%), fatigue (100%); nausea (80%), fever (25%). CNS: seizures. Hematol: ↓ WBC, ↓ Hgb. Hepatic: liver function tests ↑. Neuropathy. Penile ulcers.
Ganciclovir (Cytovene)	IV: 5 mg per kg q12h times 14 days (induction) 5 mg per kg IV q24h or 6 mg per kg 5 times per wk (maintenance) Dosage adjust. with renal dysfunction (see Table 17) (500 mg IV $45) Oral: 1.0 gm tid with food (fatty meal) (500 mg $9.60)	**Adverse effects:** Absolute neutrophil count dropped below 500 per mm³ in 15%, thrombocytopenia 21%, anemia 6%. Fever 48%. GI 50%: nausea, vomiting, diarrhea, abdominal pain 19%, rash 10%. Retinal detachment 11% (relationship to ganciclovir ?). Confusion, headache, psychiatric disturbances and seizures. Neutropenia may respond to granulocyte colony stimulating factor (G-CSF or GM-CSF). Severe myelosuppression may be ↑ with coadministration of zidovudine or azathioprine. 32% dc/interrupted rx, principally for neutropenia. Hematologic less frequent than with IV. Granulocytopenia 18%, anemia 12%, thrombocytopenia 6%. GI, skin same as with IV. Retinal detachment 8%.
Ganciclovir (Vitrasert)	intraocular implant (~$5000 per device + cost of surgery).	**Adverse effects:** Late retinal detachment (7/30 eyes). Does not prevent CMV retinitis in good eye or visceral dissemination. **Comment:** Replacement every 6 months recommended
Valganciclovir (Valcyte)	900 mg (two 450 mg tabs) po bid times 21 days for induction, followed by 900 mg po q24h. Take with food. (450 mg cap $31.70; ~$1,900 for 60 caps)	A prodrug of ganciclovir with better bioavailability. 60% with food. **Adverse effects:** Similar to ganciclovir.
Herpesvirus (non-CMV)		
Acyclovir (Zovirax or generic)	Doses: see *Table 14A* 400 mg tab G $0.30–0.70 (or $110–200/yr for chronic suppression) IV 500 mg $9.60 Suspension 200 mg per 5 mL $137 Ointment 5% 15 gm $90	**po:** Generally well-tolerated with occ. diarrhea, vertigo, arthralgia. Less frequent rash, fatigue, insomnia, fever, menstrual abnormalities, acne, sore throat, muscle cramps, lymphadenopathy. **IV:** Phlebitis, caustic with vesicular lesions with IV infiltration. CNS (1%): lethargy, tremors, confusion, hallucinations, delirium, seizures, coma (*CID 21:435, 1995*). Improve 1–2 weeks after rx stopped. Renal (5%): ↑ creatinine, hematuria. With high doses may crystallize in renal tubules → obstructive uropathy (rapid infusion, dehydration, renal insufficiency and ↑ dose ↑ risk). Adequate pre-hydration may prevent such nephrotoxicity. Hepatic: ↑ ALT, AST. Uncommon: neutropenia (*CID 20: 1557, 1995*), rash, diaphoresis, hypotension, headache, nausea.
Famciclovir (Famvir)	250 mg cap $4.70 500 mg cap $9.33	Metabolized to penciclovir. **Adverse effects:** similar to acyclovir, included headache, nausea, diarrhea, and dizziness but incidence did not differ from placebo (*JAMA 276:47, 1996*). May be taken without regard to meals. Dose should be reduced if CrCl <60 mL per min (see package insert & Table 14A, page 109 & Table 17, page 138).
Penciclovir (Denavir) Trifluridine (Viroptic)	Topical 1% cream 1.5 gm $26 1 drop 1% solution q2h (max. 9 drops per day) for max. of 21 days (7.5 mL 1% solution $105)	Apply to area of recurrence of herpes labialis with start of sx, then q2h while awake times 4 days. Well tolerated. Mild burning (5%), palpebral edema (3%), punctate keratopathy, stromal edema
Valacyclovir (Valtrex)	500 mg cap $5	An ester pro-drug of acyclovir that is well-absorbed, bioavailability 3–5 times greater than acyclovir. **Adverse effects** similar to acyclovir (see *JID 186:540, 2002*). Thrombotic thrombocytopenic purpura/hemolytic uremic syndrome reported in pts with advanced HIV disease and transplant recipients participating in clinical trials at doses of 8 gm per day.

TABLE 14B (2)

DRUG NAME(S) GENERIC (TRADE)	DOSAGE/ROUTE/COST*	COMMENTS/ADVERSE EFFECTS
Hepatitis **Adefovir dipivoxil** (Hepsera)	10 mg po q24h (with normal CrCl); see *Table 17A if renal impairment* Cost $18 ea. = $546 per month	Adefovir dipivoxil is a prodrug of adefovir. It is an acyclic nucleotide analog with activity against hepatitis B (HBV) few side at 0.2–2.5 mM (IC₅₀); see *Table 9 for Cmax & T½*. Primarily renal excretion—adjust dose. No food interactions. Remarkably few side effects. No nephrotoxic at 10 mg per day. Monitor renal function, esp. with pre-existing or other risks for renal impairment. Lactic acidosis reported with nucleoside analogs, esp. in women. Pregnancy Category C. Hepatitis may exacerbate when rx dc. 6–25% of pts developed ALT ↑ 10 times normal within 12 wks; usually responds to re-treatment or self-limited, but hepatic decompensation has occurred.
Entecavir (Baraclude)	0.5 mg q24h. If refractory to lamivudine: 1 mg per day ($714.60 per month)	A nucleoside analog active against HBV including lamivudine-resistant mutants. Minimal adverse effects reported: headache, fatigue, dizziness, & nausea reported in 22% of pts. Potential for lactic acidosis but not reported to date. Adjust dosage in renal impairment (see *Table 17, page 137*).
Interferon alfa is available as alfa-2a (Roferon-A), **alfa-2b** (Intron-A)	3 million units: (Roferon $40, Intron $39; Infergen 9 mcg $52)	**Adverse effects:** Flu-like syndrome common, esp. during 1st week of rx: fever 98%, fatigue 89%, myalgia 73%, headache 71%, GI: anorexia 46%, diarrhea 29%. CNS: dizziness 21% Rash 18%, later profound fatigue & psychiatric symptoms in up to ½ of pts (*J Clin Psych 64:708, 2003*) (depression, anxiety, emotional lability and agitation), alopecia, ↑ TSH, autoimmune thyroid disorders with hypo- or hyperthyroidism. Graves disease reported (*J Inv Med 53:26, 2005*). Hematol.: ↓ WBC 49%, ↓ Hgb 27%, ↓ platelets 35%. Consider prophylactic antidepressants in pts with history. Acute reversible hearing loss and/or tinnitus in up to 1/3 (*Ln 343:1134, 1994*). Optic neuropathy (retinal hemorrhage, cotton wool spots, ↓ in color vision) reported (*AIDS 18:1805, 2004*). Cryoglobulinemia assoc. with HCV usually responds to IFN rx but exacerbations with vasculitis also reported with rx (*Clin Rheum, e30, June 2005*). Side-effects ↑ with ↑ doses and dose reduction necessary in up to 46% receiving chronic rx for HBV.
PEG interferon alfa-2b (PEG-Intron)	0.5–1.5 mcg per kg subcut. q wk (120 mcg $391)	Attachment of IFN to polyethylene glycol (PEG) prolongs half-life and allows weekly dosing. Better efficacy data with similar adverse effects profile compared to regular formulation.
Pegylated-40k interferon alfa-2a (Pegasys)	180 mcg subcut. q wk times 48 wks (180 mcg $404)	
Lamivudine (3TC) (Epivir-HBV)	**Adverse effects:** See *Table 14D, page 122.* NOTE: 100 mg po q24h times 1 yr for HBV.	**Ribavirin:** Hemolytic anemia common but usually responds to ↓ ribavirin
Ribavirin–interferon alfa-2b combination pack (Rebetron) or **PEG IFN + ribavirin in combination**	Combination kit contains 2 wk supply of IFN and 42, 70, or 84 caps of 200 mg ribavirin. **Dose:** IFN 3 million units subcut. 3 times per wk AND ribavirin 400 mg po a.m. + 600 mg po q.p.m. (<75 kg) or 600 mg po bid (>75 kg). Rebetron (1000 mg per day ribavirin dose pack). ($9652 per 24 wk course)	dosage (see *package insert*). Ribavirin plasma level correlates with degree of anemia but also with efficacy against HBV (*JAIDS 39:401, 2005*). 1 Japanese study suggests levels between 3000 to 3500 ng per mL 8 wks after initiating rx optimal (*Intervirol 48:138, 2005*). Erythropoietin (Epoetin alfa) effective in ↑ Hgb levels & quality of life while allowing adequate dosage of ribavirin to be maintained (*Pharmacother 25:862, 2005*). Pure red cell aplasia 2° to anti-erythropoietin antibodies reported (*Am J Gastro 100:1415, 2005*). **Since ribavirin is teratogenic, drug must not be used during pregnancy or within 6 months of pregnancy.** Also should not be used in pts with endstage renal failure, severe heart disease, or hemoglobinopathies. ARDS reported (*Chest 124:406, 2003*). **Interferon alfa:** Severe psychiatric effects, esp. depression, most common (23–36%) reason for discontinuation of rx. Suicidal behavior reported. Preemptive rx with antidepressants effective in 1 open-label study (*J Hpt 42:793, 2005*). Hyper- & hypothyroidism, alopecia (30%) including reversible alopecia universalis (*J Chemother 17:212, 2005*), & pulmonary disease reported (*Mayo Clin Proc 74:367, 1999*). Uncommon side-effects include exacerbation of psoriasis (*Chemotherapy 51:167, 2005*) & other rheumatological conditions (*Rheumatol 44:1016, 2005*), sexual dysfunction with ↓ testosterone levels (*J Endo 185:345, 2005*), ↑ risk of lipoatrophy 2° to mitochondrial toxicity when administered with nucleoside analogs to HIV-HBV co-infected pts (*Antivir Ther 10:557, 2005*), & sarcoidosis (*ArDerm 141:865, 2005*).

Dose changes (for PEG IFN + ribavirin):

	Ribavirin	Interferon
Hgb: <10 <8.5	↓ to 200 mg q a.m. DC	No change DC
WBC <1500 <1000	No change DC	↓ to 1.5 million units subcut. 3 times per wk DC
Abs. PMNs <750 <500	No change DC	↓ to 1.5 million units subcut. 3 times per wk DC
Platelets: <50,000 <25,000	No change DC	↓ to 1.5 million units subcut. 3 times per wk DC

* See page 2 for abbreviations. NOTE: *All dosage recommendations are for adults (unless otherwise indicated) and assume normal renal function.*
Costs from 2005 DRUG TOPICS RED BOOK, Medical Economics. Price is average wholesale price (AWP).

TABLE 14B (3)

DRUG NAME(S) GENERIC (TRADE)	DOSAGE/ROUTE/COST*	COMMENTS/ADVERSE EFFECTS
Hepatitis *(continued)*		
Ribavirin (Rebetol)	Use with pegylated interferons (alfa-2a & 2b) for treatment of hepatitis C. Available as 200 mg capsules. Dose: <75 kg BW = 2 caps in a.m. & 3 caps in p.m., >75 kg BW 3 caps in a.m. & 3 caps in p.m. Cost: 200 mg \$10.60	Side-effects as above, esp. hemolytic anemia (during 1st 1–2 wks of rx) with hemoglobin ↓ of 3–4 gm. Should not be used with CrCl <50 mL per min & cautiously with cardiac disease.
Influenza A		
Amantadine (Symmetrel) or Rimantadine (Flumadine)	Amantadine and rimantadine doses are the same (rimantadine approved only for prophylaxis in children, not treatment). Amantadine 100 mg po bid; >65 y.o., 100 mg po q24h. G: 100 mg cap \$0.50, 100 mg per 10 mL soln. \$1.80. Rimantadine 100 mg tab/syrup \$2	**Side-effects/toxicity:** CNS (nervousness, anxiety, difficulty concentrating, and lightheadedness). Symptoms occurred in 6% on rimantadine vs 14% on amantadine. They usually ↓ after 1st week and disappear when drug dc. GI (nausea, anorexia). Some serious side-effects—delirium, hallucinations, and seizures—are associated with high plasma drug levels resulting from renal insufficiency, esp. in older pts, those with prior seizure disorders, or psychiatric disorders. In pts with impaired renal function, dosage of both drugs should be reduced (amantadine: creatinine clearance <50 mL per min; rimantadine: CrCl <10 mL per min), *see package inserts and Table 17, pages 137 & 138*. Both drugs teratogenic in animals and contraindicated during pregnancy *(Med Lett 39:72, 1997)*.
Influenza A and B—For both drugs, initiate within 48 hrs of symptom onset		
Zanamivir (Relenza) For pts ≥12 yrs of age	2 inhalations (2 times 5 mg) bid times 5 days. Powder is inhaled using specially designed breath-activated device. Each medication-containing blister contains 5 mg of zanamivir. \$60 per course	Active by inhalation against neuraminidase of both influenza A and B and inhibits release of virus from epithelial cells of respiratory tract. Approx. 4–17% of inhaled dose absorbed from plasma. Excreted by kidney but with low absorption, dose reduction not necessary in renal impairment. Minimal side-effects: <3% cough, sinusitis, diarrhea, nausea and vomiting. **Reports of respiratory adverse events in pts with or without h/o airways disease, should be avoided in pts with respiratory disease.**
Oseltamivir (Tamiflu)	75 mg po bid for treatment [pediatric suspension (12 mg per mL) approved for treatment, not prevention, in children age 1–12 at dose of 2 mg per kg (up to 75 mg) bid times 5 days]. For prevention: 75 mg po q24h for duration of peak of flu epidemic. \$73 per 5 day course	Well absorbed (80% bioavailable) from GI tract as ethyl ester of active compound GS 4071. T½ 6–10 hrs; excreted unchanged by kidney. Adverse effects in 15% include diarrhea 1.6%, nausea 0.5%, vomiting, headache *(J Am Ger Soc 50:608, 2002)*. Nausea ↓ with food. Also available as 12 mg per mL oral suspension.
Respiratory Syncytial Virus (RSV) and other		
Palivizumab (Synagis) *(See Med Lett 41:1, 1999)* Used only for prevention of RSV infection in high-risk children *Pediatrics 102:1211, 1998)*	15 mg per kg IM q month 100 mg vial (for 1 injection) \$1560	A monoclonal antibody directed against the F glycoprotein on surface of virus; side-effects are nominal, occ. ↑ ALT *(JID 176:1215, 1997)*.
Ribavirin (Virazole)	1.1 gm per day (6 gm vial for inhalation \$1574)	**Ribavirin side-effects:** Anemia, rash, conjunctivitis. Read package insert. Avoid procedures that lead to drug precipitation in ventilator tubing with subsequent dysfunction. Significant teratogenicity in animals. **Contraindicated in pregnant women and partners.** Pregnant health care workers should avoid direct care of pts receiving aerosolized ribavirin.
RSV-IV immunoglobulin (IG) (RespiGam)	100 mg per kg IV q month (50 mL \$1487)	RespiGam side-effects rare but include fatal anaphylaxis, pruritus, rash, wheezing, fever, joint pain.
Warts *(See CID 28:S37, 1999)*		
Interferon alfa-2b or alfa-n3	Apply 1 million units into lesion	Interferon alfa-2b 3 million units per 0.5 mL, interferon alfa-n3 5 million units per 1 mL. Cost: \$10
Podofilox (Condylox)	3.5 mL for topical application, \$130	**Side-effects:** Local reactions—pain, burning, inflammation in 50%. No systemic effects.
Imiquimod (Aldara)	Cream applied 3 times per week to maximum of 16 wks. 250 mg packets \$15	Mild erythema, erosions, itching and burning

TABLE 14C: ANTIRETROVIRAL THERAPY IN TREATMENT-NAIVE ADULTS

(See the 2005 SANFORD GUIDE TO HIV/AIDS THERAPY, Table 6, for additional information regarding treatment and complications of antiretroviral agents)

In 2005, guidelines and recommendations for the treatment of individuals infected with HIV-1 were updated: DHHS guidelines for the use of antiretroviral therapy (ART) in pediatrics, and recommendations for ART in pregnant women. All documents are available online at www.aidsinfo.nih.gov. New treatment recommendations by the International AIDS Society–USA Panel were also published (JAMA 292:251, 2004), as were guidelines for primary care management of HIV-infected persons provided by the HIV Medicine Association of the IDSA (CID 39:609, 2004). For additional explanation and alternatives, see www.aidsinfo.nih.gov.

A. When to start therapy? (www.aidsinfo.nih.gov)

HIV Symptoms	CD4 cells per mcL	Start Treatment	Comment
Yes	Any	Yes	
No	<200	Yes	Risk for progression to AIDS also depends on viral load; consider on individual basis
No	>200–≤350	Offer (see Comment)	Maybe if CD4 decreasing rapidly and/or viral load >100,000 copies per mL
No	>350	No (see Comment)	

• **Acute retroviral syndrome**—See page 118, section C

B. Suggested Initial Therapy Regimens for Untreated Chronic HIV Infection (For pregnancy, see below and Table 8 of the SANFORD GUIDE TO HIV/AIDS THERAPY, 2005)

1. Preferred Regimens

Regimen	Pill strength (mg)	Usual Daily Regimen (oral)	No. pills per day	Cost per month (Avg. Wholesale Price)	Comment (See also individual agents)
a. **(Zidovudine + Lamivudine) +** Efavirenz	(300 + 150) + 600	**(Combination—Combivir** 1 tab bid) + 1 tab q24h at bedtime, empty stomach (see Comment)	3	$1135	Good efficacy; low pill burden; low AE profile. **If rx stopped, dc efavirenz 1–2 wks before Combivir** (for explanation, see page 120). Avoid efavirenz in pregnancy or in women who might become pregnant **(Pregnancy Category D).** Food may ↑ serum efavirenz concentration, which can lead to ↑ adverse events.
b. **(Tenofovir + Emtricitabine) +** Efavirenz	(300 + 200) + 600	**(Combination—Truvada** 1 tab q24h) + 1 tab q24h at bedtime, empty stomach. Food may ↑ serum efavirenz concentration, which can lead to ↑ adverse events.	2	$1258	Good efficacy; low pill burden. Tenofovir: emerging reports of renal toxicity. Avoid efavirenz in pregnancy or in women who might become pregnant **(Pregnancy Category D).** Interim analysis of ongoing trial suggests superiority of emtricitabine/tenofovir/ efavirenz over 3TC/ZDV/efavirenz in rx-naive pts (3rd IAS, 2005).
c. **(Zidovudine + Lamivudine) +** Lopinavir/Ritonavir	(300 + 150) + 200/50	**(Combination—Combivir** 1 tab bid) + 2 tabs bid without regard to food		$1394	Good virologic efficacy and durable effect. Tolerable AEs. ↓ accumulation of resistance mutations than nelfinavir regimen (NEJM 346:2039, 2002). Lopinavir/ ritonavir can be given as 4 tabs once daily in rx-naive pts.

2. Alternative Regimens

a. **Didanosine EC + Lamivudine +** Efavirenz	400 + 300 + 600	1 cap q24h at bedtime, fasting + 1 tab q24h + 1 tab q24h at bedtime, empty stomach. **Didanosine dosage shown for ≥60 kg.**	3	$1071	Low pill burden. Efficacy and durability under study. Potential didanosine AEs (pancreatitis, peripheral neuritis). Avoid efavirenz in pregnancy or in women who might become pregnant **(Pregnancy Category D).** Food may ↑ serum efavirenz concentration, which can lead to ↑ adverse events. Can substitute emtricitabine 200 mg po q24h for lamivudine 300 mg po q24h.
b. **(Zidovudine + Lamivudine) + Fosamprenavir + Ritonavir**	(300 + 150) + 700 + 100	**(Combination—Combivir** 1 tab bid) + 1 tab bid fed or fasting + 1 tab bid fed or fasting	6	$1892	Take without regard to meals. Skin rash, GI symptoms. Contains sulfa moiety. Alternative fosamprenavir regimens available for rx-naive pts: fosamprenavir without ritonavir & once-daily fosamprenavir/ritonavir (see label for doses). For peds: oral solution of amprenavir available.
c. **(Zidovudine + Lamivudine) +** Nelfinavir	(300 + 150) + 625	**(Combination—Combivir** 1 tab bid) + 2 tabs bid, with food	6	$1490	Nelfinavir-associated diarrhea in 20%. Nelfinavir contraindicated with drugs highly dependent on CYP3A4 elimination where ↑ levels may cause life-threatening toxicity.
d. **(Zidovudine + Lamivudine) +** Atazanavir	(300 + 150) + 200	**(Combination—Combivir** 1 tab bid) + 2 caps q24h, with food	4	$1485	Lower potential for lipid derangement by atazanavir than other PIs. May ↑ PR interval & bilirubin.

TABLE 14C (2)

Regimen	Pill strength (mg)	Usual Daily Regimen (oral)	No. pills per day	Cost per month (Avg. Wholesale Price)	Comment (See also individual agents)
2. **Alternative Regimens** (continued)					
e. (Zidovudine + Lamivudine) + Indinavir + Ritonavir	(300 + 150) + 400 + 100	(Combination—**Combivir** 1 tab bid) + 2 caps q12h + 1 cap q12h	8	$1672	Nephrolithiasis—hydrate! GI symptoms. Metabolic effects of PI. May ↑ bilirubin.
3. **Triple nucleoside or nucleoside/nucleotide regimen: Due to inferior virologic activity, use only when preferred or alternative regimen not possible.**					
a. (Zidovudine + Lamivudine) + Abacavir	(300 + 150) + 300	(Combination—**Trizivir** 1 tab bid)	2	$1110	Reduced efficacy as compared to preferred & alternative regimens. Potential serious abacavir AEs. (See comments for individual agents)

4. **During pregnancy.** Expert consultation mandatory. Timing of rx initiation & drug choice must be individualized. Viral resistance testing should be strongly considered. Longterm effects of agents unknown. Certain drugs hazardous or contraindicated (see *SANFORD GUIDE TO HIV/AIDS THERAPY, Table 17*). See *www.aidsinfo.nih.gov* for additional information & alternative rx options, and (see *SANFORD GUIDE TO HIV/AIDS THERAPY, Table 8A*) for regimens to prevent mother-child transmission.

Regimen	Pill strength (mg)	Usual Daily Regimen (oral)	No. pills per day	Cost per month (Avg. Wholesale Price)	Comment (See also individual agents)
a. (Zidovudine + Lamivudine) + Nevirapine	(300 + 150) + 200	(Combination—**Combivir** 1 tab bid) + 1 tab bid fed or fasting [after 14-day lead-in period of 1 tab q24h]	4	$1097	See nevirapine Black Box warnings (page 120)—among others, ↑ risk of **potentially fatal hepatotoxicity** in women with CD4 >250. Avoid in this group unless benefits clearly > risks; monitor intensively if drug must be used.
b. (Zidovudine + Lamivudine) + Nelfinavir	(300 + 150) + 625	(Combination—**Combivir** 1 tab bid) + 2 tabs bid, with food	6	$1490	(See section 2.c above)
c. (Zidovudine + Lamivudine) + Saquinavir + Ritonavir	(300 + 150) + 500 + 100	(Combination—**Combivir** 1 tab bid) + 2 tabs bid + 1 cap bid	8	NA	Use saquinavir tabs only in combination with ritonavir. Certain drugs metabolized by CYP3A4 are contraindicated with saquinavir/ritonavir. (DHHS recommendations based on saquinavir softgel caps, which are no longer available, plus ritonavir. *www.aidsinfo.nih.gov*.)

C. Suggested Regimen for Acute Primary HIV Infection (See Comment)

Regimen	Pill Strength (mg)	Usual Daily Regimen (oral)	No. pills per day	Cost per month (Avg. Wholesale Price)	Comment (See also individual agents)
(Zidovudine + Lamivudine)+ Efavirenz	(300 + 150) + 600	(Combination—**Combivir** 1 tab bid) + 1 tab q24h at bedtime, empty stomach. Food may ↑ serum efavirenz concentration, which can lead to ↑ adverse advents.	3	$1135	Benefits of rx acute HIV infection uncertain; treatment is considered optional, and best undertaken in research setting. Perform resistance testing. Optimal duration of rx unknown. (See *www.aidsinfo.nih.gov*). Avoid efavirenz in pregnancy or in women who might become pregnant (**Pregnancy Category D**).

D. Some Antiretroviral Therapies Should NOT Be Offered: see *2005 SANFORD GUIDE TO HIV/AIDS THERAPY, Table 6, for details*

E. Selected Characteristics of Antiretroviral Drugs

1. Selected Characteristics of Nucleoside or Nucleotide Reverse Transcriptase Inhibitors (NRTIs)
  All agents have Black Box warning: Risk of lactic acidosis/hepatic steatosis. Also, labels note risk of fat redistribution/accumulation with ARV rx. For combinations, see warnings for component agents.

Generic/Trade Name	Pharmaceutical Prep. (Avg. Wholesale Price)	Usual Adult Dosage & Food Effect	Absorbed, %, po	Serum T½, hrs	Intracellular T½, hrs	Elimination	Major Adverse Events/Comments (See Table 14D)
Abacavir (ABC; Ziagen)	300 mg tabs or 20 mg per mL oral solution ($448 per month)	300 mg po bid or 600 mg po q24h. Food OK	83	1.5	20	Liver metab., renal excretion of metabolites, 82%. Alcohol ↑ AUC	**Hypersensitivity reaction:** fever, rash, N/V, malaise, diarrhea, abdominal pain, respiratory symptoms. (Severe reactions may be ↑ with 600 mg dose). **Do not rechallenge!** Report to 800-270-0425.

TABLE 14C (3)

1. **Selected Characteristics of Nucleoside or Nucleotide Reverse Transcriptase Inhibitors (NRTIs)** *(continued)*
All agents have Black Box warning: Risk of lactic acidosis/hepatic steatosis. Also, labels note risk of fat redistribution/accumulation with ARV rx. For combinations, see warnings for component agents.

Generic/Trade Name	Pharmaceutical Prep. (Avg. Wholesale Price)	Usual Adult Dosage & Food Effect	Absorbed, %, po	Serum T½, hrs	Intracellular T½, hrs	Elimination	Major Adverse Events/Comments (See Table 14D)
Abacavir/lamivudine/zidovudine (Trizivir)	Film-coated tabs: ABC 300 mg + 3TC 150 mg + ZDV 300 mg ($1170 per month)	1 tab po bid (not recommended for wt <40 kg or CrCl <50 mL per min or impaired hepatic function)	*(See individual components)*			*(See Comments for individual components)*	*(See Comments for individual components)* **Note: Black Box warnings** for ABC hypersensitivity reaction & others. Should only be used for regimens intended to include these 3 agents. **Black Box warning**—limited data for VL >100,000 copies per mL.
Didanosine (ddi; Videx or Videx EC) *Comment:* Potential ↑ toxicity & ↓ efficacy if used with tenofovir (see AIDS Reader 15:403, 2005).	25, 50, 100, 150, 200 mg chewable tabs; 100, 167, 250 mg powder for oral solution; 125, 200, 250, 400 enteric-coated caps Videx EC)	>60 kg: Usually 400 mg enteric-coated po q24h ½ hr before or 2 hrs after meal. **Do not crush.** <60 kg: 250 mg EC po q24h Food ↓ levels. *See Comment*	30–40	1.6	25–40	Renal excretion, 50%	**Pancreatitis**, peripheral neuropathy, lactic acidosis & hepatic steatosis (rare but life-threatening, esp. combined with stavudine in pregnancy). Retinal, optic nerve changes reported. **If ddi + TDF is used, reduce dose from 400 mg to 250 mg EC q24h (or from 250 mg EC to 200 mg EC for adults <60 kg).**
Emtricitabine (FTC, Emtriva) **Exacerbation of Hep B reported after stopping FTC**	200 mg caps; 10 mg per mL solution ($318 per month)	200 mg po q24h. Food OK	93	Approx. 10	39	Renal excretion 86%, minor biotransformation, 14% excretion in feces	Well tolerated; headache, nausea, vomiting & diarrhea occasionally, skin rash rarely. Skin hyperpigmentation. Differs only slightly in structure from lamivudine (5-fluoro substitution).
Emtricitabine/tenofovir disoproxil fumarate (Truvada)	Film-coated tabs: FTC 200 mg + TDF 300 mg ($781 per month)	1 tab po q24h for CrCl ≥50 mL per min. Food OK.	92/25	10/17	—	Primarily renal/renal	*See Comments for individual agents.* **Black Box warning**—not indicated for rx of Hep B. Exacerbation after stopping.
Lamivudine (3TC; Epivir)	150, 300 mg tabs; 10 mg per mL oral solution ($331 per month)	150 mg po bid or 300 mg po q24h. Food OK.	86	5–7	18	Renal excretion, minimal metabolism	**Use HIV dose, not Hep B dose.** Usually well-tolerated. **Risk of exacerbation of Hep B after stopping 3TC.**
Lamivudine/abacavir (Epzicom)	Film-coated tabs: 3TC 300 mg + abacavir 600 mg ($781 per month)	1 tab po q24h. Food OK. Not recommended for CrCl <50 mL per min or impaired hepatic function.	86/86	5–7/1.5	—	Primarily renal/metabolism	*See Comments for individual agents.* **Note abacavir hypersensitivity Black Box warnings** (severe reactions may be ↑ with 600 mg dose).
Lamivudine/zidovudine (Combivir)	Film-coated tabs: 3TC 150 mg + ZDV 300 mg ($722 per month)	1 tab po bid. Not recommended for CrCl <50 mL per min or impaired hepatic function. Food OK.	86/64	5–7/0.5–3	—	Primarily renal/metabolism with renal excretion of glucuronide	*See Comments for individual agents.* See **Black Box warning**—exacerbation of Hep B in pts stopping 3TC
Stavudine (d4T; Zerit)	15, 20, 30, 40 mg capsules; 1 mg per mL oral solution ($370 per month 40 mg caps)	>60 kg: 40 mg po bid <60 kg: 30 mg po bid Food OK.	86	1.2–1.6	3.5	Renal excretion, 40%	**Highest incidence of lactic acidosis of all NRTIs.** (*See Comments for didanosine.*) Pancreatitis. Peripheral neuropathy. High incidence of lipoatrophy, hyperlipidemia.
Tenofovir disoproxil fumarate (TDF; Viread)—a nucleotide **Black Box warning**—Not indicated for treatment of Hep B; **exacerbations of Hep B reported after stopping tenofovir.**	300 mg tabs ($478 per month)	CrCl ≥50 mL per min: 300 mg po q24h. Food OK; high-fat meal ↑ absorption	39 (with food); 25 (fasted)	17	>60	Renal excretion 70–80%	Headache, N/V. Cases of renal dysfunction reported: avoid concomitant nephrotoxic agents. Must adjust dose of ddi (↓) if used concomitantly (*see ddi Comments box*). Atazanavir & lopinavir/ritonavir ↑ tenofovir concentrations: monitor for adverse effects.

TABLE 14C (4) *(continued)*

1. Selected Characteristics of Nucleoside or Nucleotide Reverse Transcriptase Inhibitors (NRTIs) *(continued)*

All agents have Black Box warning: Risk of lactic acidosis/hepatic steatosis. Also, labels note risk of fat redistribution/accumulation with ARV rx. For combinations, see warnings for component agents.

Generic/Trade Name	Pharmaceutical Prep. *(Avg. Wholesale Price)*	Usual Adult Dosage & Food Effect	Absorbed, %, po	Serum T½, hrs	Intracellular T½, hrs	Elimination	Major Adverse Events/Comments *(See Table 14D)*
Zalcitabine (ddC; Hivid)	0.375, 0.75 tabs ($273 per month)	0.75 mg po q8h. Food OK	85	2	3	Renal excretion, 70%	**Peripheral neuropathy**, stomatitis, rarely life-threatening lactic acidosis, pancreatitis
Zidovudine (ZDV, AZT; Retrovir)	100 mg caps, 300 mg tabs; 10 mg per mL IV solution; 10 mg per mL oral syrup ($389 per month)	300 mg po q12h. Food OK	60	1.1	11	Metabolized to glucuronide & excreted in urine	Bone marrow suppression, GI intolerance, headache, insomnia, malaise, myopathy

2. Selected Characteristics of Non-Nucleoside Reverse Transcriptase Inhibitors (NNRTIs)

Generic/Trade Name	Pharmaceutical Prep. *(Avg. Wholesale Price)*	Usual Adult Dosage & Food Effect	Absorbed, %, po	Serum T½, hrs	Elimination	Major Adverse Events/Comments *(See Table 14D)*
Delavirdine (Rescriptor)	100, 200 mg tabs ($253 per month)	400 mg po q8h. Food OK	85	5.8	Cytochrome P450 (3A inhibitor), 51% excreted in urine (<5% unchanged), 44% in feces	Rash severe enough to stop drug in 4.3%. ↑ AST/ALT, headaches
Efavirenz (Sustiva) **Pregnancy Category D—may cause fetal harm—avoid in pregnant women or those who might become pregnant** (Note: No single method of contraception is 100% reliable)	50, 100, 200 mg capsules; 600 mg tablet ($479 per month)	600 mg po q24h at bedtime, without food. Food may ↑ serum conc., which can lead to ↑ in risk of adverse events.	42	40–55 See Comment	Cytochrome P450 (3A mixed inducer/inhibitor). 14–34% of dose excreted in urine as glucuronidated metabolites, 16–61% in feces	Rash severe enough to d/c use of drug in 1.7%. High frequency of diverse CNS AEs: somnolence, dreams, confusion, agitation. Serious psychiatric symptoms. False-pos. cannabinoid screen. Very long tissue T½. If efavirenz to be discontinued, stop efavirenz 1–2 wks before stopping companion drugs. Otherwise, risk of developing efavirenz resistance, as after 1–2 days only efavirenz in blood and/or tissue (*11th CROI 2004, Abst. 131*)
Nevirapine (Viramune) **Black Box warning—fatal hepatotoxicity.** Women with CD4 >250 esp. vulnerable, including pregnant women. Avoid in this group unless benefits clearly > risks (*www.fda.gov/cder/drug/advisory/nevirapine.htm*)	200 mg tabs; 50 mg per 5 mL oral suspension ($424 per month)	200 mg po q24h for 14 days & then 200 mg po bid (*see Comments & Black Box warning*) Food OK	>90	25–30	Cytochrome P450 (3A4, 2B6) inducer. 80% of dose excreted in urine as glucuronidated metabolites, 10% in feces	If used, intensive monitoring required. Men with CD4 >400 also at ↑ risk. Rash severe enough to stop drug in 7%, severe or life-threatening skin reactions in 2%. Do not restart if any suspicion of such reactions. 2-week dose escalation period may ↓ skin reactions. As with efavirenz, because of long T½, consider continuing companion agents for several days if nevirapine is discontinued.

3. Selected Characteristics of Protease Inhibitors (PIs).

All PIs: Glucose metabolism: new diabetes mellitus or deterioration of glucose control; fat redistribution; possible hemophilia bleeding; hypertriglyceridemia or hypercholesterolemia. Exercise caution re: potential drug interactions.

Generic/Trade Name	Pharmaceutical Prep. *(Avg. Wholesale Price)*	Usual Adult Dosage & Food Effect	Absorbed, %, po	Serum T½, hrs	Elimination	Major Adverse Events/Comments *(See Table 14D)*
Atazanavir (Reyataz)	100, 150, 200 mg capsules ($857 per month)	400 mg po q24h with food (exception is atazanavir 300 mg po q24h + ritonavir 100 mg po q24h when combined with efavirenz 600 mg po q24h or TDF 300 mg po q24h). Take with food 2 hrs pre or 1 hr post buffered ddl. Ritonavir-boosted dose also recommended for ARV rx-experienced pts.	Good oral bioavailability; food enhances bioavailability & ↓ pharmacokinetic variability. Absorption ↓ by antacids, H₂-blockers, proton pump inhibitors.	Approx. 7	Cytochrome P450 (3A4, 1A2 & 2C9 inhibitor) & UGT1A1 inhibitor. 13% excreted in urine (7% unchanged), 79% excreted in feces (20% unchanged)	No ↑ lipids in available studies. Asymptomatic unconjugated hyperbilirubinemia common. Headache, rash, GI symptoms. **Prolongation of PR interval (1st degree AV block) reported. Efavirenz & tenofovir ↓ atazanavir exposure; use atazanavir/ritonavir regimen; also, atazanavir ↑ tenofovir concentrations—watch for adverse events.**

3. Selected Characteristics of Protease Inhibitors (PIs) *(continued)*

TABLE 14C (5)

All PIs: Glucose metabolism: new diabetes mellitus or deterioration of glucose control; fat redistribution; possible hemophilia bleeding; hypertriglyceridemia or hypercholesterolemia. Exercise caution re: potential drug interactions.

Generic/Trade Name	Pharmaceutical Prep. (Avg. Wholesale Price)	Usual Adult Dosage & Food Effect	Absorbed, %, po	Serum T½, hrs	Elimination	Major Adverse Events/Comments (See Table 14D)
Fosamprenavir (Lexiva)	700 mg tablet ($632 per month if with ritonavir)	1400 mg (two 700 tabs) po bid OR With ritonavir: [1400 mg fosamprenavir (2 tabs) + ritonavir 200 mg] po q24h OR [700 mg fosamprenavir (1 tab) + ritonavir 100 mg] po bid	Bioavailability not established. Food OK	7.7	Hydrolyzed to amprenavir, then Cytochrome P450 (3A4 substrate, inhibitor, inducer)	Amprenavir prodrug. *(See amprenavir adverse events, Table 14D(2).)* Once-daily regimen: (1) not recommended for PI-experienced pts. (2) additional ritonavir needed if given with efavirenz *(see label)*. Boosted twice-daily regimen is recommended for PI-experienced pts.
Indinavir (Crixivan)	100, 200, 333, 400 mg capsules ($546 per month) Store in original container with desiccant	Two 400 mg caps (800 mg) po q8h. Without food or with light meal. Can take with ritonavir (e.g., 800 mg indinavir + 100 mg ritonavir po bid), no food restrictions)	65	1.2–2	Cytochrome P450 (3A4 inhibitor)	**Maintain hydration. Nephrolithiasis**, nausea, inconsequential ↑ of indirect bilirubin, ↑ AST/ALT, headache, asthenia, blurred vision, metallic taste, hemolysis. ↑ urine WBC (>100 per hpf) has been assoc. with nephritis/medullary calcification, cortical atrophy.
Lopinavir + ritonavir (Kaletra)	(200 mg lopinavir + 50 mg ritonavir) tablets. Tabs do not need refrigeration. Oral solution: (80 mg lopinavir + 20 mg ritonavir) per mL. (**Note:** *drug content of tabs is **not** equal to that of previous 133.3/33.3 mg capsules.*)	(400 mg lopinavir + 100 mg ritonavir)—2 tabs po bid. Higher dose may be needed in non-rx-naive pts when used with efavirenz, nevirapine, amprenavir (caps), or unboosted fosamprenavir (tabs). *(See Table 22B & C & pkg labeling for specific agents.)*	No food effect with tablets. *(Earlier capsule formulation required food.)*	5–6	Cytochrome P450 (3A4 inhibitor)	Nausea, vomiting, diarrhea, ↑ AST/ALT, pancreatitis. Oral solution 42% alcohol. Lopinavir + ritonavir can be taken as single daily dose of 4 tabs (total 800 mg lopinavir + 200 mg ritonavir), except in rx-experienced pts or those taking concomitant efavirenz, nevirapine, amprenavir, or nelfinavir.
Nelfinavir (Viracept)	625, 250 mg tabs; 50 mg per gm oral powder ($726 per month)	2 625 mg tabs (1250 mg) po bid, with food	20–80 Food ↑ exposure & ↓ variability	3.5–5	Cytochrome P450 (3A4 inhibitor)	Diarrhea. Coadministration of drugs with life-threatening toxicities & which are cleared by CYP3A4 is contraindicated.
Ritonavir (Norvir)	100 mg capsules; 600 mg per 7.5 mL solution. Refrigerate caps but not solution. Room temperature times 1 mo. OK. ($10.29 per capsule)	Full dose: 6 caps (600 mg) po bid, with food. Escalate to full dose: 300 mg po bid times 2 days; 400 mg bid times 3 days; 500 mg bid times 7 days; then full dose. "Booster drug"—see Comment	Erratic, 4 (saquinavir alone) Food ↑ absorption	3–5	Cytochrome P450. Potent 3A4 & 2D6 inhibitor	Nausea/vomiting/diarrhea, extremity & circumoral paresthesias, hepatitis, pancreatitis, taste perversion, ↑ CPK & uric acid. **Used to enhance pharmacokinetics of other PIs, using lower ritonavir doses. Black Box warning**—potentially fatal drug interactions. Many drug interactions—see Table 22A–C, pages 149 & 152
Saquinavir (**Invirase—hard gel caps or tabs**) + ritonavir	Saquinavir 200 mg caps, 500 mg film-coated tablets; ritonavir 100 mg caps ($718 per month)	2 625 mg tabs (1250 mg) po [2 tabs saquinavir (1000 mg)] OR (5 caps saquinavir (1000 mg)) + 1 cap ritonavir (100 mg)] po bid with food		1–2	Cytochrome P450 (3A4 inhibitor)	Nausea, diarrhea, headache, ↑ AST/ALT. Avoid rifampin with saquinavir + ritonavir: ↑ hepatitis risk (www.fda.gov/oashi/aids/new.html, accessed 2/26/05). **Black Box warning**—Invirase to be used only with ritonavir.
Tipranavir (Aptivus) For rx-experienced pts or PI-resistant strains	250 mg capsules. Refrigerate unopened bottles. Use opened bottles within 2 months.	[500 mg (two 250 mg caps) + ritonavir 200 mg] po bid, with food	Absorption low, ↑ with high fat meal, ↓ from Al+++ & Mg++ antacids	5.5–6	Cytochrome 3A4, but with ritonavir most of drug is eliminated in feces	Contains sulfa moiety. **Black Box warning**—hepatitis, fatal hepatic failure. Use cautiously in pts with liver disease, esp. Hep B or C; contraindicated in Child-Pugh class B–C. Monitor LFTs. Coadministration of certain drugs contraindicated (see Drug-Drug Interactions, Table 22).

TABLE 14C (6)

4. Selected Characteristics of Fusion Inhibitors

Generic/Trade Name	Pharmaceutical Prep. (Avg. Wholesale Price)	Usual Adult Dosage & Food Effect	Absorbed, %	Serum T½, hrs	Elimination	Major Adverse Events/Comments (See Table 14D)
Enfuviritide (T20, Fuzeon) Hypersensitivity reactions reported (fever, rash, chills, N/V, ↓BP, &/or ↑AST/ ALT)—do not restart if occur.	Single-use vials of 90 mg per mL when reconstituted. Vials should be stored at room temperature. Reconstituted vials can be refrigerated for 24 hrs only. ($23,990 per year)	90 mg (1 mL) subcut. bid. Rotate injection sites, avoiding those currently inflamed.	84	3.8	Catabolism to its constituent amino acids with subsequent recycling of the amino acids in the body pool. Elimination pathway(s) have not been performed in humans. Does not alter the metabolism of CYP3A4, CYP2D6, CYP1A2, CYP2C19 or CYP2E1 substrates.	Local reaction site reactions 98%, 4% discontinue; erythema/induration ~80–90%, nodules/cysts ~80%, including background regimens, peripheral neuropathy 8.9%, insomnia 11.3%, ↓ appetite 6.3%, myalgia 5%, lymphadenopathy 2.3%, eosinophilia ~10%. ↑ incidence of bacterial pneumonias. Alone offers little benefit to a failing regimen (NEJM 348:2249, 2003).

TABLE 14D: ANTIRETROVIRAL DRUGS AND ADVERSE EFFECTS (www.aidsinfo.nih.gov—accessed February 2005)

DRUG NAME(S): GENERIC (TRADE)	ADVERSE EFFECTS
Nucleoside Reverse Transcriptase Inhibitors (NRTI) (Black Box warning for all nucleoside/nucleotide RTIs: lactic acidosis/hepatic steatosis, potentially fatal. Also carry Warnings that fat redistribution has been observed)	
Abacavir (Ziagen)	**Most common:** Headache 7–13%, nausea 7–19% diarrhea 7%, malaise 7–12% **Most significant: Black Box warning—Hypersensitivity reaction** in 8% with malaise, fever, GI upset, rash, lethargy, & respiratory symptoms most commonly reported; myalgia, arthralgia, edema, paresthesia less commonly reported. Severe hypersensitivity reaction may be more common with once-daily dosing. **Rechallenge contraindicated; may be life-threatening.**
Didanosine (ddI) (Videx)	**Most common:** Diarrhea 28%, nausea 6%, rash 9%, headache 7%, fever 12%, hyperuricemia 2% **Most significant: Pancreatitis 1–9%. Black Box warning—Cases of fatal and nonfatal pancreatitis** have occurred in pts receiving ddI, especially when used in combination with d4T or d4T + hydroxyurea. Fatal lactic acidosis in pregnancy with ddI + d4T. Peripheral neuropathy in 20%, 12% required dose reduction. Rarely, retinal changes.
Emtricitabine (FTC, Emtriva)	**Most common:** Headache 20%, diarrhea, nausea, rash, skin hyperpigmentation **Most significant:** Potential for lactic acidosis (as with other NRTIs); **exacerbation of hepatitis B on stopping drug**
Lamivudine (3TC) (Epivir)	Well tolerated. Headache 35%, nausea 33%, diarrhea 18%, abdominal pain 9%, insomnia 11% (all in combination with ZDV). Pancreatitis more common in pediatrics (15%). **Black Box warning.** Make sure to use HIV dosage, not Hep B dosage. **Exacerbation of hepatitis B on stopping drug.**
Stavudine (d4T) (Zerit)	**Most common:** Diarrhea, nausea, vomiting, headache **Most significant: Peripheral neuropathy** 15–20%. Pancreatitis 1%. Appears to produce lactic acidosis more commonly than other NRTIs. **Black Box warning— Fatal & nonfatal pancreatitis with d4T + ddI + hydroxyurea. Fatal lactic acidosis/steatosis in pregnant women receiving d4T + ddI.** Motor weakness in the setting of lactic acidosis mimicking the clinical presentation of Guillain-Barré syndrome (including respiratory failure) (rare)
Zalcitabine (ddC) (Hivid)	**Most common:** Oral ulcers 13%, rash 8% **Most significant: Black Box warning—Pancreatitis** <1%, **peripheral neuropathy** 22–35%. Severe continuous pain, slowly reversible when ddC is discontinued, ↑ risk with diabetes mellitus. **Hepatic failure in pts with Hep B.**
Zidovudine (ZDV, AZT) (Retrovir)	**Most common:** Nausea 50%, anorexia 20%, vomiting 17%, **headache 62%** Also reported: asthenia, insomnia, myalgias, nail pigmentation. Macrocytosis expected with all dosage regimens. **Most significant: Black Box warning—hematologic toxicity, myopathy. Anemia** (<8 gm, 1%), **granulocytopenia** (<750, 1.8%). Anemia may respond to epoetin alfa if endogenous serum erythropoietin levels are ≤500 million units per mL.
Nucleotide Reverse Transcriptase Inhibitor (NtRTI) (Black Box warning for all nucleoside/nucleotide RTIs: lactic acidosis/hepatic steatosis, potentially fatal. Also carry Warnings that fat redistribution has been observed)	
Tenofovir (TDF) (Viread)	**Most common:** Diarrhea 11%, nausea 8%, vomiting 5% (generally well tolerated) **Most significant: Black Box Warning—Severe exacerbations of hepatitis B reported in pts who stop tenofovir.** Not indicated to treat Hep B. Monitor carefully if drug is stopped; anti-HBV rx may be warranted if TDF stopped. Possible ↑ bone demineralization. Reports of Fanconi syndrome & renal injury induced by tenofovir (CID 37:e174, 2003; JAIDS 35:269, 2004). Modest decline in Ccr with TDF may be greater than with NRTIs (CID 40:1194, 2005).
Non-Nucleoside Reverse Transcriptase Inhibitors (NNRTI)	
Delavirdine (Rescriptor)	**Most common:** Nausea, diarrhea, vomiting, headache **Most significant: Skin rash** has occurred in 18%, can continue or restart drug in most cases. Stevens-Johnson syndrome and erythema multiforme have been reported rarely. ↑ in liver enzymes in <5% of patients.

DRUG NAME(S): GENERIC (TRADE)	ADVERSE EFFECTS
Non-Nucleoside Reverse Transcriptase Inhibitors (NNRTI) *(continued)*	
Efavirenz (Sustiva)	**Most common: CNS side-effects 52%;** symptoms include dizziness, insomnia, somnolence, impaired concentration, psychiatric sx, and abnormal dreams; symptoms are worse after 1st or 2nd dose and improve over 2-4 weeks; discontinuation rate 2.6%. Rash 26%; improves with oral antihistamines; discontinuation rate 1.7%. Can cause false-positive urine test results for cannabinoid with CEDIA DAU multi-level THC assay. **Most significant:** Serious neuropsychiatric symptoms, including severe depression 2.4% & suicidal ideation 0.7%. Elevation in liver enzymes. **Teratogenicity reported in primates; pregnancy category D—may cause fetal harm, avoid in pregnant women or those who might become pregnant** (see *2005 SANFORD GUIDE TO HIV/AIDS THERAPY, Table 8*). NOTE: No single method of contraception is 100% reliable. Contraindicated with certain drugs metabolized by CYP3A4.
Nevirapine (Viramune)	**Most common: Rash 37%:** occurs during 1st 6 wks of therapy. Follow recommendations for 14-day lead-in period to ↓ risk of rash (*see Table 14D*). Women experience 7-fold ↑ in risk of severe rash (*CID 32:124, 2001*). 50% resolve within 2 wks of dc drug and 80% by 1 month. 6.7% discontinuation rate. **Most significant: Black Box warning—Severe life-threatening skin reactions reported:** Stevens-Johnson syndrome, toxic epidermal necrolysis, and hypersensitivity reaction or drug rash with eosinophilia and systemic symptoms (DRESS) (*ArIM 161:2501, 2001*). For severe rashes, dc drug immediately and do not restart. In a clinical trial, the use of prednisone ↑ the risk of rash. **Black Box warning—Life-threatening hepatitis reported:** 2/3 during the first 12 wks of rx. Overall 1% develop hepatitis. Pts with pre-existing ↑ in ALT or AST and/or history of chronic Hep B or C ↑ susceptible (*Hpt. 35:182, 2002*). Women with CD4 >250, including pregnant women, at ↑ risk. Avoid in this group unless no other option. Men with CD4 >400 also at ↑ risk. Monitor pts intensively (clinical and LFTs), esp. during the first 12 wks of rx. If clinical hepatotoxicity occurs, dc drug and never rechallenge.
Protease inhibitors (PI)	Abnormalities in glucose metabolism, dyslipidemias, fat redistribution syndromes are potential problems. Pts taking PI may be at increased risk for developing osteopenia/osteoporosis. Spontaneous bleeding episodes have been reported in HIV+ pts with hemophilia being treated with PI. Rheumatoid complications have been reported with use of PIs (*An Rheum Dis 61:82, 2002*). **Caution for all Pts—**Coadministration with certain drugs dependent on CYP3A for elimination & for which ↑ levels can cause serious toxicity may be contraindicated.
Amprenavir (Agenerase)	**Most common:** Nausea 43-74%, vomiting 24-34%, diarrhea 39-60%, paresthesias 26-31%, ↑ ALT/AST. Contains sulfa moiety. **Most significant:** Skin rash 28%. Most maculopapular of mild-moderate intensity, some with pruritus. Severe or life-threatening rash, including Stevens-Johnson syndrome, in 1% of pts. Skin rash onset 7-73 days, median 11 days. **Black Box warning**—potential propylene glycol toxicity with oral solution. Do not use in pregnancy, children <4 yrs old, renal/hepatic failure, with disulfiram or metronidazole.
Atazanavir (Reyataz)	**Most common:** Asymptomatic unconjugated hyperbilirubinemia in up to 60% of pts, jaundice in 7-9%. Moderate to severe events: Diarrhea 1-3%, nausea 6-14%, abdominal pain 4%, headache 6%, rash 5-7%. **Most significant:** Prolongation of PR interval (1st degree AV block) reported; rarely 2° AV block. One case acute interstitial nephritis (*Am J Kidney Dis 44:E81, 2004*).
Fosamprenavir (Lexiva)	**Most common:** Skin rash 20-30% (moderate or worse in 3-8%), nausea, headache, diarrhea. **Most significant:** Rarely Stevens-Johnson syndrome, hemolytic anemia.
Indinavir (Crixivan)	**Most common:** ↑ in indirect bilirubin 10-15% (≥2.5 mg per dL), due to a drug-induced Gilbert's syndrome (of no clinical significance). Nausea 12%, vomiting 4%, diarrhea 5%. Paronychia of big toe reported (*CID 32:140, 2001*). **Most significant: Kidney stones** Due to indinavir crystals in collecting system. Nephrolithiasis in 12% of adults, higher in pediatrics. Prevent (minimize) by good hydration (at least 48 oz. water per day) (*AAC 42:332, 1998*). Tubulointerstitial nephritis/renal cortical atrophy reported in association with asymptomatic ↑ urine WBC. Severe hepatitis reported in 3 cases (*Ln 349:924, 1997*). Hemolytic anemia reported.
Lopinavir/Ritonavir (Kaletra)	**Most common:** GI: **diarrhea** 14-24%, nausea 2-16%, lipid abnormalities in up to 20-40%. More diarrhea with q24h dosing. **Most significant:** Pancreatitis, inflammatory edema of the legs (*AIDS 16:673, 2002*).
Nelfinavir (Viracept)	**Most common:** Mild-moderate **diarrhea** 20%. For diarrhea: Oat bran tabs, calcium, or oral anti-diarrheal agents (e.g., loperamide, diphenoxylate/atropine sulfate).
Ritonavir (Norvir)	**Most common:** GI: bitter aftertaste (↓ by taking with chocolate milk, Ensure, or Advera; nausea 23%, ↓ by initial dose escalation (titration) regimen; vomiting 13%, diarrhea 15%. Circumoral paresthesias 5-6%. ↑ dose >100 mg q12h assoc. with ↑ GI side-effects & ↑ in lipid abnormalities. **Black Box warning** relates to many important drug-drug interactions—inhibits P450 CYP3A & CYP2D6 system—may be life-threatening (*see Table 22*). Rarely Stevens-Johnson syndrome, anaphylaxis.
Saquinavir (Invirase: hard cap, tablet)	**Most common: Diarrhea,** abdominal discomfort, nausea, headache. **Black Box Warning—**Invirase & Fortovase are not bioequivalent. (NOTE: Fortovase discontinued in 2006.) **Use Invirase only with ritonavir.**
Tipranavir (Aptivus)	**Most common:** Nausea & vomiting, diarrhea, abdominal pain. Rash in 8-14%, more common in women, & 33% in women taking ethinyl estradiol. Major lipid effects. Diarrhea 32%, nausea 23%, fatigue 20%. **Most serious: Black Box warning—**associated with hepatitis & fatal hepatic failure. Risk of hepatotoxicity ↑ in HepB or HepC co-infection. Potential for major drug interactions.
Fusion Inhibitor: Enfuvirtide (T20, Fuzeon)	**Most common:** local injection site reactions (98% at least 1 local ISR, 4% dc because of ISR) (pain & discomfort, induration, erythema, nodules & cysts, pruritus, & ecchymosis). **Most significant:** ↑ rate of bacterial pneumonia (6.7 pneumonia events per 100 pt yrs), hypersensitivity reactions ≤1% (rash, fever, nausea & vomiting, chills, rigors, hypotension, & ↑ serum liver transaminases).

TABLE 15A: ANTIMICROBIAL PROPHYLAXIS FOR SELECTED BACTERIAL INFECTIONS*

CLASS OF ETIOLOGIC AGENT/DISEASE/CONDITION	PROPHYLAXIS: AGENT/DOSE/ROUTE/DURATION	COMMENTS
Group B streptococcal disease (GBS), neonatal: Approaches to management [CDC Guidelines, MMWR 51(RR-11):1, 2002]:		
Pregnant women—intrapartum antimicrobial prophylaxis procedures: 1. Screen all pregnant women with vaginal & rectal swab for GBS at 35-37 wks gestation (unless other indications for prophylaxis exist: GBS bacteriuria during this pregnancy or previously delivered infant with invasive GBS disease; even then cultures may be useful for susceptibility testing). Use transport medium; GBS survive at room temp. up to 96 hrs. **Rx during labor if swab culture positive.** 2. Rx during labor if previously delivered infant with invasive GBS infection, or if any GBS bacteriuria during this pregnancy (MMWR 53:506, 2004). 3. Rx if GBS status unknown but if any of the following are present: (a) delivery at <37 wks gestation [see MMWR 51(RR-11):1, 2002 algorithm for threatened preterm delivery]; or (b) duration of ruptured membranes ≥18 hrs; or (c) intrapartum temp. ≥100.4°F (≥38.0°C).	**Prophylactic regimens during labor:** **Pen G** 5 million units IV (load) then 2.5 million units IV q4h. Alternative rx: **Ampicillin** 2 gm IV (load) then give 1 gm IV q4h. **Pen-allergic: Pts not at high risk for anaphylaxis: Cefazolin** 2 gm IV initial dose, then 1 gm IV q8h. **Pts at high risk for anaphylaxis:** GBS susceptible to clinda & erythro: **Clindamycin** 900 mg IV q8h or **erythromycin** 500 mg IV q6h. Vancomycin for pts at high risk for anaphylaxis when alternative to clindamycin or erythromycin needed (e.g., GBS-resistant or unknown susceptibility). Continue treatment until delivery.	
Neonate of mother given prophylaxis	Careful observation of signs & symptoms. 95% of infants will show clinical signs of infection during the 1st 24 hrs whether mother received intrapartum antibiotics or not (Pediatrics 106:244, 2000). For gestational age <35 wks or intrapartum antibiotics <4 hrs, lab evaluation (CBC, diff, blood culture) & ≥48 hr observation recommended. See algorithm: MMWR 51(RR-11):1, 2002	
Preterm, premature rupture of the membranes in Group B strep-negative women	(IV **ampicillin** 2 gm q6h + IV **erythromycin** 250 mg q6h) for 48 hrs followed by po **amoxicillin** 250 mg q8h + po **erythromycin** base 333 mg q8h times 5 days. Decreases infant morbidity. (JAMA 278:989, 1997)	Antibiotic rx reduced infant respiratory distress syndrome (50.6% to 40.8%, p = 0.03), necrotizing enterocolitis (5.8% to 2.3%, p = 0.03) and prolonged pregnancy (2.9 to 6.1 days, p < 0.001) vs placebo. In 1 large study (4809 pts), po erythromycin improved neonatal outcomes vs placebo (11.2% vs 14.4% poor outcomes, p=0.02 for single births) but not co-AM-CL or both drugs in combination (both assoc. with ↑ necrotizing enterocolitis) (Ln 357:979, 2001). (See ACOG discussion, Ob Gyn 102:875, 2003)
Post-splenectomy bacteremia Likely agents: Pneumococci (90%), meningococci, H. influenzae type b (also at ↑ risk of fatal malaria, severe babesiosis) Ref.: 2003 Red Book, 26th Ed., Amer Acad Pediatrics	**Immunizations:** Ensure admin. of pneumococcal vaccine, H. influenzae B, & quadrivalent meningococcal vaccines at recommended ages. In addition, asplenic children with sickle cell anemia, thalassemia, & perhaps others, daily antimicrobial prophylaxis until at least age 5—see Comments.	Antimicrobial prophylaxis until age 5: Amox 20 mg per kg once per day or Pen V-K 125 mg bid. Over age 5: Consider Pen V-K 250 mg bid for at least 1 yr in children post-splenectomy. Maintain immunizations plus self-administer AM-CL with any febrile illness while seeking physician assistance. Pen. allergy: TMP-SMX or clarithro. May need to consider other alternatives if pen-resistant S. pneumo prevalence increases.
Sexual Exposure		
Sexual assault survivor [likely agents and risks, see NEJM 332:234, 1995; MMWR 51(RR-6):1, 2002]	(**Ceftriaxone** 125 mg IM) + (**metronidazole** 2 gm po single dose) + (**azithromycin** 1 gm po single dose) or (**doxycycline** 100 mg po bid times 7 days) [MMWR 51 (RR-6):1, 2002]	Obtain expert advice re: forensic exam & specimens, pregnancy, physical trauma, psychological issues. At initial exam: Culture for gonococci & chlamydia (if available), wet mount for T. vaginalis (& culture vaginal swab). Serologic evaluation for syphilis, Hep B, HIV, others as appropriate. Initiate post-exposure protocols for HIV & hepatitis B as appropriate (see Table 15D). Follow-up exam for STD at 1-2 wks. Retest syphilis & HIV serology at 6, 12, 24 wks if negative earlier.
Sexual contacts, likely agents: N. gonorrhoeae, C. trachomatis	[(**Ceftriaxone** 125 mg IM once) + (**doxycycline** 100 mg bid, po times 7 days)] or [(**cefixime** 400 mg po) + (**azithromycin** 1 gm po), each as single dose]	Be sure to check for syphilis since all regimens may not eradicate incubating syphilis. Identify & rx contacts as appropriate to suspected STD [see MMWR 51(RR-6):1, 2002 for other etiologies & rx options].
Syphilis exposure		Presumptive rx for exposure within 3 mos., as tests may be negative. See Table 1, page 18. Make effort to dx syphilis
Sickle-cell disease. Likely agent: S. pneumoniae (see post-splenectomy, above) Ref.: 2003 Red Book, 26th Ed., Amer Acad Pediatrics	Children <5 yrs: **Penicillin V** 125 mg po bid ≥5 yrs: **Penicillin V** 250 mg po bid. (Alternative in children: Amoxicillin 20 mg po per kg per day)	Start prophylaxis by 2 mos. (Pediatrics 106:367, 2000; http://aapredbook.aappublications.org). Age-appropriate vaccines, including pneumococcal ,Hib, influenza ± meningococcal. Treating infections, consider possibility of penicillin non-susceptible pneumococci.

TABLE 15B: SURGICAL ANTIBIOTIC PROPHYLAXIS* (*EID 7:220, 2001; CID 38:1706, 2004; Am J Surg 189:395, 2005*)

Surgical Procedures: To be optimally effective, **antibiotics must be started in the interval: 2 hrs before time of surgical incision** (*NEJM 326:281, 1992*). For most procedures the number of doses needed for optimal coverage is not defined. Most applications employ a single dose (*Med Lett 43:92, 2001*) although FDA-approved product labeling is often for 2 or more doses. If the surgical procedure lasts >3 hrs, additional intraoperative doses of rapidly eliminated drugs should be given at approx. 3-hr intervals. A recent consensus statement from the National Surgical Infection Prevention Project (*CID 38:1706, 2004*) advises antibiotic prophylaxis be started within 1 hr before incision (except vancomycin & quinolones). The dose/route/durations listed below for single dose regimens, the dosage & route are the same.) See Table 15C for regimens to reduce risk of endocarditis.
General Comments: In some centers, ↑ resistance may render certain regimens (e.g., quinolones) unacceptable. Pharmacokinetic considerations suggest that typical prophylaxis dosing may yield suboptimal serum/tissue levels in pts with high BMI (see *Surgery 136:738, 2004* for cefazolin; *Eur J Clin Pharm 54:632, 1998* for vancomycin), although clinical implications uncertain.

TYPE OF SURGERY	PROPHYLAXIS	COMMENTS
Cardiovascular Surgery Antibiotic prophylaxis in cardiovascular surgery has been proven beneficial only in the following procedures: • Reconstruction of abdominal aorta • Any vascular procedure that inserts prosthesis/foreign body • Procedures on the leg that involve a groin incision • Lower extremity amputation for ischemia • Cardiac surgery • Perhaps permanent pacemakers (*see Comment*)	**Cefazolin** 1–2 gm IV as a single dose or q8h for 1–2 days or **cefuroxime** 1.5 gm IV as a single dose or q12h for total of 6 gm **or vancomycin** 1 gm IV as single dose or q12h for 1–2 days. Consider **intranasal mupirocin** evening before, day of surgery & bid for 5 days post-op in pts with pos. nasal culture for S. aureus.	Single injection just before surgery probably as effective as multiple doses. Not recommended for cardiac catheterization. For prosthetic heart valves, customary to stop prophylaxis either after removal of retrosternal drainage catheters or just a 2nd dose after coming off bypass. Vancomycin may be preferable in hospitals with ↑ frequency of MRSA or in high-risk pts (*CID 38: 1555, 2004*), or those colonized with MRSA (*CID 38:1706, 2004*); however, does not cover Gm-neg. bacilli, therefore would add cefazolin for groin incisions. Meta-analysis failed to demonstrate overall superiority of vancomycin over β-lactam prophylaxis for cardiac surgery (*CID 38: 1357, 2004*). A meta-analysis of 7 placebo-controlled randomized studies of antimicrobial prophylaxis for implantation of permanent pacemakers, sig. ↓ in incidence of infection (*Circulation 97: 1796, 1998*). Intranasal mupirocin ↓ sternal wound infections from S. aureus in 1850 pts; used historical controls (*An Thor Surg 71:1572, 2001*); in another trial, it reduced nosocomial S. aureus infections only in nasal carriers (*NEJM 346:1871, 2002*).
Gastric, Biliary and Colonic Surgery **Gastroduodenal/Biliary** Gastroduodenal, includes percutaneous endoscopic gastrostomy (high-risk only; *see Comments*) Biliary, includes laparoscopic cholecystectomy (high-risk only; *see Comments*)	**Cefazolin** or **cefoxitin** or **cefotetan** or **ceftizoxime** or **ceftizoxime** 1.5 gm IV as a single dose (some give additional doses q12h for 2–3 days). In biliary surgery, cefazolin 1 gm & ceftizoxime 1 gm (± repeat dosing at 12 & 24 hrs) were equivalent (*AAC 40:70, 1996*).	Gastroduodenal: High-risk is marked obesity, obstruction, ↓ gastric acid or ↓ GI motility. Biliary: Cephalosporins not active vs enterococci yet clinically effective as prophylaxis in biliary surgery. With cholangitis, treat as infection, not prophylaxis: TC-CL 3.1 gm q4–6h IV or (PIP-TZ 3.375 gm q6h or 4.5 gm q8h IV) or AM-SB 3.0 gm q6h IV. Biliary high-risk: age >70, acute cholecystitis, non-functioning gallbladder, obstructive jaundice or common duct stones. Meta-analysis supports use in percutaneous endoscopic gastrostomy (*Am J Gastro 95:3133, 2000*).
Endoscopic retrograde cholangiopancreatography Controversial: No benefit from single dose piperacillin in randomized placebo-controlled trial. *AnIM 125:442, 1996* (see *Comment*)	No rx without obstruction. If obstruction: **Ciprofloxacin** 500–750 mg po 2 hrs prior to procedure or **Ceftizoxime** 1.5 gm IV 1 hr prior to procedure or **Piperacillin** 4 gm IV 1 hr prior to procedure	Most studies show that achieving **adequate drainage** will prevent postprocedural cholangitis or sepsis and no further benefit from prophylactic antibiotics. With inadequate drainage antibiotics may be of value. American Society for GI Endoscopy recommends use for known or suspected biliary obstruction. Oral CIP as effective as cephalosporins in 2 studies & less expensive (*CID 23:380, 1996*).
Colorectal, includes appendectomy Elective surgery Emergency surgery	**Neomycin + erythromycin** po (*see Comment for dose*). [**Cefazolin** 1–2 gm IV + **metronidazole** 0.5 gm IV (single dose)] or **cefoxitin** or **cefotetan** 1–2 gm IV	Elective colorectal prep: Pre-op day: (1) 10 am 4 L polyethylene glycol electrolyte solution (Colyte, GoLYTELY) po over 2 hr. (2) Clear liquid diet only. (3) 1 pm, 2 pm and 11 pm, neomycin 1 gm + erythro base 1 gm po. (4) NPO after midnight. There are alternative regimens which have been less well studied: GoLYTELY 1–6 pm; then neomycin 2 gm po + metronidazole 2 gm po at 7 pm and 11 pm. Oral regimen as effective as parenteral; parenteral in addition to oral not required. For emergency colorectal surgery, use parenteral. (*CID 15 Suppl. 1:S313, 1992*).

Ruptured viscus: See *Peritonitis, Secondary, Table 1, page 34.*

* *See page 2 for abbreviations*

TABLE 15B (2)

TYPE OF SURGERY	PROPHYLAXIS	COMMENTS
Head and Neck Surgery (*Ann Otol Rhinol Laryngol 101 Suppl:16, 1992*) Antimicrobial prophylaxis in head & neck surgery appears efficacious only for procedures involving oral/pharyngeal mucosa (e.g. laryngeal or pharyngeal tumor) but even with prophylaxis, wound infection rate high (41% in 1 center) (*Head Neck 23:447, 2001*). Uncontaminated head & neck surgery does not require prophylaxis.		
Clean, non-implant; e.g., craniotomy	**Cefazolin** 1 gm IV once. Alternative: **vanco** 1 gm IV once	Reference: *Ln 344:547, 1994*
Clean, contaminated (cross sinuses, or naso/oropharynx)	**Clindamycin** 900 mg IV (single dose)	British recommend amoxicillin-clavulanate 1.2 gm IV[ᴺᴮ] or (cefuroxime 1.5 gm IV + metronidazole 0.5 gm IV).
CSF shunt surgery: controversial (Meta-analysis: *CID 17:98, 1993*)	**Vancomycin** 10 mg into cerebral ventricles + **gentamicin** 3 mg into cerebral ventricles (*Ln 344:547, 1994*)	Efficacy when infection rate >15%. Alternative: TMP (160 mg) + SMX (800 mg) IV pre-op and q12h times 3 doses
Obstetric/Gynecologic Surgery		
Vaginal or abdominal hysterectomy	**Cefazolin** 1–2 gm or **cefoxitin** 1–2 gm or **cefotetan** 1–2 gm or **cefuroxime** 1.5 gm all IV 30 min. before surgery.	1 study found cefotetan superior to cefazolin (*CID 20:677, 1995*). For prolonged procedures, doses can be repeated q4–8h for duration of procedure.
Cesarean section for premature rupture of membranes or active labor	**Cefazolin** once, administer IV as soon as umbilical cord clamped.	Prophylaxis decreases risk of endometritis/wound infection in elective as well as non-elective C-section; single dose equivalent to multiple dose regimens (*Cochrane Database System Rev 2002, issue 3, & 1999, issue 1*).
Abortion	1st trimester: aqueous **pen G** 2 mU IV or **doxycycline** 300 mg po. 2nd trimester: **Cefazolin** 1 gm IV	Meta-analysis showed benefit of antibiotic prophylaxis in all risk groups. One regimen was doxy 100 mg orally 1 hr before procedure, then 200 mg after procedure (*Ob Gyn 87:884, 1996*).
Orthopedic Surgery [Most pts with prosthetic joints do not require prophylaxis for routine dental procedures, but individual considerations prevail for high-risk procedures & prostheses (*J Am Dental Assn 134:895, 2003; Med Lett 47:59, 2005*)].		
Hip arthroplasty,[1] spinal fusion	Same as cardiac	Customarily stopped after "Hemovac" removed. NSIPP workgroup recommends stopping prophylaxis within 24 hrs of surgery (*CID 38:1706, 2004*).
Total joint replacement (other than hip)	**Cefazolin** 1–2 gm IV pre-op (± 2nd dose) or **vancomycin** 1 gm IV on call to OR	Post-op: some would give no further rx (*Med Lett 39:98, 1997*). NSIPP workgroup recommends stopping prophylaxis within 24 hrs of surgery (*CID 38:1706, 2004*).
Open reduction of closed fracture with internal fixation	**Ceftriaxone** 2 gm IV or IM once	3.6% vs 8.3% (for placebo) infection found in Dutch trauma trial (*Ln 347:1133, 1996*).
Peritoneal Dialysis Catheter Placement	**Vancomycin** single 1000 mg dose 12 hrs prior to procedure	Effectively reduced peritonitis during 14 days post-placement in 221 pts: vanco 1%, cefazolin 7%, placebo 12% (p=0.02) (*Am J Kidney Dis 36:1014, 2000*).
Urologic Surgery/Procedures Antimicrobials not recommended in pts with sterile urine. Pts with pre-operative bacteriuria should be treated.	Recommended antibiotic rx in pts with pre-operative bacteriuria: **Cefazolin** 1 gm IV q8h times 1–3 doses perioperatively, followed by oral antibiotics. (**nitrofurantoin** or **TMP-SMX**) until catheter is removed or for 10 days. Modify based on susceptibility test results.	
Transrectal prostate biopsy	**Ciprofloxacin** 500 mg po 12 hrs prior to biopsy and repeated 12 hrs after 1st dose	Bacteremia 7% with CIP vs 37% gentamicin (*Urology 38:84, 1991; review in JAC 39:115, 1997*). Levo 500 mg 30–60 min. before procedure was effective in low-risk pts; additional doses were given for ↑ risk (*J Urol 168:1021, 2002*).
Other		
Breast surgery, herniorrhaphy	**P Ceph 1,2**, dosage as Gynecologic Surgery, above	Meta-analysis did not show clear evidence of benefit from prophylaxis in elective inguinal hernia repair (*Cochrane Database System Rev 2004, issue 4*).

---

[1] Gentamicin (12.5 mg per gm of acrylic bone cement) is released for at least 3 weeks. Usefulness not proven.

TABLE 15C: ANTIMICROBIAL PROPHYLAXIS FOR THE PREVENTION OF BACTERIAL ENDOCARDITIS IN PATIENTS WITH UNDERLYING CARDIAC CONDITIONS*
[These are the recommendations of the American Heart Association (*JAMA 277:1794, 1997*). *However, a population-based prospective case-controlled study brings into serious question whether dental procedures predispose to endocarditis and whether antibiotic prophylaxis is of any value* [see *AnlM 129:761, 1998; Brit Dent J 189:610, 2000*)]

ENDOCARDITIS PROPHYLAXIS RECOMMENDED	ENDOCARDITIS PROPHYLAXIS NOT RECOMMENDED
Cardiac conditions associated with endocarditis **High-risk conditions:**[1] 　Prosthetic valves—bioprosthetic and homograft, as well as mechanical 　Previous bacterial endocarditis 　Complex cyanotic congenital heart disease, e.g., single ventricle, transposition, tetralogy of Fallot 　Surgically constructed systemic pulmonic shunts or conduits **Moderate-risk conditions:** 　Most other congenital heart abnormalities or acquired valvular disease; hypertrophic cardiac myopathy; mitral prolapse with regurgitation	Negligible-risk (same as general population): 　Atrial septal defect (secundum) or repaired ASD/VSD, or PDA (beyond 6 months) 　Previous CABG; mitral prolapse without MI (*see discussion JAMA 277:1794, 1997*) 　Physiologic, functional, or innocent heart murmurs 　Previous Kawasaki or rheumatic fever without valve dysfunction 　Cardiac pacemakers (all) and implanted defibrillators
ENDOCARDITIS PROPHYLAXIS RECOMMENDED	**ENDOCARDITIS PROPHYLAXIS NOT RECOMMENDED**
Dental and other procedures where prophylaxis is considered for patients with moderate- or high-risk cardiac conditions Dental: Extractions, periodontal procedures[1] 　Implants, root canal, subgingival antibiotic fibers/strips 　Initial orthodontic bands (not brackets); intraligamentary local anesthetic 　Cleaning of teeth/implants if bleeding anticipated Respiratory: T&A, surgery on respiratory mucosa, rigid bronchoscopy GI: Sclerotherapy of esophageal varices; dilation of esophageal stricture; ERCP with biliary obstruction GU: Prostate surgery; cystoscopy, urethral dilatation	Dental: Filling cavities with local anesthetic 　Placement of rubber dams, suture removal, orthodontic removal 　Orthodontic adjustments, dental x-rays 　Shedding of primary teeth Respiratory: Intubation, flexible bronchoscopy[2], tympanostomy tube GI: Transesophageal cardiac echo[2], EGD without biopsy[2] GU: Vaginal hysterectomy[2], vaginal delivery[2], C-section 　If uninfected, Foley catheter, uterine D&C, therapeutic abortion, tubal ligation, insert/remove IUD Other: Cardiac cath, balloon angioplasty, implanted pacemaker, defibrillators, coronary stents 　Skin biopsy, circumcision

Abbreviations: T&A = tonsillectomy/adenoidectomy, ERCP = endoscopic retrograde cholangiography, ASD/VSD = atrial septal defect/ventricular septal defect, PDA = patent ductus arteriosus, EGD = esophagogastroduodenoscopy, D&C = dilation and curettage

PROPHYLACTIC REGIMENS FOR DENTAL, ORAL, RESPIRATORY TRACT, OR ESOPHAGEAL PROCEDURES

SITUATION	AGENT	REGIMEN[3]
Standard general prophylaxis	Amoxicillin	Adults 2 gm; children 50 mg per kg orally 1 hr before procedure
Unable to take oral medications	Ampicillin	Adults 2 gm IM or IV; children 50 mg per kg IM or IV within 30 min. before procedure
Allergic to penicillin	Clindamycin　OR (Cephalexin[4] or cefadroxil[4]_OR Azithromycin or clarithromycin	Adults 600 mg; children 20 mg per kg orally 1 hr before procedure Adults 2 gm; children 50 mg per kg orally 1 hr before procedure Adults 500 mg; children 15 mg per kg orally 1 hr before procedure
Allergic to penicillin and unable to take oral medications	Clindamycin　OR Cefazolin[4]	Adults 600 mg; children 20 mg per kg IV within 30 min. before procedure Adults 1 gm; children 25 mg per kg IM or IV within 30 min. before procedure

[1] Some now recommend that for adults, prophylaxis prior to dental procedures should **only** be used for **extractions** and **gingival surgery** (including implant replacement) and **only** for patients with **prosthetic cardiac valves** or **previous endocarditis** (*AnlM 129:829, 1998*). If any of these 4 conditions exist = prophylactic antibiotics according to American Heart Association are recommended.
[2] Prophylaxis optional for high-risk patients
[3] Total children's dose should not exceed adult dose
[4] Cephalosporins should not be used in individuals with immediate-type hypersensitivity reaction (urticaria, angioedema, or anaphylaxis) to penicillins.

* *See page 2 for abbreviations*

TABLE 15C (2)

PROPHYLACTIC REGIMENS FOR GENITOURINARY/GASTROINTESTINAL (EXCLUDING ESOPHAGEAL) PROCEDURES

SITUATION	AGENT	REGIMEN[1]
High-risk patients	Ampicillin + gentamicin	**Adults: ampicillin** 2 gm IM or IV + **gentamicin** 1.5 mg per kg (not to exceed 120 mg) within 30 min. of starting the procedure; 6 hr later, **ampicillin** 1 gm IM/IV or **amoxicillin** 1 gm orally. **Children: ampicillin** 50 mg per kg IM or IV (not to exceed 2 gm) + **gentamicin** 1.5 mg per kg within 30 min. of starting the procedure; 6 hrs later, **ampicillin** 25 mg per kg IM/IV or **amoxicillin** 25 mg per kg orally
High-risk patients allergic to ampicillin or amoxicillin	Vancomycin + gentamicin	**Adults: vancomycin** 1 gm IV over 1–2 hrs + **gentamicin** 1.5 mg per kg IV/IM (not to exceed 120 mg); complete injection/infusion within 30 min. of starting the procedure. **Children: vancomycin** 20 mg per kg IV over 1–2 hrs + **gentamicin** 1.5 mg per kg IV/IM; complete injection/ infusion within 30 min. of starting the procedure
Moderate-risk patients	Amoxicillin or ampicillin	**Adults: amoxicillin** 2 gm orally 1 hr before procedure, or **ampicillin** 2 gm IM/IV within 30 min. of starting the procedure **Children: amoxicillin** 50 mg per kg orally 1 hr before procedure, or **ampicillin** 50 mg per kg IM/IV within 30 min. of starting the procedure
Moderate-risk patients allergic to ampicillin or amoxicillin	Vancomycin	**Adults: vancomycin** 1 gm IV over 1–2 hrs; complete infusion within 30 min. of starting the procedure **Children: vancomycin** 20 mg per kg IV over 1–2 hrs; complete infusion within 30 min. of starting the procedure

[1] Total children's dose should not exceed adult dose

TABLE 15D: MANAGEMENT OF EXPOSURE TO HIV-1 AND HEPATITIS*

OCCUPATIONAL EXPOSURE TO BLOOD, PENILE/VAGINAL SECRETIONS OR OTHER POTENTIALLY INFECTIOUS BODY FLUIDS OR TISSUES WITH RISK OF TRANSMISSION OF HEPATITIS B/C AND/OR HIV-1 (E.G., NEEDLESTICK INJURY)

[Adapted from *MMWR 50(RR-11):1, 2001* and *NEJM 348:826, 2003.*]

Free consultation for occupational exposures, call (PEPline) 1-888-448-4911.

General steps in management:
1. Wash clean wounds/flush mucous membranes immediately (use of caustic agents or squeezing the wound is discouraged; data lacking regarding antiseptics).
2. Assess risk by doing the following: (a) Characterize exposure; (b) Determine/evaluate source of exposure by medical history, risk behavior, & testing for hepatitis B/C, HIV; (c) Evaluate and test exposed individual for hepatitis B/C & HIV

Hepatitis B Exposure *[Adapted from CDC recommendations: MMWR 50(RR-11), 2001]*

Exposed Person	Exposure Source		
	HBs Ag+	HBs Ag–	Status Unknown
Unvaccinated	Give HBIG 0.06 mL per kg IM & initiate HB vaccine	Initiate HB vaccine	Initiate HB vaccine and If possible, check HBs Ag of source person
Vaccinated (antibody status unknown)	Do anti-HBs on exposed person: If titer ≥10 milli-International units per mL, no rx If titer <10 milli-International units per mL, give HBIG + 1 dose HB vaccine*	No rx necessary	Do anti-HBs on exposed person: If titer ≥10 milli-International units per mL, no rx If titer <10 milli-International units per mL, give 1 dose of HB vaccine (plus 1 dose HBIG if source high risk)*

For known vaccine series responder (titer ≥10 milli-International units per mL), monitoring of levels or booster doses not currently recommended. Known non-responder (<10 milli-International units per mL) to 1° series HB vaccine & exposed to either HBsAg+ source or suspected high-risk source—rx with HBIG & re-initiate vaccine series **or** give 2 doses HBIG 1 month apart. For non-responders after a 2nd vaccine series, 2 doses HBIG 1 month apart is preferred approach to new exposure *[MMWR 40(RR-13):21; 2001].*

* Follow-up to assess/address vaccine response.

Hepatitis C Exposure
Determine antibody to hepatitis C for both exposed person and, if possible, exposure source. If source +, follow-up HCV testing advised. **No recommended prophylaxis**; immune serum globulin not effective. Monitor for early infection, as therapy may ↓ risk of progression to chronic hepatitis. *See Table 12 and discussion in Clin. Micro Rev 16:546, 2003.*

* See page 2 for abbreviations

TABLE 15D (2)

HIV: Occupational exposure management

- The decision to initiate post-exposure prophylaxis (PEP) for HIV is a clinical judgment that should be made in concert with the exposed healthcare worker (HCW). It is based on:
  1. Likelihood of the source patient having HIV infection: ↑ with history of high-risk activity—injection drug use, sexual activity with known HIV+ person, unprotected sex with multiple partners (either hetero- or homosexual), receipt of blood products 1978–1985. ↑ with clinical signs suggestive of advanced HIV (unexplained wasting, night sweats, thrush, seborrheic dermatitis, etc.). Remember, the vast majority of persons are **not** infected with HIV (1/200 women infected in larger U.S. cities) and likelihood of infection is low if not in above risk groups.
  2. Type of exposure (approx. 1 in 300–400 needlesticks from infected source will transmit HIV).
  3. Limited data regarding efficacy of PEP (PEP with ZDV alone reduced transmission by >80% in 1 retrospective case-controlled study—*NEJM 337:1485, 1997*).
  4. Significant adverse effects of PEP drugs.

- If source person is **known positive for HIV** or **likely to be infected** and **status of exposure warrants PEP**, antiretroviral drugs should be started **immediately** (ASAP or within hours). If source person is HIV antibody negative, drugs can be stopped **unless source is suspected of having acute HIV infection**. The HCW should be re-tested at **3–4 weeks, 3 & 6 months whether PEP is used or not** (the vast majority of seroconversions will occur by 3 months; delayed conversions after 6 months are exceedingly rare). Tests for HIV RNA should not be used for dx of HIV infection because of false-positives (esp. at low titers) & these tests are only approved for established HIV infection [a possible exception is if pt develops signs of acute HIV (mononucleosis-like) syndrome within the 1st 4–6 wks of exposure when antibody tests might still be negative.]

- PEP for HIV is usually given for **4 weeks** and monitoring of adverse effects recommended: baseline **complete blood count, renal and hepatic panel** to be **repeated at 2 weeks**. 50–75% of HCW on PEP demonstrate mild side-effects (nausea, diarrhea, myalgias, headache, etc.) but in up to ½ severe enough to discontinue PEP *(Antivir Ther 3:195, 2000)*. Consultation with infectious diseases/ HIV specialist valuable when questions regarding PEP arise. **Seek expert help in special situations, such as pregnancy, renal impairment, treatment-experienced source.**

3 Steps to HIV Post-Exposure Prophylaxis (PEP) After Occupational Exposure: *[For latest CDC recommendations, see MMWR 54(RR-9), 2005]*

Step 1: Determine the exposure code (EC)

Is source material blood, bloody fluid, semen/vaginal fluid or other normally sterile fluid or tissue?

Yes → What type of exposure occurred?
No → No PEP

What type of exposure occurred?

- Mucous membrane or skin integrity compromised (e.g., dermatitis, open wound) → Volume
- Percutaneous exposure → Severity
- Intact skin → No PEP

Volume:
- Small: Few drops → EC1
- Large: Major splash and/or long duration → EC2

Severity:
- Less severe: Solid needle, scratch → EC2
- More severe: Large-bore hollow needle, deep puncture, visible blood, needle used in blood vessel of source (risk 1:300/400) → EC3

Step 2: Determine the HIV Status Code (HIV SC)

What is the HIV status of the exposure source?

- HIV negative → No PEP
- HIV positive:
  - Low titer exposure: asymptomatic, low VL (<1500 copies per mL), low CD4 count, & high CD4 count → HIV SC 1
  - High titer exposure: advanced AIDS, primary HIV, high viral load or low CD4 count → HIV SC 2
- Status unknown → HIV SC unknown
- Source unknown → HIV SC unknown

* Exceptions can be considered when there has been prolonged, high-volume contact.

* See page 2 for abbreviations

TABLE 15D (3)

Step 3: Determine Post-Exposure Prophylaxis (PEP) Recommendation

EC	HIV SC	PEP
1	1	Consider basic regimen[1] [a]
1	2	Recommend basic regimen[1] [a,b]
2	1	Recommend basic regimen[1] [b]
2	2	Recommend expanded regimen[1]
3	1 or 2	Recommend expanded regimen[1]
1, 2, 3	Unknown	If exposure setting suggests risks of HIV exposure, consider basic regimen[1] [c]

[a] Based on estimates of ↓ risk of infection after mucous membrane exposure in occupational setting compared with needlestick.

Modification of CDC recommendations:
[b] Or, consider expanded regimen[1].
[c] In high risk circumstances, consider expanded regimen[1] on case-by-case basis.

Around the clock, urgent expert consultation available from:
National Clinicians' Post-Exposure Prophylaxis Hotline
(PEPline) at 1-888-448-4911 (1-888-HIV-4911)

[1] **Regimens:** (Treat for 4 weeks; monitor for drug side-effects every 2 weeks)
Basic regimen: ZDV + 3TC, or FTC + TDF, or possibly d4T + 3TC.
Expanded regimen: Basic regimen + one of the following: lopinavir/ritonavir, nelfinavir, indinavir/ritonavir, fosamprenavir/ritonavir, atazanavir (or atazanavir/ritonavir); efavirenz can be considered (except in pregnancy or potential for pregnancy—**Pregnancy Category D**), but CNS symptoms might be problematic. [**Do not use nevirapine**: serious adverse reactions including hepatic necrosis reported in healthcare workers (MMWR 49:1153, 2001).]
Other regimens can be designed. If possible, use 2 antiretroviral drugs that source pt (if known) is not currently taking or for which resistance is unlikely based on susceptibility data or treatment history. Seek expert consultation if ARV-experienced source or in pregnancy or potential for pregnancy.
NOTE: Some authorities feel that an expanded regimen should be employed whenever PEP is indicated (NEJM 349:1091, 2003; Eur J Epidemiol 19:577, 2004, & NY State AIDS Institute, 2004). For example, the latter recommends ZDV + 3TC + tenofovir (www.hivguidelines.org/public_html/center/clinical-guidelines/pep_guidelines/pep_guidelines. htm). Expanded regimens are likely to be advantageous with ↑ numbers of ART-experienced source pts or when there is doubt about exact extent of exposures in decision algorithm. Mathematical model suggests that under some conditions, completion of full course basic regimen is better than prematurely discontinued expanded regimen (CID 39:395, 2004). However, while expanded PEP regimens have ↑ adverse effects, there is not necessarily ↑ discontinuation (CID 40:205, 2005).

POST-EXPOSURE PROPHYLAXIS FOR NON-OCCUPATIONAL EXPOSURES TO HIV
From MMWR 54(RR-2):1, 2005—DHHS recommendations

Because the risk of transmission of HIV via sexual contact or sharing needles by injection drug users may reach or exceed that of occupational needlestick exposure, it is reasonable to consider PEP in persons who have had a non-occupational exposure to blood or other potentially infected fluids (e.g., genital/rectal secretions, breast milk) from an HIV+ source. Risk of HIV acquisition per exposure varies with the act (for needle sharing and receptive anal intercourse, ≥0.5%; approximately 10-fold lower with insertive vaginal or anal intercourse, 0.05–0.07%). Overt or occult traumatic lesions may ↑ risk in survivors of sexual assault.

For pts at risk of HIV acquisition through non-occupational exposure to HIV+ source material having occurred ≤72 hours before evaluation, DHHS recommendation is to treat for 28 days with an anti-retroviral **expanded regimen**, using preferred regimens [efavirenz *(not in pregnancy or pregnancy risk—**Pregnancy Category D**)* + (3TC or FTC) + (ZDV or TDF)] **or** [lopinavir/ritonavir + (3TC or FTC) + ZDV] or one of several alternative regimens [see Table 14C section B & MMWR 54(RR-2):1, 2005].

Areas of uncertainty: (1) expanded regimens are not proven to be superior to 2-drug regimens, (2) while PEP not recommended for exposures >72 hours before evaluation, it may possibly be effective in some cases, (3) when HIV status of source patient is unknown, decision to treat and regimen selection must be individualized based on assessment of specific circumstances.

Evaluate for exposures to Hep B, Hep C. (See *Occupational PEP above*), and bacterial sexually-transmitted diseases [see Table 15A, & MMWR 51(RR-6):1, 2002] and treat as indicated.

*See page 2 for abbreviations

TABLE 15E: PREVENTION OF OPPORTUNISTIC INFECTION IN HUMAN STEM CELL TRANSPLANTATION (HSCT) OR SOLID ORGAN TRANSPLANTATION (SOT) FOR ADULTS WITH NORMAL RENAL FUNCTION*

General comments: See Table 15F, page 132 for typical timing of infections post-transplant. References.: *MMWR 49(RR-10):1, 2000; CID 33:S26, 2001; COID 17:353, 2004*

OPPORTUNISTIC INFECTION (at risk)	TYPE OF TRANSPLANT	PROPHYLACTIC REGIMENS	COMMENTS/REFERENCES
Herpes simplex (seropositive)	HSCT	Acyclovir 200 mg po 3 times per day from conditioning to engraftment or resolution of mucositis	Do not need acyclovir if receiving CMV prophylaxis
	SOT	Acyclovir 200 mg po 3 times per day—start early post-transplant	
CMV (Recipient + OR Donor +/-Recipient –)	HSCT	**Preemptive therapy:** Monitor ≥ once weekly (days 10-100) for CMV-antigenemia or viremia by PCR test (Note: culture alone not sufficiently sensitive) & start rx when positive. [Ganciclovir 5 mg per kg IV 12h for 7–14 days, then 5 mg per kg IV q24h 5 days per week to day 100 or ≥3 wks (whichever is longer) [*MMWR 49(RR-10):1, 2000*]. Some use oral ganciclovir 1 gm q8h after the 7–14 day IV induction phase. Some use shorter courses; however, monitoring tests should be negative before stopping rx (*CID 35:999, 2002*). OR **Prophylaxis:** (for high-risk pts, see *CID 35:999, 2002*, or where CMV detection tests not available) From engraftment to day 100, rx with ganciclovir 5 mg per kg q12h for 7 days, then 5 mg per kg q24h 5–6 days per week.	
		General Comments: Review in *CMR 16:647, 2003.* Role of valganciclovir in CMV prevention is under investigation.	
	SOT	**Kidney, kidney/pancreas, heart:** Valganciclovir 900 mg po q24h; start by day 10 & continue through day 100 of transplant. **Liver:** Ganciclovir 1 gm po q8h, start by day 10 & continue through day 100. **Lung:** Ganciclovir 5 mg per kg q12h for 5–7 days, then valganciclovir 900 mg po q24h for 6 months (or at least 3 mos.) PLUS consider CMV immune globulin 150 mg per kg within 72 hrs of transplant, & at 2, 4, 6, & 8 wks post-transplant, then 100 mg per kg at wk 12 & 16. **Comments:** Regimens are evolving & institutional protocols vary. For recommendations by American & Canadian transplantation societies, see *Am J Transpl 4(Suppl.10):51, 2004 & 5:218, 2005.* For lung, see *Transpl 80:157, 2005.* The universal prophylaxis approach (above) is favored by most, but there are proponents of preemptive therapy in liver transplantation (*CID 40:704 & 709, 2005; Transpl 79:85 & 1428, 2005*). Valganciclovir not approved by FDA for liver transplantation, but some use it. Some add CMV Ig for other high-risk SOTs also.	
Hepatitis B-induced cirrhosis	Liver	See Table 14A, page 107	
Candida sp. (*CID 38:161, 2004*)	Liver	Fluconazole 200–400 mg IV/po 1 time per day starting before transplant & continuing up to 3 mos. in high-risk pts. Optimal duration unknown. Concerns for ↑ non-albicans candida with fluconazole prophylaxis (*Transpl 75:2023, 2003*).	
	HSCT	Fluconazole 400 mg po 1 time per day from day 0 to engraftment or ANC >1000	
Aspergillus sp.	Lung/Heart-lung	No controlled trials to determine optimal management, but regimens of an aerosolized ampho B preparation & an oral anti-aspergillus agent have been used [*Am J Transpl 4(Suppl.10):110, 2004*]. Randomized trial suggested nebulized ABLC better tolerated than nebul. ampho B deoxycholate (*Transpl 77:232, 2004*).	
	HSCT	Itraconazole solution led to non-significant ↓ invasive aspergillus (*AnIM 138:705, 2003*) or significant ↓ infection with ↑ toxicity/intolerance (*Blood 103:1527, 2003*). Study of voriconazole vs fluconazole to prevent invasive fungal infections in progress (*CID 39:S176, 2004*). Vori assoc. with ↑ risk of zygomycosis (*JID 191:1350, 2005*).	
Coccidioides immitis	All	Reasonable: Fluconazole 400 mg po q24h (*Transpl Inf Dis 5:3, 2003*)	
Pneumocystis carinii (P. jiroveci) & Toxoplasma gondii	All	TMP-SMX-SS or -DS, 1 tab po q24h. Duration: 6 mos.–1 yr renal; ≥6 mos. for allogenic HSCT; ≥1 yr to lifetime for heart, lung, liver [*Am J Transpl 4(Suppl.10):135, 2004*]. Breakthrough pneumocystis infections reported with atovaquone doses <1500 mg per day (*CID 38:e76, 2004*). For toxo D+/R– heart transplants, 3 mos. pyrimethamine/sulfa prior to lifetime TMP-SMX prophylaxis has been suggested [*see Am J Transpl 4(Suppl.10):142, 2004*] for intensive pyri-sulfa regimen & alternatives]	
Trypanosoma cruzi	Heart	If known Chagas' disease in donor or recipient, contact CDC for nifurtimox	

* See page 2 for abbreviations

132

TABLE 15F
TEMPORAL APPROACH TO DIFFERENTIAL DIAGNOSIS OF INFECTION AFTER ORGAN TRANSPLANTATION*

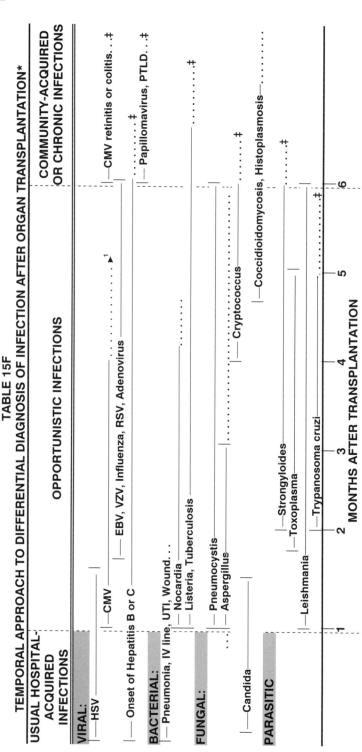

* Adapted from Fishman and Rubin, *NEJM 338:1741, 1998*. For hematopoietic stem cell transplant recipients, see *MMWR 49:RR-10, 2000*.
‡ Solid lines indicate usual time period for onset of infection; dotted lines indicate risk at reduced level

[1] Symptomatic CMV antigenemia may be delayed in patients receiving 3-mo. ganciclovir prophylaxis (*Transpl Inf Dis 6:3, 2004*).

TABLE 16: PEDIATRIC DOSAGES OF SELECTED ANTIBACTERIAL AGENTS*

[Adapted from: (1) Nelson's Pocket Book of Pediatric Antimicrobial Therapy, 2002-2003, 15th Ed., J. Bradley & J. Nelson, eds., Lippincott Williams and Wilkins, and (2) 2003 Red Book, 26th Ed., American Academy of Pediatrics, pages 700–718]

DRUG	DOSES IN MG PER KG PER DAY OR MG PER KG AT FREQUENCY INDICATED[1]				
	BODY WEIGHT <2000 gm		BODY WEIGHT >2000 gm		>28 DAYS OLD
	0–7 days old	8–28 days old	0–7 days old	8–28 days old	
Aminoglycosides, IV or IM (check levels; some dose by gestational age + wks of life; see Nelson's Pocket Book, p. 19)					
Amikacin	7.5 q18–24h	7.5 q12h	10 q12h	10 q12h	10 q8h
Gent/tobra	2.5 q18–24h	2.5 q12h	2.5 q12h	2.5 q12h	2.5 q8h
Aztreonam, IV	30 q12h	30 q8h	30 q8h	30 q6h	30 q6h
Cephalosporins					
Cefaclor					20–40 div tid
Cefadroxil					30 div bid (max 2 gm per day)
Cefazolin	20 q12h	20 q12h	20 q12h	20 q8h	20 q8h
Cefdinir					7 q12h or 14 q24h
Cefepime					150 div q8h
Cefixime					8 as q24h or div bid
Cefotaxime	50 q12h	50 q8h	50 q12h	50 q8h	50 q6h (75 q6h for meningitis)
Cefoxitin		20 q12h			80–160 div q6h
Cefpodoxime					10 div bid (max 400 mg per day)
Cefprozil					15–30 div bid (max 1 gm per day)
Ceftazidime	30 q12h	30 q8h	30 q12h	30 q8h	50 q8h
Ceftibuten					4.5 bid
Ceftizoxime					33–66 q8h
Ceftriaxone	50 q24h	50 q24h	50 q24h	75 q24h	50–75 q24h (meningitis 100)
Cefuroxime IV	50 q12h	50 q8h	50 q8h	50 q8h	50 q8h (80 q8h for meningitis)
po					10–15 bid (max 1 gm per day)
Cephalexin					25–50 div q6h (max 4 gm per day)
Loracarbef					15–30 div bid (max 0.8 gm per day)
Chloramphenicol IV	25 q24h	25 q24h	25 q24h	15 q12h	12.5–25 q6h (max 2–4 gm per day)
Clindamycin IV	5 q12h	5 q8h	5 q8h	5 q6h	7.5 q6h
po					5–6 q6h
Ciprofloxacin po[2]					20–30 div bid (max 1.5 gm per day)
Ertapenem IV	No data	No data	No data	No data	15 q12h
Imipenem[3] IV		25 q12h		25 q8h	15–25 q6h (max 2 gm per day)
Linezolid	No data	10 q8h	No data	10 q8h	10 q8h to age 12
Macrolides					
Erythro IV & po	10 q12h	10 q8h	10 q12h	13 q8h	10 q6h
Azithro po					10–12 day 1, then 5 per day[4]
Clarithro po					7.5 q12h (max. 1 gm per day)
Meropenem IV	20 q12h	20 q8h	20 q12h	20 q8h	60–120 div q8h (120 for meningitis)
Metro IV & po	7.5 q24h	7.5 q12h	7.5 q12h	15 q12h	7.5 q6h
Penicillins					
Ampicillin	50 q12h	50 q8h	50 q8h	50 q6h	50 q6h
AMP-sulbactam					100–300 div q6h
Amoxicillin po				30 div bid	25–50 div tid
Amox-Clav po	30 div bid	30 div bid	30 div bid	30 div bid	45 or 90 (AM/CL-HD) div bid if over 12 wks of age
Dicloxacillin					12–25 div q6h
Mezlocillin	75 q12h	75 q8h	75 q12h	75 q8h	75 q6h
Nafcillin, oxacillin IV	25 q12h	25 q8h	25 q8h	37 q6h	37 q6h (to max. 8–12 gm per day)
Piperacillin, PIP-tazo IV	75 mg per kg q12h	75 mg per kg q12h	75 mg per kg q8h	75 mg per kg q8h	100–300 div q4–6h
Ticarcillin, T.clav IV	75 q12h	75 q8h	75 q8h	75 q6h	75 q6h
Tinidazole					> Age 3: 50 mg per kg for 1 dose
Penicillin G, **U/kg** IV	50,000 q12h	75,000 q8h	50,000 q8h	50,000 q6h	50,000 units per kg per day
Penicillin V					25–50 mg per kg per day div q6–8h
Rifampin po		10, single dose	20, single dose	20, single dose (max. 600 mg)	
Sulfisoxazole po				120–150	120–150 mg per kg per day div q4–6h
TMP-SMX po, IV; UTI: 8–12 TMP component div bid; Pneumocystis: 20 TMP component div q6h					
Tetracycline po (age 8 or older)					25–50 div q6h
Doxycycline po, IV (age 8 or older)					2–4 div bid
Vancomycin IV	12.5 q12h	15 q12h	18 q12h	22 q12h	40–60 div q6h

[1] May need higher doses in patients with meningitis: see CID 39:1267, 2004
[2] With exception of cystic fibrosis, not approved for use under age 18.
[3] Not recommended in children with CNS infections due to risk of seizures.
[4] Dose for otitis; for pharyngitis, 12 mg per kg times 5 days
* See page 2 for abbreviations

TABLE 17A: DOSAGE OF ANTIMICROBIAL DRUGS IN ADULT PATIENTS WITH RENAL IMPAIRMENT

Adapted from DRUG PRESCRIBING IN RENAL FAILURE, 4th Ed., Aronoff et al (Eds.), American College of Physicians, 1999 and Berns et al, Renal Aspects of Antimicrobial Therapy for HIV Infection. In: P. Kenimel & J. Berns, Eds., HIV INFECTION AND THE KIDNEY, Churchill-Livingstone, 1995, pp. 195-236.

UNLESS STATED, ADJUSTED DOSES ARE % OF DOSE FOR NORMAL RENAL FUNCTION.

Drug adjustments are based on the patient's estimated endogenous creatinine clearance, which can be calculated as:

$$\frac{(140-age)(\text{ideal body weight in kg})}{(72)(\text{serum creatinine, mg per dL})}\ \text{for men (x 0.85 for women)}$$

Ideal body weight for men: 50.0 kg + 2.3 kg per inch over 5 feet
Ideal body weight for women: 45.5 kg + 2.3 kg per inch over 5 feet

For alternative method to calculate estimated CrCl, see *AnIM* 130:461, 1999.

NOTE: For summary of drugs requiring NO dosage adjustment with renal insufficiency, see Table 17B, page 139.

ANTIMICROBIAL	HALF-LIFE (NORMAL/ESRD) hr	DOSE FOR NORMAL RENAL FUNCTION§	METHOD* (see footnote)	ADJUSTMENT FOR RENAL FAILURE — Estimated creatinine clearance (CrCl), mL per min >50-90	10-50	<10	SUPPLEMENT FOR HEMODIALYSIS, CAPD+ (see footnote)	COMMENTS ± DOSAGE FOR CAVH‡
ANTIBACTERIAL ANTIBIOTICS								
Aminoglycoside Antibiotics:		Traditional multiple daily doses—adjustment for renal disease						
Amikacin	1.4-2.3/17-150	7.5 mg per kg q12h	D&I	60-90% q12h	30-70% q12-18h Same dose for CAVH‡	20-30% q24-48h	HEMO: Extra ½ of normal renal function dose AD‡ CAPD: 15-20 mg lost per L dialysate per day (see Comment)	High flux hemodialysis membranes lead to unpredictable aminoglycoside clearance, measure post-dialysis drug levels for efficacy and toxicity. With CAPD, pharmacokinetics highly variable—**check serum levels**. Usual method for CAPD: 2 liters of dialysis fluid placed qid or 8 liters per day (give 8L×20 mg lost per L = 160 mg of amikacin supplement IV per day)
Gentamicin, Tobramycin	2-3/20-60	1.7 mg per kg q8h	D&I	60-90% q8-12h	30-70% q12h Same dose for CAVH‡	20-30% q24-48h	HEMO: Extra ½ of normal renal function dose AD‡ CAPD: 3-4 mg lost per L dialysate per day	
Netilmicin[NUS]	2-3/35-72	2.0 mg per kg q8h	D&I	50-90% q8-12h	20-60% q12h Same dose for CAVH‡	10-20% q24-48h	HEMO: Extra ½ of normal renal function dose AD‡ CAPD: 3-4 mg lost per L dialysate per day	Adjust dosing weight for obesity: [ideal body weight + 0.4(actual body weight – ideal body weight)] (CID 25:112, 1997).
Streptomycin	2-3/30-80	15 mg per kg (max. of 1.0 gm) q24h	I	50% q24h	q24-72h Same dose for CAVH‡	q72-96h	HEMO: Extra ½ of normal renal function dose AD‡ CAPD: 20-40 mg lost per L dialysate per day	

ONCE-DAILY AMINOGLYCOSIDE THERAPY: ADJUSTMENT IN RENAL INSUFFICIENCY (see Table 10D for OD dosing/normal renal function)

Drug / Creatinine Clearance (mL per min.)	>80	60-80	40-60	30-40	20-30	10-20	<10-0
	Dose q24h (mg per kg)				Dose q48h (mg per kg)		Dose q72h and AD+
Gentamicin/Tobramycin	5.1	4	3.5	2.5	4	3	3
Amikacin/kanamycin/streptomycin	15	12	7.5	4	7.5	4	3
Isepamicin[NUS]	8	8	8	8	8	8 q72h	8 q96h
Netilmicin[NUS]	6.5	5	4	2	2.5	2	2

ANTIMICROBIAL	HALF-LIFE (NORMAL/ESRD) hr	DOSE FOR NORMAL RENAL FUNCTION§	METHOD*	>50-90	10-50	<10	SUPPLEMENT FOR HEMODIALYSIS, CAPD+	COMMENTS ± DOSAGE FOR CAVH‡
Carbapenem Antibiotics								
Ertapenem	4/>4	1.0 gm q24h	D	1.0 gm q24h	0.5 gm q24h (CrCl <30)	0.5 gm q24h	HEMO: Dose as for CrCl <10; if dosed <6 hrs prior to HD, give 150 mg supplement AD‡	
Imipenem (see Comment)	1/4	0.5 gm q6h	D&I	250-500 mg q6-8h	250 mg q6-12h Dose for CAVH‡: 0.5-1 gm bid (AAC 49:2421, 2005)	125-250 mg q12h	HEMO: Dose AD‡ CAPD: Dose for CrCl <10	↑ potential for seizures if recommended doses exceeded in pts with CrCl <20 mL per min. See pkg insert, esp. for pts <70 kg
Meropenem	1/6-8	1.0 gm q8h	D&I	1.0 gm q8h	1.0 gm q12h Same dose for CAVH‡	0.5 gm q24h	HEMO: Dose AD‡ CAPD: Dose for CrCl <10	

‡ **CAVH** = continuous arteriovenous hemofiltration (*NEJM* 336:1303, 1997) usually results in CrCl of approx. 30 mL per min.; + **AD** = after dialysis. **"Dose AD" refers to timing of dose.** Supplement is to replace drug lost via dialysis; extra drug beyond continuation of regimen used for CrCl <10 mL per min.
See page 2 for abbreviations.

TABLE 17A (2)

ANTIMICROBIAL	HALF-LIFE (NORMAL/ESRD) hr	DOSE FOR NORMAL RENAL FUNCTION§	METHOD* (see footnote)	ADJUSTMENT FOR RENAL FAILURE Estimated creatinine clearance (CrCl), mL per min			SUPPLEMENT FOR HEMODIALYSIS, CAPD+ (see footnote)	COMMENTS ± DOSAGE FOR CAVH‡
				>50-90	10-50	<10		
Cephalosporin Antibiotics: DATA ON SELECTED PARENTERAL CEPHALOSPORINS								
Cefazolin	1.9/40-70	1.0-2.0 gm q8h	I	q8h	q12h **Same dose for CAVH‡**	q24-48h	HEMO: Extra 0.5-1 gm AD+ CAPD: 0.5 gm q12h	
Cefepime	2.2/18	2.0 gm q8h (max. dose)	D&I	2 gm q8h	2 gm q12-24h **Same dose for CAVH‡**	1 gm q24h	HEMO: Extra 1 gm AD+ CAPD: 1-2 gm q48h	CAVH‡ dose: As for CrCl 10-50
Cefotaxime, Ceftizoxime	1.7/15-35	2.0 gm q8h	I	q8-12h	q12-24h **Same dose for CAVH‡**	q24h	HEMO: Extra 1 gm AD+ CAPD: 0.5-1 gm q24h	Active metabolite of cefotaxime in ESRD. ↓ dose further for hepatic & renal failure.
Cefotetan	3.5/13-25	1-2 gm q12h	D	100%	50%	25%	HEMO: Extra 1 gm AD+ CAPD: 1 gm q24h	CAVH‡ dose: 750 mg q12h
Cefoxitin	0.8/13-23	2.0 gm q8h	I	q8h	q8-12h **Same dose for CAVH‡**	q24-48h	HEMO: Extra 1 gm AD+ CAPD: 1 gm q24h	May falsely increase serum creatinine by interference with assay.
Ceftazidime	1.2/13-25	2 gm q8h	I	q8-12h	q24-48h **Same dose for CAVH‡**	q48h	HEMO: Extra 1 gm AD+ CAPD: 0.5 gm q24h	Volume of distribution increases with infection.
Cefuroxime sodium	1.2/17	0.75-1.5 gm q8h	I	q8h	q8-12h	q24h	HEMO: Dose AD+ CAPD: Dose for CrCl <10	CAVH‡ dose: 1.5 gm, then 750 mg IV q24h
Fluoroquinolone Antibiotics								
Ciprofloxacin	4/6-9	500-750 mg po (or 400 mg IV) q12h	D	100%	50-75%	50%	HEMO: 250 mg po or 200 mg IV q12h CAPD: 250 mg po or 200 mg IV q8h	CAVH‡ dose: 200 mg IV q12h
Gatifloxacin	7-14/36	400 mg po/IV q24h	D	400 mg q24h	400 mg, then 200 mg q24h **Same dose for CAVH‡**	400 mg, then 200 mg q24h	HEMO: 200 mg q24h AD+ CAPD: 200 mg q24h	CAVH‡ dose: As for CrCl 10-50
Gemifloxacin	7/>7	320 mg po q24h	D	320 mg q24h	160 mg q24h	160 mg q24h	HEMO: 160 mg q24h AD+ CAPD: 160 mg q24h	
Levofloxacin	6-51/76	750 mg q24h IV, PO	D&I	750 mg q24h	750 mg once, then 500 q48h	750 mg once, then 500 q48h	HEMO/CAPD: Dose for CrCl <10	CAVH‡ dose: As for CrCl 10-50
Macrolide Antibiotics								
Clarithromycin	5-7/22	0.5-1.0 gm q12h	D	100%	75%	50-75%	HEMO: Dose AD+ CAPD: None	ESRD dosing recommendations based on extrapolation
Erythromycin	1.4/5-6	250-500 mg q6h	D	100%	100%	50-75%	HEMO/CAPD/CAVH‡: None	Ototoxicity with high doses in ESRD
Miscellaneous Antibacterial Antibiotics								
Colistin	<6/≥48	80-160 mg q8h	D	160 mg q12h	160 mg q24h	160 mg q36h	HEMO: 80 mg AD+	
Daptomycin	9.4/30	4 mg per kg per day	I	4 mg per kg per day	CrCl <30, 4 mg per kg q48h	4 mg per kg q48h	HEMO & CAPD: 4 mg per kg q48h (after dialysis if possible)	
Linezolid	6.4/7.1	600 mg po/IV q12h	None	600 mg q12h	600 mg po/IV q12h **Same dose for CAVH‡**	600 mg q12h AD+	HEMO: As for CrCl <10 CAPD: No data	CAVH‡: Accumulation of 2 metabolites—risk unknown (JAC 56:172, 2005)
Metronidazole	6-14/7-21	7.5 mg per kg q6h	D	100%	100% **Same dose for CAVH‡**	50%	HEMO: Dose AD+ CAPD: Dose for CrCl <10	Hemo clears metronidazole and its metabolites (AAC 29:235, 1986)
Nitrofurantoin	0.5/1	50-100 mg	D	100%	Avoid	Avoid	Not applicable	
Sulfamethoxazole	10/20-50	1.0 gm q8h	I	q12h	q18h **Same dose for CAVH‡**	q24h	HEMO: Extra 1 gm AD+ CAPD: 1 gm q24h	
Teicoplanin[nus]	45/62-230	6 mg per kg per day	I	q24h	q48h **Same dose for CAVH‡**	q72h	HEMO: Dose for CrCl <10 CAPD: Dose for CrCl <10	
Telithromycin	10/15	800 mg per day	D	800 mg q24h	600 mg q24h (<30 mL per min.) **Same dose for CAVH‡**	600 mg q24h	HEMO: 600 mg q24h CAPD: No data	

‡ **CAVH** = continuous arteriovenous hemofiltration (NEJM 336:1303, 1997) usually results in CrCl of approx. 30 mL per min. + **AD** = after dialysis. **"Dose AD" refers to timing of dose.**
Supplement is to replace drug lost via dialysis; extra drug beyond continuation of regimen used for CrCl <10 mL per min.
See page 138 for other footnotes and page 2 for abbreviations.

TABLE 17A (3)

ANTIMICROBIAL	HALF-LIFE (NORMAL/ESRD) hr	DOSE FOR NORMAL RENAL FUNCTION§	METHOD* (see footnote)	>50-90	10-50	<10	SUPPLEMENT FOR HEMODIALYSIS, CAPD⁺ (see footnote)	COMMENTS ± DOSAGE FOR CAVH‡
Miscellaneous Antibacterial Antibiotics (continued)								
Trimethoprim	11/20-49	100-200 mg q12h	I	q12h	q18h **Same dose for CAVH‡**	q24h	HEMO: Dose AD⁺ / CAPD: q24h	CAVH‡ dose: q18h
Trimethoprim-sulfamethoxazole-DS								
Treatment	As above	5 mg per kg IV q8h	D	100%	50%	Not recommended		
Prophylaxis	As above	1 tab po q24h or 3 times per week	No change	100%	100%	100%		
Vancomycin	6/200-250	1 gm q12h	D&I	1 gm q12h	1 gm q24-96h	1 gm q4-7 days	HEMO/CAPD: Dose for CrCl <10	CAVH‡ 500 mg q24-48h. New hemodialysis membranes ↑ clear. of vanco; **check levels**
Penicillins								
Amoxicillin	1.0/5-20	250-500 mg q8h	–	q8h	q8-12h	q24h	HEMO: Dose AD⁺ / CAPD: 250 mg q12h	IV amoxicillin not available in the U.S.
Ampicillin	1.0/7-20	250 mg-2 gm q6h	–	q6h	q6-12h	q12-24h	HEMO: 250 mg q12h / CAPD: As for CrCl <10; extra dose after dialysis	
Amoxicillin/ Clavulanate[1]	1.3 AM/1.0, 5-20/4.0	500/125 mg q8h (see Comments)	D&I	500/125 mg q8h	250-500 mg AM component q8h	250-500 mg AM component q24h	HEMO: Dose AD⁺ / CAPD: Dose for CrCl <10	**If CrCl ≤30 per mL, do not use 875/125 or 1000/62.5 AM/CL**
Ampicillin (AM)/ Sulbactam(SB)	1.0 (AM)/1.0 (SB), 9.0 (AM)/10.0 (SB)	2 gm AM + 1.0 gm SB q6h	D&I	q6h	q8-12h	q24h	HEMO: Dose AD⁺ / CAPD: 2 gm AM/1 gm SB q24h	CAVH‡ dose: 1.5 AM/0.75 SB q12h
Aztreonam	2.0/6-8	2 gm q8h	D	100%	50-75% **Same dose for CAVH‡**	25%	HEMO: Extra 0.5 gm AD⁺ / CAPD: Dose for CrCl <10	Technically is a β-lactam antibiotic.
Penicillin G	0.5/6-20	0.5-4 million U q4h	D	100%	75% **Same dose for CAVH‡**	20-50%	HEMO: Dose AD⁺ / CAPD: Dose for CrCl <10	1.7 mEq potassium per million units. ↑ potential of seizure. 6 million units per day max. dose in ESRD.
Piperacillin	1.0/3.3-5.1	3-4 gm q4-6h	I	q4-6h	q6-8h **Same dose for CAVH‡**	q8h	HEMO: Dose AD⁺ / CAPD: Dose for CrCl <10	1.9 mEq sodium per gm
Pip (P)/Tazo(T)	1.0 P/1.0 T, 3.0 P/4.0 T	3.375 gm q6h	D&I	3.375 gm q6h	2.25 gm q6h	2.25 gm q8h	HEMO: Dose for CrCl <10 + 0.75 gm AD⁺ / CAPD: Dose for CrCl <10	
Ticarcillin	1.2/13	3 gm q4h	D&I	1-2 gm q4h	1-2 gm q8h **Same dose for CAVH‡**	1-2 gm q12h	HEMO: Extra 3.0 gm AD⁺ / CAPD: Dose for CrCl <10	5.2 mEq sodium per gm
Ticarcillin/ Clavulanate[1]	1.0 (TC)/1.0 (CL), 13 (TC)/4.0 (CL)	3.1 gm q4h	D&I	3.1 gm q4h	2.0 gm q4-8h **Same dose for CAVH‡**	2.0 gm q12h	HEMO: Extra 3.1 gm AD⁺ / CAPD: 3.1 gm q12h	See footnote 2
Tetracycline Antibiotics								
Tetracycline	6-10/57-108	250-500 mg qid	I	q8-12h	q12-24h **Same dose for CAVH‡**	q24h	HEMO/CAPD/CAVH‡: None	Avoid in ESRD
ANTIFUNGAL ANTIBIOTICS								
Amphotericin B & ampho B lipid complex	24/unchanged	Non-lipid: 0.4-1.0 mg per kg per day; ABCC: 3-6 mg per kg per day; ABLC: 5 mg per kg per day; LAB: 3-5 mg per kg per day	I	q24h	q24h **Same dose for CAVH‡**	q24-48h	HEMO: None / CAPD: Dose for CrCl <10	For ampho B, toxicity lessened by saline loading; risk amplified by concomitant cyclosporine A, aminoglycosides, or pentamidine
Fluconazole	37/100	200-400 mg q24h	D	200-400 mg q24h	100-200 mg q24h **Same dose for CAVH‡**	100-200 mg q24h	HEMO: 100% of recommended dose AD⁺ / CAPD: Dose for CrCl <10	
Flucytosine	3-6/75-200	37.5 mg per kg q6h	I	q12h	q12-24h	q24h	HEMO: Dose AD⁺ / CAPD: 0.5-1.0 gm q24h	Goal is peak serum level >25 mcg per mL and <100 mcg per mL

* Clavulanate cleared by liver, not kidney. Hence as dose of combination decreased, a deficiency of clavulanate may occur (JAMA 285:386, 2001).

‡ **CAVH** = continuous arteriovenous hemofiltration (NEJM 336:1303, 1997) usually results in CrCl of approx. 30 mL per min. + **AD** = after dialysis. **Supplement is to replace drug lost via dialysis; extra drug beyond continuation of regimen used for CrCl <10 mL per min.**

See page 138 for other abbreviations and page 2 for abbreviations.

TABLE 17A (4)

ANTIMICROBIAL	HALF-LIFE (NORMAL/ESRD) hr	DOSE FOR NORMAL RENAL FUNCTION§	METHOD* (see footnote)	ADJUSTMENT FOR RENAL FAILURE — Estimated creatinine clearance (CrCl), mL per min >50–90	10–50	<10	SUPPLEMENT FOR HEMODIALYSIS, CAPD† (see footnote)	COMMENTS ± DOSAGE FOR CAVH‡
ANTIFUNGAL ANTIBIOTICS *(continued)*								
Itraconazole, po soln.	35/–	100–200 mg q12h	–	100%	100%	100%		HEMO/CAPD/CAVH‡: No adjustment with oral solution
Itraconazole, IV	35/–	200 mg IV q12h	–		200 mg IV bid		Do not use IV itra if CrCl <30 due to accumulation of carrier: cyclodextrin	
Terbinafine	36–200/?	250 mg po per day	–		q24h		Use has not been studied. Recommend avoidance of drug.	
Voriconazole, **IV**	Non-linear kinetics	6 mg per kg IV q12h times 2, then 4 mg per kg q12h	–		No change		If CrCl <50 mL per min., accum. of IV vehicle (cyclodextrin). Switch to po or DC	
ANTIPARASITIC ANTIBIOTICS								
Pentamidine	29/118	4 mg per kg per day	I	q24h	q24h	q24–36h	HEMO/CAPD/CAVH‡: None	
Quinine	5–16/5–16	650 mg q8h	I	650 mg q8h	650 mg q8–12h **Same dose for CAVH‡**	650 mg q24h	HEMO: Dose AD⁺ CAPD: Dose for CrCl <10	Marked tissue accumulation
ANTITUBERCULOUS ANTIBIOTICS *(Excellent review: Nephron 64:169, 1993)*								
Ethambutol	4/7–15	15–25 mg per kg q24h	I	q24h **Same dose for CAVH‡**	q24–36h	q48h	HEMO: Dose AD⁺ CAPD: Dose for CrCl <10	25 mg per kg 4–6 hr prior to 3 times per wk dialysis. Streptomycin instead of ethambutol in renal failure.
Ethionamide	2.1/?	250–500 mg q12h	D	100%	100%	50%	HEMO/CAPD/CAVH‡: None	
Isoniazid	0.7–4/8–17	5 mg per kg per day (max. 300 mg)	D	100%	100%	100%	HEMO: Dose AD⁺ CAPD/CAVH‡: Dose for CrCl <10	
Pyrazinamide	9/26	25 mg per kg q24h (max. dose 2.5 gm q24h)	D	25 mg per kg q24h	25 mg per kg q24h	12–25 mg per kg q24h	HEMO: 25–35 mg per kg after each dialysis CAPD: No reduction; CAVH‡: No data	
Rifampin	1.5–5/1.8–11	600 mg per day	D	600 mg q24h	300–600 mg q24h	300–600 mg q24h	HEMO: None CAPD/CAVH‡: Dose for CrCl <10	Biologically active metabolite
ANTIVIRAL AGENTS								
Acyclovir, IV	2.5/20	5–12.4 mg per kg q8h	D&I	5–12.4 mg per kg q8h	5–12.4 mg per kg q12–24h	2.5 mg per kg q24h	HEMO: Dose AD⁺ CAPD: Dose for CrCl <10	Rapid IV infusion can cause ↑ Cr. CAVH‡ dose: 3.5 mg per kg per day
Adefovir	7.5/–	10 mg po q24h	I	10 mg q24h	10 mg q48–72h	No data	HEMO: q7d AD⁺	
Amantadine	12/500	100 mg po bid	I	q24–48h	q48–72h	q7days	HEMO/CAPD/CAVH‡: None	
Cidofovir: Complicated dosing—see package insert								
Induction	2.5/unknown	5 mg per kg once per wk for 2 wks	–	5 mg per kg once per wk	0.5–2 mg per kg once per wk	0.5 mg per kg once per wk	No data	Major toxicity is renal. No efficacy, safety, or pharmacokinetic data in pts with moderate/severe renal disease.
Maintenance	2.5/unknown	5 mg per kg q2wks	–	5 mg per kg q2wks	0.5–2 mg per kg q2wks	0.5 mg per kg q2wks	No data	
Didanosine tablets¹	0.6–1.6/4.5	125–200 mg q12h buffered tabs	D	200 mg q12h	200 mg q24h	<60 kg: 150 mg q24h >60 kg: 100 mg q24h	HEMO: Dose AD⁺ CAPD/CAVH‡: Dose for CrCl <10	Based on incomplete data. Data are estimates.
		400 mg q24h enteric-coated tabs	D	400 mg q24h	125–200 mg q24h	**Do not use EC tabs**	HEMO/CAPD: Dose for CrCl <10	**If <60 kg & CrCl <10 mL per min, do not use EC tabs**
Emtricitabine	10/>10	200 mg q24h	I	200 mg q24h	200 mg q48–72h	200 mg q96h	HEMO: Dose for CrCl <10	
Entecavir	128–149/?	0.5 mg q24h	D	0.5 mg q24h	0.15–0.25 mg q24h	0.05 mg q24h	HEMO/CAPD: 0.05 mg q24h	Give after dialysis on dialysis days

¹ Ref. for NRTIs and NNRTIs: Kidney International 60:821, 2001

‡ **CAVH** = continuous arteriovenous hemofiltration (NEJM 336:1303, 1997) usually results in CrCl of approx. 30 mL per min.; ⁺ **AD** = after dialysis. **"Dose AD"** refers to timing of dose. **Supplement is to replace drug lost via dialysis; extra drug beyond continuation of regimen used for CrCl <10 mL per min.**

See page 138 for other footnotes and page 2 for abbreviations.

TABLE 17A (5)

ANTIMICROBIAL	HALF-LIFE (NORMAL/ESRD) hr	DOSE FOR NORMAL RENAL FUNCTION§	METHOD* (see footnote)	ADJUSTMENT FOR RENAL FAILURE — Estimated creatinine clearance (CrCl), mL per min >50-90	10-50	<10	SUPPLEMENT FOR HEMODIALYSIS, CAPD+ (see footnote)	COMMENTS ± DOSAGE FOR CAVH‡
ANTIVIRAL AGENTS *(continued)*								
Famciclovir	2.3–3.0/10–22	500 mg q8h	D&I	500 mg q8h	500 mg q12–24h Same dose for CAVH‡	250 mg q24h	HEMO: Dose AD+ CAPD: No data	CAVH‡ dose: As for CrCl 10–50
Foscarnet (CMV dosage) Dosage adjustment based on est. CrCl (mL per min) div. by pt's kg	Normal half-life (T½) 3 hrs with terminal T½ of 18–88 hrs. T½ very long with ESRD	Induction: 60 mg per kg x2–3 wks IV; Maintenance: 90–120 mg per kg per day IV	D&I	*CrCl as mL per min per kg body weight—ONLY FOR FOSCARNET:* >1.4: 60 q8h / 120 q24h; >1.0–1.4: 45 q24h / 90 q24h; >0.8–1.0: 50 q12h / 105 q48h; >0.6–0.8: 40 q12h / 105 q48h; >0.5–0.6: 60 q24h / 80 q48h; >0.4–0.5: 50 q24h / 65 q48h; <0.4: Do not use / Do not use			HEMO: Dose AD+ CAPD: No data	See package insert for further details
Ganciclovir	2.9/30 — IV; po	Induction 5 mg per kg q12h IV; Maintenance 5 mg per kg q24h IV; 1.0 gm tid po	D&I; D&I; D&I	5 mg per kg q12h; 2.5–5.0 mg per kg q24h; 0.5–1 gm tid	1.25–2.5 mg per kg q24h; 0.6–1.25 mg per kg q24h; 0.5–1.0 gm q24h	1.25 mg per kg 3 times per wk; 0.625 mg per kg 3 times per wk; 0.5 gm 3 times per week	HEMO: Dose AD+ CAPD: Dose for CrCl <10; HEMO: 0.6 mg per kg AD+ CAPD: Dose for CrCl <10; HEMO: 0.5 gm AD+	
Lamivudine[1]	5–7/15–35	300 mg po q24h	D&I	300 mg po q24h	50–150 mg q24h	25–50 mg q24h	HEMO: Dose AD+; CAPD/CAVH‡: No data	
Oseltamivir	1–3/no data	75 mg po bid	I	75 mg q12h	75 mg q24h	No data	No data	
Ribavirin	13–65/Prolonged	100 mg bid po		Use with caution in patients with creatinine clearance <10 mL per min				Use with caution, little data
Rimantadine	1–1.4/5.5–8	100 mg bid po		100 mg bid	100 mg q24h–bid	100 mg q24h	HEMO/CAPD: No data	
Stavudine, po[1]	1–1.4/5.5–8	30–40 mg q12h	D&I	100%	50% q12–24h Same dose for CAVH‡	>60 mg: 20 mg per day <60 kg:15 mg per day	HEMO: Dose as for CrCl <10 AD+ CAPD: No data	CAVH‡ dose: As for CrCl 10–50
Tenofovir, po		300 mg q24h	D&I	300 mg q24h	300 mg q24h (CrCl 30–50); 2 times per wk (CrCl 10–30)	No data	HEMO: Give 300 mg po after every 3rd hemodialysis	
Valacyclovir	2.5–3.3/14	1.0 gm q8h	D&I	1.0 gm q8h	1.0 gm q12–24h Same dose for CAVH‡	0.5 gm q24h	HEMO: Dose AD+ CAPD: Dose for CrCl <10	CAVH‡ dose: As for CrCl 10–50
Valganciclovir	4/67	900 mg po bid	D&I	900 mg po bid	450 mg q24h to 450 mg every other day	DO NOT USE	CAPD: No data	
Zalcitabine[1]	2.0/>8	0.75 mg q8h	D&I	0.75 mg q8h	0.75 mg q12h Same dose for CAVH‡	0.75 mg q24h	HEMO: Dose AD+ CAPD: No data	CAVH‡ dose: As for CrCl 10–50
Zidovudine[1]	1.1–1.4/1.4–3	300 mg q12h	D&I	300 mg q12h	300 mg q12h	100 mg q6–8h; if hemo, AD+	HEMO: Dose for CrCl <10 CAPD: Dose for CrCl <10	CAVH‡ dose: 100 mg q8h

* **CAVH** = continuous arteriovenous hemofiltration (*NEJM 336:1303, 1997*); + **AD** = after dialysis.
‡ **CAVH** = continuous arteriovenous hemofiltration (*NEJM 336:1303, 1997*). **Supplement is to replace drug lost via dialysis; extra drug beyond continuation of regimen used for CrCl <10 mL per min. "Dose AD" refers to timing of dose.**
§ Dosages are for life-threatening infections. * **D** = dosage reduction, **I** = interval extension; ** Per cent refers to % change from dose for normal renal function.

† Ref. for NRTIs and NNRTIs: *Kidney International 60:821, 2001*

TABLE 17B: NO DOSAGE ADJUSTMENT WITH RENAL INSUFFICIENCY, BY CATEGORY:*

Antibacterials		Antifungals	Anti-TBc	Antivirals	
Azithromycin	Linezolid	Caspofungin	Rifabutin	Abacavir	Lopinavir
Ceftriaxone	Minocycline	Itraconazole oral solution	Rifapentine	Atazanavir	Nelfinavir
Chloramphenicol	Moxifloxacin	Micafungin		Delavirdine	Nevirapine
Ciprofloxacin XL	Nafcillin	Voriconazole, **po only**		Efavirenz	Ribavirin
Clindamycin	Pyrimethamine			Fosamprenavir	Saquinavir
Dirithromycin	Rifaximin			Indinavir	Tipranavir
Doxycycline	Tigecycline				

TABLE 18: ANTIMICROBIALS AND HEPATIC DISEASE DOSAGE ADJUSTMENT*

The following alphabetical list indicates antibacterials excreted/metabolized by the liver **wherein a dosage adjustment may be indicated** in the presence of hepatic disease. Space precludes details; consult the PDR or package inserts for details. List is **not** all-inclusive:

Antibacterials		Antifungals	Antivirals§	
Ceftriaxone	Nafcillin	Caspofungin	Abacavir	Indinavir
Chloramphenicol	Rifabutin	Itraconazole	Atazanavir	Lopinavir/ritonavir
Clindamycin	Rifampin	Voriconazole	Delavirdine	Nelfinavir
Fusidic acid	Synercid**		Efavirenz	Nevirapine
Isoniazid	Tigecycline		Enfuvirtide	Rimantadine
Metronidazole	Tinidazole		Fosamprenavir	Ritonavir

§ Ref. on antiretrovirals: *CID 40:174, 2005*   ** Quinupristin/dalfopristin

TABLE 19: TREATMENT OF CAPD PERITONITIS IN ADULTS[1]*
(*Periton Dial Intl 20:396, 2000*)

EMPIRIC Intraperitoneal Therapy:[2] Culture Results Pending

Drug		Residual Urine Output	
		<100 mL per day	>100 mL per day
Cefazolin +	Can mix in same bag	1 gm per bag, q24h	20 mg per kg BW per bag, q24h
Ceftazidime		1 gm per bag, q24h	20 mg per kg BW per bag, q24h

Drug Doses for SPECIFIC Intraperitoneal Therapy—Culture Results Known. NOTE: Few po drugs indicated

Drug	Intermittent Dosing (once per day)		Continuous Dosing (per liter exchange)	
	Anuric	Non-Anuric	Anuric	Non-Anuric
Gentamicin	0.6 mg per kg	↑ dose 25%	MD 8 mg	↑ MD by 25%
Cefazolin	15 mg per kg	20 mg per kg	LD 500 mg, MD 125 mg	LD 500 mg, ↑ MD 25%
Ceftazidime	1000–1500 mg	ND	LD 250 mg, MD 125 mg	ND
Ampicillin	250–500 mg po bid	ND	250–500 mg po bid	ND
Ciprofloxacin	500 mg po bid	ND	LD 50 mg, MD 25 mg	ND
Vancomycin	15–30 mg per kg q5–7 days	↑ dose 25%	MD 30–50 mg per L	↑ MD 25%
Metronidazole	250 mg po bid	ND	250 mg po bid	ND
Amphotericin B	NA	NA	MD 1.5 mg	NA
Fluconazole	200 mg q24h	ND	200 mg q24h	ND
Itraconazole	100 mg q12h	100 mg q12h	100 mg q12h	100 mg q12h
Amp-sulbactam	2 gm q12h	ND	LD 1.0 gm, MD 100 mg	ND
TMP-SMX	320/1600 mg po q1–2 days	ND	LD 320/1600 mg po, MD 80/400 mg po q24h	ND

[1] **All doses IP unless indicated otherwise.**
   LD = loading dose, **MD** = maintenance dose, **ND** = no data; **NA** = not applicable—dose as normal renal function. **Anuric** = <100 mL per day, **non-anuric** = >100 mL per day
[2] **Does not provide treatment for MRSA.** If Gram-positive cocci on Gram stain, include vancomycin.
* *See page 2 for other abbreviations*

TABLE 20A: RECOMMENDED CHILDHOOD AND ADOLESCENT IMMUNIZATION SCHEDULE[1]: UNITED STATES, 2005 *(MMWR 54:Q1, 2005) (For overall recommendations, see MMWR 51:RR-2, 2002)*

	Range of recommended ages			Catch-up vaccination				Preadolescent assessment			
VACCINE	Birth	1 mo	2 mos	4 mos	6 mos	12 mos	15 mos	18 mos	24 mos	4–6 yrs	11–12 yrs	13–18 yrs
Hepatitis B[2]	HepB #1 only if mother HBsAg(–)	HepB #2			HepB #3						HepB series	
Diphtheria, Tetanus, Pertussis[3]			DTaP	DTaP	DTaP		DTaP			DTaP	Td	Td
Haemophilus influenzae Type b[4]			Hib	Hib	Hib[4]	Hib						
Inactivated Poliovirus			IPV	IPV	IPV					IPV		
Measles, Mumps, Rubella[5]						MMR #1				MMR #2	MMR #2	
Varicella[6]						Varicella				Varicella		
Pneumococcal[7]			PCV	PCV	PCV	PCV			PCV			
									PPV			
Influenza[8]					Influenza (yearly)					Influenza (yearly)		
— — — — —Vaccines below this line are for selected populations— — — —												
Hepatitis A[9]										HepA series		

[1] This schedule indicates the recommended ages for routine administration of currently licensed childhood vaccines, as of Dec. 1, 2004, for children aged ≤18 yrs. Any dose administered at the recommended age should be administered at any subsequent visit when indicated and feasible. ▓ indicates age groups that warrant special effort to administer those vaccines not previously administered. Additional vaccines might be licensed & recommended during the year. Licensed combination vaccines may be used whenever any components of the combination are indicated & other components of the vaccine are not contraindicated. Providers should consult package inserts for detailed recommendations. Clinically significant adverse events that follow immunization should be reported to the Vaccine Adverse Event Reporting System; guidance is available at www.vaers.org or by telephone, 800-822-7967.

[2] **Hepatitis B (HepB) vaccine.** All infants should receive the 1st dose of HepB vaccine soon after birth & before hospital discharge; the 1st dose may also be administered by age 2 months if the mother is hepatitis B surface antigen (HBsAg) negative. Only monovalent HepB may be used for the birth dose. Monovalent or combination vaccine containing HepB may be used to complete the series. Four doses of vaccine may be administered when a birth dose is administered. The 2nd dose should be administered at least 4 weeks after the 1st dose, except for combination vaccines, which cannot be administered before age 6 weeks. The 3rd dose should be administered at least 16 weeks after the 1st dose & at least 8 weeks after the 2nd dose. The final dose in the vaccination series (3rd or 4th dose) should not be administered before age 24 weeks. **Infants born to HBsAg-positive mothers** should receive HepB and 0.5 mL of hepatitis B immune globulin (HBIG) at separate sites within 12 hours of birth. The 2nd dose is recommended at age 1–2 months. The final dose in the immunization series should not be administered before age 24 weeks. These infants should be tested for HBsAg and antibody to HBsAg at age 9–15 months. **Infants born to mothers whose HBsAg status is unknown** should receive the 1st dose of the HepB series within 12 hours of birth. Maternal blood should be drawn as soon as possible to determine the mother's HBsAg status; if the HBsAg test is positive, the infant should receive HBIG as soon as possible (no later than age 1 week). The 2nd dose is recommended at age 1–2 months. The last dose in the immunization series should not be administered before age 24 weeks.

[3] **Diphtheria and tetanus toxoids and acellular pertussis (DTaP) vaccine.** The 4th dose of DTaP may be administered as early as age 12 months, provided 6 months have elapsed since the 3rd dose and the child is unlikely to return at age 15–18 months. The final dose in the series should be administered at age ≥4 years. **Tetanus and diphtheria toxoids (Td)** is recommended at age 11–12 years if at least 5 years have elapsed since the last dose of tetanus & diphtheria toxoid-containing vaccine. Subsequent routine Td boosters are recommended every 10 years.

[4] **Haemophilus influenzae type b (Hib) conjugate vaccine.** Three Hib conjugate vaccines are licensed for infant use. If PRP-OMP [PedvaxHIB® or ComVax® (Merck)] is administered at ages 2 & 4 months, a dose at age 6 months is not required. DTaP/Hib combination products should not be used for primary immunization in infants at ages 2, 4, or 6 months but can be used as boosters after any Hib vaccine. The final dose in the series should be administered at age ≥12 months.

[5] **Measles, mumps, and rubella (MMR) vaccine.** The 2nd dose of MMR is recommended routinely at age 4–6 years but may be administered during any visit, provided at least 4 weeks have elapsed since the 1st dose & both doses are administered beginning at or after age 12 months. Those who have not previously received the 2nd dose should complete the schedule by age 11–12 years.

[6] **Varicella vaccine** is recommended at any visit at or after age 12 months for susceptible children (i.e., those who lack a reliable history of chickenpox). Susceptible persons aged ≥13 years should receive 2 doses administered at least 4 weeks apart.

[7] **Pneumococcal vaccine.** The heptavalent **pneumococcal conjugate vaccine (PCV)** is recommended for all children aged 2–23 months & for certain children aged 24–59 months. The final dose in the series should be administered at age ≥12 months. **Pneumococcal polysaccharide vaccine (PPV)** is recommended in addition to PCV for certain groups at high risk. *See MMWR 49(RR-9), 2000.*

[8] **Influenza vaccine** is recommended annually for children aged ≥6 months with certain risk factors (including, but not limited to, asthma, cardiac disease, sickle cell disease, HIV, & diabetes), health-care workers, & other persons (including household members) in close contact with persons in groups at high risk *[see MMWR 53(RR-6), 2004]*. In addition, healthy children aged 6–23 months & close contacts of healthy children aged 0–23 months are recommended to receive influenza vaccine because children in this age group are at substantially increased risk for influenza-related hospitalizations. For healthy persons aged 5–49 years, the intranasally administered, live, attenuated influenza vaccine (LAIV) is an acceptable alternative to the intramuscular trivalent inactivated influenza vaccine (TIV). *See MMWR 53(RR-6), 2004.* Children receiving TIV should be administered a dosage appropriate for their age (0.25 mL if aged 6–35 months or 0.5 mL if aged ≥3 years). Children aged ≤8 years who are receiving influenza vaccine for the first time should receive 2 doses (separated by at least 4 weeks for TIV & at least 6 weeks for LAIV).

[9] **Hepatitis A vaccine** is recommended for children and adolescents in selected states & regions & for certain groups at high risk; consult your local public health authority. Children & adolescents in these states, regions, & groups who have not been immunized against hepatitis A can begin the hepatitis A immunization series during any visit. The 2 doses in the series should be administered at least 6 months apart. *See MMWR 48(RR-12), 1999.*

TABLE 20A (2)

Catch-Up Schedule For Children Aged 4 Months–6 Years

Vaccine	Minimum age for dose 1	Minimum interval between doses			
		Dose 1 to dose 2	Dose 2 to dose 3	Dose 3 to dose 4	Dose 4 to dose 5
DTaP[1]	6 wks	4 wks	4 wks	6 mos.	6 mos.[1]
IPV[2]	6 wks	4 wks	4 wks	4 wks[2]	
HepB[3]	Birth	4 wks	8 wks (& 16 wks after 1st dose)		
MMR[4]	12 mos	4 wks[4]			
Varicella	12 mos				
Hib[5]	6 wks	4 wks: if 1st dose given at age <12 mos / 8 wks (as final dose): if 1st dose given at age 12–24 mos / No further doses needed if 1st dose given at age ≥15 mos.	4 wks[6]: if current age <12 mos / 8 wks (as final dose)[6]: if current age ≥12 mos & 2nd dose given at age <15 mos / No further doses needed if previous dose given at age ≥15 mos	8 wks (as final dose): this dose only necessary for children aged 12 mos–5 yrs who received 3 doses before age 12 mos	
PCV[7]	6 wks	4 wks: if 1st dose given at age <12 mos & current age <24 mos / 8 wks (as final dose): if 1st dose given at age ≥12 mos or current age 24–59 mos / No further doses needed for healthy children if 1st dose given at age ≥24 mos	4 wks: if current age <12 mos / 8 wks (as final dose): if current age ≥12 mos / No further doses needed for healthy children if previous dose given at age ≥24 mos.	8 wks (as final dose): this dose only necessary for children aged 12 mos.–5 yrs who received 3 doses before age 12 mos	

Catch-Up Schedule for Children Aged 7–18 Years

Vaccine	Minimum interval between doses		
	Dose 1 to dose 2	Dose 2 to dose 3	Dose 3 to booster dose
Td[8]	4 wks	6 mos	6 mos[8]: if 1st dose given at age <12 mos & current age <11 yrs / 5 yrs[8]: if 1st dose given at age ≥12 mos & 3rd dose given at age <7 yrs & current age ≥11 yrs / 10 yrs[8]: if 3rd dose given at age ≥7 yrs
IPV[9]	4 wks	4 wks	IPV[2,9]
HepB	4 wks	8 wks (& 16 wks after 1st dose)	
MMR	4 wks[4]		
Varicella[10]	4 wks		

Note: A vaccine series does not require restarting, regardless of the time that has elapsed between doses.
[1] **Diphtheria and tetanus toxoids and acellular pertussis (DTaP) vaccine:** The 5th dose is not necessary if the 4th dose was given after the 4th birthday.
[2] **Inactivated poliovirus (IPV) vaccine:** For children who received an all-IPV or all-oral poliovirus (OPV) series, a 4th dose is not necessary if 3rd dose was given at age ≥4 yrs. If both OPV and IPV were given as part of a series, a total of ⟨ doses should be given, regardless of the child's current age.
[3] **Hepatitis B (HepB) vaccine:** All children and adolescents who have not been immunized against hepatitis B should begin the HepB immunization series during any visit. Providers should make special efforts to immunize children who were born in, or whose parents were born in, areas of the world where hepatitis B virus infection is moderately or highly endemic.
[4] **Measles, mumps, and rubella (MMR) vaccine:** The 2nd dose of MMR is recommended routinely at age 4–6 yrs, but may be given earlier if desired.
[5] **Haemophilus influenzae type b (Hib) vaccine:** Vaccine is not generally recommended for children aged ≥5 years.
[6] **Hib vaccine:** If current age is <12 months and the first 2 doses were PRP-OMP [PedVaxHIB® or ComVax (Merck)®], the 3rd (and final) dose should be given at age 12–15 months and at least 8 weeks after the 2nd dose.
[7] **Pneumococcal conjugate (PCV) vaccine:** Vaccine is not generally recommended for children aged ≥5 years.
[8] **Tetanus and diphtheria toxoids (Td):** For children aged 7–10 years, the interval between the 3rd & booster dose is determined by the age when the 1st dose was given. For adolescents aged 11–18 years, the interval is determined by the age when the 3rd dose was administered.
[9] **IPV:** Vaccine is not generally recommended for persons aged ≥18 years.
[10] **Varicella vaccine:** Administer the 2-dose series to all susceptible adolescents aged ≥13 years.

Conjugate pneumococcal vaccine (PCV): For all infants <2 years old & high-risk children (e.g., HIV, asplenia, nephrotic syndrome, sickle cell anemia) between 2 and 5 years of age (Med Lett 42:25, 2000; PIDJ 19:181, 2000; PIDJ 19: 371ff, 2000). Also approved for prevention of otitis media (Med Lett 45:27, 2003) & for cochlear implant recipients (MMWR 52: 739, 2003). Use of vaccine associated with decline in invasive pneumococcal disease (NEJM 348:1737, 2003).
Immunization schedule: (see Schedule, page 140)

Age at first dose (0.5 mL)	Total number of doses	Timing
Infants	4	2, 4, 6, and 12–15 months
7–11 months	3	2 doses at least 4 wks apart; 3rd dose after 1 year birthday, separated from 2nd dose by at least 2 months
12–23 months	2	2 doses at least 2 months apart
≥24 months	1*	

* For children ≥24 months old who are chronically ill or immunosuppressed, ICIP recommends 2 doses of PCV admin. 2 mos. apart, followed by 1 dose of a 23-valent pneumococcal vaccine 2 or 3 mos. after 2nd PCV dose (MMWR 50:10, 2001).

TABLE 20B: MENINGOCOCCAL VACCINE *[MMWR 54(RR-7), 2005]*

Population	Age Group (years)				
	<2	2–10	11–19	20–55	>55
General	None	None	Single dose MCV4	None	None
Increased risk groups: College freshmen (in dorms) Traveler's epidemic area Microbiologists/Military recruits	None	Single dose MPSV4	Single dose MCV4	Single dose MCV4	Single dose MCV4
Anatomic/functional asplenia*					
Terminal complement deficiency*					

MCV4 = Meningococcal protein conjugate vaccine (Menactra); **MPSV4** = Meningococcal polysaccharide vaccine (Menomune)
* Revaccinate every 3–5 years. **NOTE:** 5 cases Guillain-Barré after MCV4; causal relationship unknown

TABLE 20C: ADULT IMMUNIZATION IN THE UNITED STATES *(MMWR 53:Q1, 2004)*
(Travelers: see Med Lett 38:17, 1996)
Recommended Adult Immunization Schedule—United States, 2004–2005

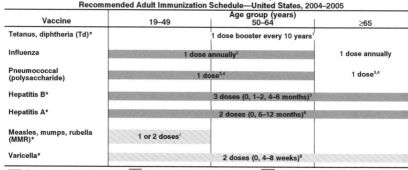

Vaccine	Age group (years)		
	19–49	50–64	≥65
Tetanus, diphtheria (Td)*	1 dose booster every 10 years[1]		
Influenza	1 dose annually[2]		1 dose annually
Pneumococcal (polysaccharide)	1 dose[3,4]		1 dose[3,4]
Hepatitis B*	3 doses (0, 1–2, 4–6 months)[5]		
Hepatitis A*	2 doses (0, 6–12 months)[6]		
Measles, mumps, rubella (MMR)*	1 or 2 doses[7]		
Varicella*	2 doses (0, 4–8 weeks)[8]		

☐ For all persons in this group   ■ For persons at risk (i.e., with medical exposure/indications)   ▨ For persons lacking documentation of vaccination or evidence of disease

* Covered by the Vaccine Injury Compensation Program.

[1] **Tetanus and diphtheria (Td).** *See Table 20D.* Adults, including pregnant women with uncertain history of a complete primary vaccination series, should receive a primary series of Td. A primary series for adults is 3 doses; give the 1st 2 doses at least 4 weeks apart & the 3rd dose 6–12 months after the 2nd. Give 1 dose if the person received the primary series & if the last vaccination was received ≥10 years previously. The American College of Physicians Task Force on Adult Immunization supports a 2nd option for Td use in adults: a single Td booster at age 50 years for persons who have completed the full pediatric series, including the teenage/young adult booster.

[2] **Influenza vaccination.** Medical indications: chronic disorders of the cardiovascular or pulmonary systems, including asthma; chronic metabolic diseases, including diabetes mellitus, renal dysfunction, hemoglobinopathies, or immunosuppression (including immunosuppression caused by medications or by HIV; and pregnancy during the influenza season. Occupational indications: health-care workers & employees of long-term-care & assisted living facilities. Other indications: residents of nursing homes & other long-term-care facilities; persons likely to transmit influenza to persons at high risk (i.e., in-home caregivers to persons with medical indications, household/close contacts & out-of-home caregivers of children aged 0–23 months, household members & caregivers of elderly persons & adults with high-risk conditions); & anyone who wishes to be vaccinated. For healthy persons aged 5–49 years without high-risk indications who are not contacts of severely immunocompromised persons in special care units, either the inactivated vaccine or the intranasally administered influenza vaccine (FluMist®) may be given *[see MMWR 53(RR-6), 2004]*.

[3] **Pneumococcal polysaccharide vaccination.** Medical indications: chronic lung disease (excluding asthma); cardiovascular diseases; diabetes mellitus; chronic liver diseases, including alcohol-induced cirrhosis; chronic renal failure or nephrotic syndrome; functional or anatomic asplenia; immunosuppression (e.g., congenital immunodeficiency, HIV infection, leukemia/lymphoma/multiple myeloma/Hodgkins disease, or organ or bone marrow transplantation); chemotherapy, long-term systemic corticosteroids; or cochlear implants. Geographic/other indications: Alaska Natives and certain American Indian populations. Other indications: residents of nursing homes & other long-term-care facilities *(MMWR 52:739, 2003)*.

[4] **Revaccination with pneumococcal polysaccharide vaccine.** One-time revaccination after 5 years for persons with chronic renal failure or nephrotic syndrome; functional or anatomic asplenia (e.g., sickle cell disease or splenectomy); immunosuppressive conditions (e.g., congenital immunodeficiency, HIV infection, leukemia/lymphoma/multiple myeloma/Hodgkins disease, generalized malignancy, or organ or bone marrow transplantation); chemotherapy, or long-term systemic corticosteroids. For persons aged ≥65 years, one-time revaccination if they were vaccinated ≥5 years previously & were aged <65 years at the time of primary vaccination *[see MMWR 46(RR-8), 1997]*.

[5] **Hepatitis B vaccination.** Medical indications: hemodialysis or patients who receive clotting factor concentrates. Occupational indications: health-care & public safety workers with exposure to blood, & students of medicine, dentistry, nursing, & other allied health professions. Behavioral indications: injection-drug users; persons with more than 1 sex partner during the previous 6 months; persons with a recent STD; all clients in STD clinics; & men who have sex with men. Other indications: household contacts & sex partners of persons with chronic HBV infection; clients & staff members of institutions for the developmentally disabled; inmates of correctional facilities; or travelers to countries with high prevalence of chronic HBV infection for *(www.cdc.gov/travel/diseases/hbv.htm)*. **If no HBsAb response** (<10 million units per mL), try 0.25 mL of adult vaccine intradermal week 0, repeat 9n 2 wks, & measure HBsAb 2 wks later. If still no response, repeat intradermals.

[6] **Hepatitis A vaccination.** Medical indications: clotting factor disorders or chronic liver disease. Behavioral indications: men who have sex with men or users of illegal drugs. Occupational indications: persons working with hepatitis A virus (HAV)-infected primates. Other indications: persons traveling to or working in countries with high endemic HepA. If the combined HepA & HepB vaccine is used, administer 3 doses at 0, 1, & 6 months *(www.cdc.gov/travel/diseases/hav.htm) [see MMWR 48(RR-12), 1999]*.

[7] **Measles, mumps, rubella (MMR) vaccination.** Measles component: adults born before 1957 are considered immune to measles. Adults born during or after 1957 should receive ≥1 dose of MMR unless they have a medical contraindication, documentation of ≥1 dose, or other acceptable evidence of immunity. A 2nd dose of MMR is recommended for adults who (1) were recently exposed to measles or in an outbreak setting, (2) were previously vaccinated

TABLE 20C (2)

with killed measles vaccine, (3) were vaccinated with an unknown vaccine during 1963-67, (4) are students in post-secondary educational institutions, (5) work in health-care facilities, or (6) plan to travel internationally. Mumps component: 1 dose of MMR vaccine should be adequate for protection. Rubella component: Give 1 dose of MMR vaccine to women whose rubella vaccination history is unreliable & counsel women to avoid becoming pregnant for 4 weeks after vaccination. For women of childbearing age, regardless of birth year, routinely determine rubella immunity & counsel women regarding congenital rubella syndrome. Do not vaccinate pregnant women or those planning to become pregnant during the next 4 weeks. For women who are pregnant & susceptible, vaccinate as early in the postpartum period as possible [see MMWR 47(RR-8), 1998 & MMWR 50:1117, 2001].

[8] **Varicella vaccination.** Recommended for all persons lacking reliable clinical history of varicella infection or serologic evidence of varicella zoster virus (VZV) infection who might be at high risk for exposure or transmission. This includes health-care workers & family contacts of immunocompromised persons; persons who live or work in environments where transmission is likely (e.g., teachers of young children, child care employees, & residents & staff members in institutional settings); persons who live or work in environments where VZV transmission can occur (e.g., college students, inmates, & staff members of correctional institutions, & military personnel); adolescents aged 11–18 years & adults living in households with children; women who are not pregnant but who might become pregnant; & international travelers who are not immune to infection. **Note**: Approx. 95% of U.S.-born adults are immune to VZV. Do not vaccinate pregnant women or those planning to become pregnant during the next 4 weeks. For women who are pregnant & susceptible, vaccinate as early in the postpartum period as possible [see MMWR 48(RR-6), 1999].

> This schedule (above) indicates the recommended age groups for routine administration of currently licensed vaccines for persons aged ≥19 years. Licensed combination vaccines may be used whenever any components of the combination are indicated & when the vaccine's other components are not contraindicated. Providers should consult manufacturers' package inserts for detailed recommendations. Report all clinically significant postvaccination reactions to the Vaccine Adverse Event Reporting System (VAERS). Reporting forms & instructions on filing a VAERS report are available by telephone, 800-822-7967, or from www.vaers.org. Additional information about the vaccines listed above & contraindications for immunization are available at www.cdc.gov/nip or from the National Immunization Hotline, 800-232-2522 (English) or 800-232-0233 (Spanish). Approved by the ACIP, the ACOG, & the AAFP.

Recommended Immunizations for Adults with Medical Conditions & Other Indications—U.S., 2004–2005

Indication	Vaccine						
	Tetanus, diphtheria (Td)*,[1]	Influenza[2]	Pneumo-coccal (polysac-charide)[3,4]	Hepatitis B*,[5]	Hepatitis A*,[6]	Measles, mumps, rubella (MMR)*,[7]	Vari-cella*,[8]
Pregnancy							
Diabetes, heart disease, chronic pulmonary disease, chronic liver disease (including chronic alcoholism)		A, B	B		I		
Congenital immunodeficiency, cochlear implants, leukemia, lymphoma, generalized malignancy, rx with alkylating agents, antimetabolites, CSF § leaks, radiation, or large amounts of corticosteroids			D				K
Renal failure/endstage renal disease & recipients of hemodialysis or clotting factor concentrates			D	H			
Asplenia including elective splenectomy & terminal complement-component deficiencies		C	D,E,F				
HIV infection			D,G			J	
Health-care workers							

▨ For all persons in this group   ▧ For persons at risk (i.e., with medical/exposure indications)   ▥ For persons lacking documentation of vaccination or evidence of disease   ▨ Contraindicated

[1] Covered by the Vaccine Injury Compensation Program

§ Cerebrospinal fluid

TABLE 20C (3)

Special Notes for Medical and Other Indications

A Although chronic liver disease & alcoholism are not indications for influenza vaccination, administer 1 dose annually if the patient is aged ≥50 years, has other indications for influenza vaccine, or requests vaccination.
B Asthma is an indication for influenza vaccination but not for pneumococcal vaccination.
C No data exist specifically on the risk for severe or complicated influenza infections among persons with asplenia. However, influenza is a risk factor for secondary bacterial infections that can cause severe disease among persons with asplenia.
D For persons aged <65 years, revaccinate once after ≥5 years have elapsed since initial vaccination.
E Administer meningococcal vaccine & consider Haemophilus influenzae type b vaccine (see Table 20B).
F For persons undergoing elective splenectomy, vaccinate ≥2 weeks before surgery.
G Vaccinate as soon after diagnosis as possible.
H For hemodialysis patients, use special formulation of vaccine (40 mcg per mL) or two 20 mcg per mL doses administered at one body site. Vaccinate early in the course of renal disease. Assess antibody titers to hepatitis B surface antigen (anti-HB) levels annually. Administer additional doses if anti-HB levels decline to <10 million units per mL.
I For all persons with chronic liver disease
J Withhold MMR or other measles-containing vaccines from HIV-infected persons with evidence of severe immunosuppression [see MMWR 47(RR-8:21), 1998 & MMWR 51(RR-2):22, 2002].
K Persons with impaired humoral immunity but intact cellular immunity may be vaccinated [see MMWR 48(RR-6), 1999].

Administration schedule for vaccines: Review package insert for specific product being administered

TABLE 20D/1: ANTI-TETANUS PROPHYLAXIS, WOUND CLASSIFICATION, IMMUNIZATION

WOUND CLASSIFICATION			IMMUNIZATION SCHEDULE				
Clinical Features	**Tetanus Prone**	**Non-Tetanus Prone**	**History of Tetanus Immunization**	**Dirty, Tetanus-Prone Wound**		**Clean, Non-Tetanus Prone Wound**	
Age of wound	> 6 hours	≤ 6 hours		Td[1,2]	TIG	Td	TIG
Configuration	Stellate, avulsion	Linear	Unknown or < 3 doses	Yes	Yes	Yes	No
Depth	> 1 cm	≤ 1 cm	3 or more doses	No[3]	No	No[4]	No
Mechanism of injury	Missile, crush, burn, frostbite	Sharp surface (glass, knife)	[1] Td = Tetanus & diphtheria toxoids adsorbed (adult) TIG = Tetanus immune globulin (human) [2] Yes if wound >24 hours old.				
Devitalized tissue	Present	Absent	For children <7 years, DPT (DT if pertussis vaccine contraindicated); For persons ≥7 years, Td preferred to tetanus toxoid alone.				
Contaminants (dirt, saliva, etc.)	Present	Absent	[3] Yes if >5 years since last booster [4] Yes if >10 years since last booster				
(From ACS Bull. 69:22,23, 1984, No. 10)			[From MMWR 39:37, 1990; MMWR 46(SS-2):15, 1997]				

TABLE 20D/2: RABIES POST-EXPOSURE PROPHYLAXIS[1]. All wounds should be cleaned immediately and thoroughly with soap and water. This has been shown to protect 90% of experimental animals!
Post-Exposure Prophylaxis Guide, United States, 2000 (CID 30:4, 2000; NEJM 351:2626, 2004)

Animal Type	Evaluation and Disposition of Animal	Recommendations for Prophylaxis
Dogs, cats, ferrets	Healthy and available for 10-day observation	Don't start unless animal develops sx, then immediately begin HRIG + HDCV or RVA
	Rabid or suspected rabid	Immediate vaccination
	Unknown (escaped)	Consult public health officials
Skunks, raccoons, bats,* foxes, coyotes, most carnivores	Regard as rabid	Immediate vaccination
Livestock, rodents, rabbits; includes hares, squirrels,, hamsters, guinea pigs, gerbils, chipmunks, rats, mice, woodchucks		Almost never require anti-rabies rx. Consult public health officials.

* Most recent cases of human rabies in U.S. due to contact (not bites) with silver-haired bats or rarely big brown bats (MMWR 46:770, 1997; AnIM 128:922, 1998). For more detail, see CID 30:4, 2000; JAVMA 219:1687, 2001; CID 37:96, 2003 (travel medicine advisory); Ln 363:959, 2004.

Post-Exposure Rabies Immunization Schedule
IF NOT PREVIOUSLY VACCINATED

Treatment	Regimen[2]
Local wound cleaning	All post-exposure treatment should begin with immediate, thorough cleaning of all wounds with soap and water.
Human rabies immune globulin (HRIG)	20 units per kg body weight given once on day 0. If anatomically feasible, the full dose should be infiltrated around the wound(s), the rest should be administered IM in the gluteal area. HRIG should **not** be administered in the **same syringe**, **or** into the **same anatomical site** as vaccine, or more than 7 days after the initiation of vaccine. Because HRIG may partially suppress active production of antibody, no more than the recommended dose should be given.[3]
Vaccine	Human diploid cell vaccine (HDCV), rabies vaccine adsorbed (RVA), or purified chick embryo cell vaccine (PCEC) 1.0 mL **IM** (**deltoid area**[4]), one each on days 0, 3, 7, 14, & 28.

TABLE 20D/2 (2)

IF PREVIOUSLY VACCINATED[5]	
Treatment	**Regimen[2]**
Local wound cleaning	All post-exposure treatment should begin with immediate, thorough cleaning of all wounds with soap and water.
HRIG	HRIG should **not** be administered
Vaccine	HDCV, RVA or PCEC, 1.0 mL **IM** (**deltoid area[4]**), one each on days 0 and 3

CORRECT VACCINE ADMINISTRATION SITES

Age Group	**Administration Site**
Children and adults	**DELTOID[4]** only (**NEVER** in gluteus)
Infants and young children	Outer aspect of thigh (anterolateral thigh) may be used (**NEVER** in gluteus)

[1] From *MMWR 48:RR-1, 1999; CID 30:4, 2000;* B.T. Matyas, Mass. Dept. of Public Health
[2] These regimens are applicable for all age groups, including children.
[3] In most reported post-exposure treatment failures, only identified deficiency was failure to infiltrate wound(s) with HRIG *(CID 22:228, 1996)*. However, several failures reported from SE Asia in patients in whom WHO protocol followed *(CID 28:143, 1999)*.
[4] The **deltoid** area is the **only** acceptable site of vaccination for adults and older children. For infants and young children, the outer aspect of the thigh (anterolateral thigh) may be used. Vaccine should **NEVER** be administered in the gluteal area.
[5] Any person with a history of pre-exposure vaccination with HDCV, RVA, PCEC; prior post-exposure prophylaxis with HDCV, RVA, PCEC; or previous vaccination with any other type of rabies vaccine and a documented history of antibody response to the prior vaccination

TABLE 21: SELECTED DIRECTORY OF RESOURCES

ORGANIZATION	PHONE/FAX	WEBSITE(S)
ANTIPARASITIC DRUGS and PARASITOLOGY INFORMATION *(CID 37:694, 2003)*		
CDC	Weekdays: 404-639-3670	www.cdc.gov/ncidod/srp/drugs/drug-service.html
	Evenings, weekends, holidays: 404-639-2888	
DPDx: Lab ID of parasites		www.dpd.cdc.gov/dpdx/default.htm
Gorgas Course Tropical Medicine		http://info.dom.uab.edu/gorgas
Panorama Compound. Pharm.	800-247-9767/818-787-7256	www.uniquerx.com
Parasites and Health		www.dpd.cdc.gov/dpdx/HTML/Para_Health.htm
BIOTERRORISM		
Centers for Disease Control & Prevention	770-488-7100	www.bt.cdc.gov
Infectious Diseases Society of America	703-299-0200/	www.idsociety.org
	703-299-0204	
Johns Hopkins Center Civilian Biodefense		www.jhsph.edu
Center for Biosecurity of the Univ. of Pittsburgh Med. Center		www.upmc-biosecurity.org
US Army Medical Research Institute of Inf. Dis.		www.usamriid.army.mil
HEPATITIS C *(CID 35:754, 2002)*		
CDC		www.cdc.gov/ncidod/diseases/hepatitis/C
Individual		http://hepatitis-central.com
Medscape		www.medscape.com
HIV		
General		
HIV InSite		http://hivinsite.ucsf.edu
Johns Hopkins AIDS Service		www.hopkins-aids.edu
Drug Interactions		
Johns Hopkins AIDS Service		www.hopkins-aids.edu
Liverpool HIV Pharm. Group		www.hiv-druginteractions.org
Other		http://AIDS.medscape.com
Prophylaxis/Treatment of Opportunistic Infections; HIV Treatment		www.aidsinfo.nih.gov
IMMUNIZATIONS *(CID 36:355, 2003)*		
CDC, Natl. Immunization Program	404-639-8200	www.cdc.gov/nip
FDA, Vaccine Adverse Events	800-822-7967	www.fda.gov/cber/vaers/vaers.htm
National Network Immunization Info.	877-341-6644/	www.immunizationinfo.org
	703-299-0204	
Influenza vaccine, CDC	404-639-8200	www.cdc.gov/nip/flu
Institute for Vaccine Safety		www.vaccinesafety.edu
OCCUPATIONAL EXPOSURE, BLOOD-BORNE PATHOGENS (HIV, HEPATITIS B & C)		
National Clinicians' Post-Exposure Hotline	888-448-4911	www.ucsf.edu/hivcntr
Q-T$_c$ INTERVAL PROLONGATION BY DRUGS		www.qtdrugs.com
SEXUALLY TRANSMITTED DISEASES		www.cdc.gov/std/treatment/TOC2002TG.htm
	Slides: http://www.phac-aspc.gc.ca/slm-maa/slides/index.html	
TRAVELERS' INFO: Immunizations, Malaria Prophylaxis, More		
Amer. Soc. Trop. Med. & Hyg.		www.astmh.org
CDC, general	877-394-8747/888-232-3299	www.cdc.gov/travel/index.htm
CDC, Malaria:		www.cdc.gov/malaria
Prophylaxis	888-232-3228	www.cdc.gov/travel
Treatment	770-488-7788	www.who.int/health_topics/malaria
MD Travel Health		www.mdtravelhealth.com
Pan American Health Organization		www.paho.org
World Health Organization (WHO)	(41-22)-791-2122/	www.who.int/home-page
	(00-41-22)-691-0746	
VACCINE AND IMMUNIZATION RESOURCES *(CID 36:355, 2003)*		
American Academy of Pediatrics		www.cispimmunize.org
CDC, National Immunization Program		www.cdc.gov/nip
National Network for Immunization Information		www.immunizationinfo.org

TABLE 22: ANTI-INFECTIVE DRUG-DRUG INTERACTIONS
Significance/Certainty: ± = theory/anecdotal; + = of probable importance; ++ = of definite importance

ANTI-INFECTIVE AGENT (A)	OTHER DRUG (B)	EFFECT	SIGNIFICANCE/ CERTAINTY
Amantadine (Symmetrel)	Alcohol	↑ CNS effects	+
	Anticholinergic and anti-Parkinson agents (ex. Artane, scopolamine)	↑ effect of B: dry mouth, ataxia, blurred vision, slurred speech, toxic psychosis	+
	Trimethoprim	↑ levels of A & B	+
	Digoxin	↑ levels of B	±
Aminoglycosides— parenteral (amikacin, gentamicin, kanamycin, netilmicin, sisomicin, streptomycin, tobramycin) *NOTE: Capreomycin is an aminoglycoside, used as alternative drug to treat mycobacterial infections.*	Amphotericin B	↑ nephrotoxicity	++
	Cis platinum (Platinol)	↑ nephro & ototoxicity	+
	Cyclosporine	↑ nephrotoxicity	+
	Neuromuscular blocking agents	↑ apnea or respiratory paralysis	+
	Loop diuretics (e.g., furosemide)	↑ ototoxicity	++
	NSAIDs	↑ nephrotoxicity	+
	Non-polarizing muscle relaxants	↑ apnea	+
	Radiographic contrast	↑ nephrotoxicity	+
	Vancomycin	↑ nephrotoxicity	+
Aminoglycosides— oral (kanamycin, neomycin)	Oral anticoagulants (dicumarol, phenindione, warfarin)	↑ prothrombin time	+
Amphotericin B and ampho B lipid formulations	Antineoplastic drugs	↑ nephrotoxicity risk	+
	Digitalis	↑ toxicity of B if K⁺ ↓	+
	Nephrotoxic drugs: aminoglycosides, cidofovir, cyclosporine, foscarnet, pentamidine	↑ nephrotoxicity of A	++
Ampicillin, amoxicillin	Allopurinol	↑ frequency of rash	++
Amprenavir and fosamprenavir	Antiretrovirals—see Table 22B & C		
	Contraceptives, oral	↓ levels of A; use other contraception	++
	Lovastatin/simvastatin	**↑ levels of B—avoid**	++
	Methadone	↓ levels of A & B	++
	Rifabutin	↑ levels of B (↓ dose by 50–75%)	++
	Rifampin	**↓ levels of A—avoid**	++
Atazanavir	See protease inhibitors and Table 22B & C		
Atovaquone	Rifampin (perhaps rifabutin)	↓ serum levels of A; ↑ levels of B	+
	Metoclopramide	↓ levels of A	+
	Tetracycline	↓ levels of A	++

Azole Antifungal Agents[1] [*Flu* = fluconazole, *Itr* = itraconazole, *Ket* = ketoconazole, *Vor* = voriconazole, + = occurs, **blank space** = either studied & no interaction OR no data found (may be in pharm. co. databases)]

Flu	Itr	Ket	Vor	OTHER DRUG (B)	EFFECT	SIG./CERT.
+	+			Amitriptyline	↑ levels of B	+
+	+	+	+	Calcium channel blockers	↑ levels of B	++
	+		+	Carbamazepine (vori contraindicated)	↓ levels of A	++
+	+	+	+	Cyclosporine	↑ levels of B, ↑ risk of nephrotoxicity	+
	+	+		Didanosine	↓ absorption of A	+
	+	+	+	Efavirenz	↓ levels of A, ↑ levels of B	++ (avoid)
	+	+		H₂ blockers, antacids, sucralfate	↓ absorption of A	+
+	+	+	+	Hydantoins (phenytoin, Dilantin)	↑ levels of B, ↓ levels of A	++
	+	+		Isoniazid	↓ levels of A	+
	+		+	Lovastatin/simvastatin	Rhabdomyolysis reported; ↑ levels of B	++
+	+	+	+	Midazolam/triazolam, po	↑ levels of B	++
+	+	+	+	Oral anticoagulants	↑ effect of B	++
+	+		+	Oral hypoglycemics	↑ levels of B	++
			+	Pimozide	↑ levels of B	++
	+	+	+	Protease inhibitors	↑ levels of B	++
	+	+	+	Proton pump inhibitors	↓ absorption of A, ↑ levels of B	++
+	+	+	+	Rifampin/rifabutin (vori contraindicated)	↑ levels of B, ↓ serum levels of A	++
			+	Sirolimus (vori contraindicated)	↑ levels of B	++
+		+	+	Tacrolimus	↑ levels of B with toxicity	++
+	+			Theophyllines	↑ levels of B	+
		+		Trazodone	↑ levels of B	++
+				Zidovudine	↑ levels of B	+
Caspofungin				Cyclosporine	↑ levels of A	++
				Tacrolimus	↓ levels of B	++
				Carbamazepine, dexamethasone, efavirenz, nevirapine, phenytoin, rifamycin	↓ levels of A; ↑ dose of caspofungin to 70 mg/d	++
Cephalosporins with methyltetrathiozole- thiol side-chain				Oral anticoagulants (dicumarol, warfarin), heparin, thrombolytic agents, platelet aggregation inhibitors	↑ effects of B, bleeding	+
Chloramphenicol				Hydantoins	↑ toxicity of B, nystagmus, ataxia	++
				Iron salts, Vitamin B12	↓ response to B	++
				Protease inhibitors—HIV	↑ levels of A & B	++

[1] Major interactions given; unusual or minor interactions manifest as toxicity of non-azole drug due to ↑ serum levels: Caffeine (Flu), digoxin (Itr), felodipine (Itr), fluoxetine (Itr), indinavir (Ket), lovastatin/simvastatin, quinidine (Ket), tricyclics (Flu), vincristine (Itr), and ↓ effectiveness of oral contraceptives.

TABLE 22 (2)

ANTI-INFECTIVE AGENT (A)	OTHER DRUG (B)	EFFECT	SIGNIFICANCE/ CERTAINTY
Clindamycin (Cleocin)	Kaolin	↓ absorption of A	+
	Muscle relaxants, e.g., atracurium, baclofen, diazepam	↑ frequency/duration of respiratory paralysis	+
Cycloserine	Ethanol	↑ frequency of seizures	+
	INH, ethionamide	↑ frequency of drowsiness/dizziness	+
Dapsone	Didanosine	↓ absorption of A	+
	Oral contraceptives	↓ effectiveness of B	+
	Pyrimethamine	↑ in marrow toxicity	+
	Rifampin/Rifabutin	↓ serum levels of A	+
	Trimethoprim	↑ levels of A & B (methemoglobinemia)	+
	Zidovudine	May ↑ marrow toxicity	+
Daptomycin	HMG-CoA inhibitors (statins)	DC statin while on dapto	+ +
Delavirdine (Rescriptor)	*See non-nucleoside reverse transcriptase inhibitors (NNRTIs) and Table 22C*		
Didanosine (ddI) (Videx)	Cisplatin, dapsone, INH, metronidazole, nitrofurantoin, stavudine, vincristine, zalcitabine	↑ risk of peripheral neuropathy	+
	Ethanol, lamivudine, pentamidine	↑ risk of pancreatitis	+
	Fluoroquinolones	↓ absorption 2° to chelation	+
	Drugs that need low pH for absorption: dapsone, indinavir, itra/ketoconazole, pyrimethamine, rifampin, trimethoprim	↓ absorption	+
	Methadone	↓ levels of A	+ +
	Ribavirin	↑ levels ddI metabolite—**avoid**	+ +
	Tenofovir	↑ levels of A **(reduce dose of A)**	+ +
Doxycycline	Aluminum, bismuth, iron, Mg++	↓ absorption of A	+
	Barbiturates, hydantoins	↓ serum t/2 of A	+
	Carbamazepine (Tegretol)	↓ serum t/2 of A	+
	Digoxin	↑ serum levels of B	+
	Warfarin	↑ activity of B	+ +
Efavirenz (Sustiva)	*See non-nucleoside reverse transcriptase inhibitors (NNRTIs) and Table 22C*		
Ertapenem (Invanz)	Probenecid	↑ levels of A	+ +
Ethambutol (Myambutol)	Aluminum salts (includes didanosine buffer)	↓ absorption of A & B	+

Fluoroquinolones (*Cipro* = ciprofloxacin; *Gati* = gatifloxacin; *Gemi* = gemifloxacin; *Levo* = levofloxacin; *Lome* = lomefloxacin; *Moxi* = moxifloxacin; *Oflox* = ofloxacin)

NOTE: Blank space = either studied and no interaction OR no data found (pharm. co. may have data)

Cipro	Gati	Gemi	Levo	Lome	Moxi	Oflox			
+		+		+	+		**Antiarrhythmics (procainamide, amiodarone)**	↑ Q-T interval (torsade)	+ +
+	+		+	+	+	+	Insulin, oral hypoglycemics	↑ & ↓ blood sugar	+ +
+							Caffeine	↑ levels of B	+
+			+		+		Cimetidine	↑ levels of A	+
+			+		+		Cyclosporine	↑ levels of B	±
+	+		+	+	+	+	Didanosine	↓ absorption of A	+ +
+	+	+	+	+	+	+	**Cations: Al+++, Ca++, Fe++, Mg++, Zn++ (antacids, vitamins, dairy products), citrate/citric acid**	↓ absorption of A (some variability between drugs)	+ +
+							Foscarnet	↑ risk of seizures	+
+			+		+		Methadone	↑ levels of B	+ +
+			+	+		+	**NSAIDs**	↑ risk CNS stimulation/seizures	+ +
+							Phenytoin	↑ or ↓ levels of B	+
+	+	+		+		+	Probenecid	↓ renal clearance of A	+
+	+	+	+	+		+	Sucralfate	↓ absorption of A	+ +
+							Theophylline	↑ levels of B	+ +
+			+	+		+	Tizanidine	↑ levels of B	+ +
+							Warfarin	↑ prothrombin time	+

Foscarnet (Foscavir)	Ciprofloxacin	↑ risk of seizures	+
	Nephrotoxic drugs: aminoglycosides, ampho B, cis-platinum, cyclosporine	↑ risk of nephrotoxicity	+
	Pentamidine IV	↑ risk of severe hypocalcemia	+ +
Ganciclovir (Cytovene)	Imipenem	↑ risk of seizures reported	+
	Probenecid	↑ levels of A	+
	Zidovudine	↓ levels of A, ↑ levels of B	+
Gentamicin	*See Aminoglycosides—parenteral*		
Indinavir	*See protease inhibitors and Table 22B & C*		
Isoniazid	**Alcohol, rifampin**	**↑ risk of hepatic injury**	+ +
	Aluminum salts	↓ absorption (take fasting)	+ +
	Carbamazepine, phenytoin	↑ levels of B with nausea, vomiting, nystagmus, ataxia	+ +
	Itraconazole, ketoconazole	↓ levels of B	+
	Oral hypoglycemics	↓ effects of B	+
Lamivudine	Zalcitabine	**Mutual interference—do not combine**	+ +

TABLE 22 (3)

ANTI-INFECTIVE AGENT (A)	OTHER DRUG (B)	EFFECT	SIGNIFICANCE/ CERTAINTY
Linezolid (Zyvox)	Adrenergic agents	Risk of hypertension	++
	Aged, fermented, pickled or smoked foods —↑ tyramine	Risk of hypertension	+
	Serotonergic drugs (SSRIs)	Risk of serotonin syndrome	+
Lopinavir	*See protease inhibitors*		

Macrolides   *[**Ery** = erythromycin, **Azi** = azithromycin, **Clr** = clarithromycin; **Dir** = dirithromycin, + = occurs, **blank space** = either studied and no interaction OR no data (pharm. co. may have data)]*

Ery	Dir	Azi	Clr	OTHER DRUG (B)	EFFECT	SIGNIFICANCE/ CERTAINTY
+	+		+	Carbamazepine	↑ serum levels of B, nystagmus, nausea, vomiting, ataxia	++ (avoid with erythro)
+			+	Cimetidine, **ritonavir**	↑ levels of B	+
+				Clozapine	↑ serum levels of B, CNS toxicity	+
			+	**Colchicine**	**↑ levels of B (potent, fatal)**	++ (avoid)
+				Corticosteroids	↑ effects of B	+
+	+	+	+	Cyclosporine	↑ serum levels of B with toxicity	+
+	+	+	+	Digoxin, digitoxin	↑ serum levels of B (10% of cases)	+
			+	Efavirenz	↓ levels of A	++
+	+		+	Ergot alkaloids	↑ levels of B	++
+	+		+	Lovastatin/simvastatin	↑ levels of B; rhabdomyolysis	++
+				Midazolam, triazolam	↑ levels of B, ↑ sedative effects	+
+	+		+	Phenytoin	↑ levels of B	+
+	+	+	+	Pimozide	**↑ Q-T interval**	++
+				Rifampin, rifabutin	↓ levels of A	+
+			+	Tacrolimus	↑ levels of B	++
+			+	Theophyllines	↑ serum levels of B with nausea, vomiting, seizures, apnea	++
+	+		+	Valproic acid	↑ levels of B	+
+	+		+	Warfarin	May ↑ prothrombin time	+
			+	Zidovudine	↓ levels of B	+

ANTI-INFECTIVE AGENT (A)	OTHER DRUG (B)	EFFECT	SIGNIFICANCE/ CERTAINTY
Mefloquine	ß-adrenergic blockers, calcium channel blockers, quinidine, quinine	↑ arrhythmias	+
	Divalproex, valproic acid	↓ level of B with seizures	++
	Halofantrine	Q-T prolongation	++ (avoid)
Methenamine mandelate or hippurate	Acetazolamide, sodium bicarbonate, thiazide diuretics	↓ antibacterial effect 2° to ↑ urine pH	++
Metronidazole	**Alcohol**	Disulfiram-like reaction	+
	Cyclosporin	↑ levels of B	++
	Disulfiram (Antabuse)	Acute toxic psychosis	+
	Lithium	↑ levels of B	++
	Oral anticoagulants	↑ anticoagulant effect	++
	Phenobarbital, hydantoins	↑ levels of B	++
Nelfinavir	*See protease inhibitors and Table 22B & C*		
Nevirapine (Viramune)	*See non-nucleoside reverse transcriptase inhibitors (NNRTIs) and Table 22C*		
Nitrofurantoin	Antacids	↓ absorption of A	+

Non-nucleoside reverse transcriptase inhibitors (NNRTIs): For interactions with protease inhibitors, *see Table 22C*.   **Del** = delavirdine, **Efa** = efavirenz, **Nev** = nevirapine

Del	Efa	Nev	OTHER DRUG (B)	EFFECT	SIGNIFICANCE/ CERTAINTY
			Co-administration contraindicated:		
+			Anticonvulsants: carbamazepine, phenobarbital, phenytoin		++
+			Antimycobacterials: rifabutin, rifampin		++
+			Antipsychotics: pimozide		++
+	+		Benzodiazepines: alprazolam, midazolam, triazolam		++
+	+		Ergotamine		++
+	+		HMG-CoA inhibitors (statins): lovastatin, simvastatin, atorvastatin, pravastatin		++
+			St. John's wort		++
			Dose change needed:		
+			Amphetamines	↑ levels of B—**caution**	++
+		+	Antiarrhythmics: amiodarone, lidocaine, others	↓ or ↑ levels of B—**caution**	++
+	+	+	Anticonvulsants: carbamazepine, phenobarbital, phenytoin	↓ levels of A and/or B	++
+	+	+	Antifungals: itraconazole, ketoconazole, voriconazole	Potential ↓ levels of B, ↑ levels of A	++ (avoid)
+			Antipsychotics: pimozide		++
+		+	Antirejection drugs: cyclosporine, rapamycin, sirolimus, tacrolimus	↑ levels of B	++
		+	Benzodiazepines: *as above*	↑ levels of B	++
+		+	Calcium channel blockers	↑ levels of B	++
+		+	Clarithromycin	↑ levels of B metabolite	++
+		+	Cyclosporine	↑ levels of B	++
+			Dexamethasone	↓ levels of A	++
+	+	+	Sildenafil, vardenafil, tadalafil	↑ levels of B	++
+		+	Fentanyl, methadone	↑ levels of B	++

TABLE 22 (4)

ANTI-INFECTIVE AGENT (A)			OTHER DRUG (B)	EFFECT	SIGNIFICANCE/CERTAINTY

Non-nucleoside reverse transcriptase inhibitors (NNRTIs) *(continued)*: For interactions with protease inhibitors, *see Table 22B.* **Del** = delavirdine, **Efa** = efavirenz, **Nev** = nevirapine

Del	Efa	Nev	Co-administration contraindicated:		
+			Gastric acid suppression: antacids, H-2 blockers, proton pump inhibitors	↓ levels of A	+ +
+			HMG-CoA inhibitors (statins)		
	+	+	Methadone	↓ levels of B	+ +
	+	+	Oral contraceptives	↑ or ↓ levels of B	+ +
+	+	+	Protease inhibitors—*see Table 22C*		
+	+	+	Rifabutin, rifampin	↑ or ↓ levels of rifabutin; ↓ levels of A—**caution**	+ +
+	+	+	St. John's wort	↓ levels of A	
+		+	Warfarin	↑ levels of B	+ +

Pentamidine, IV	Amphotericin B	↑ risk of nephrotoxicity	+
	Foscarnet	↑ risk of hypocalcemia	+
	Pancreatitis-associated drugs, e.g., alcohol, valproic acid	↑ risk of pancreatitis	+
Piperacillin	Cefoxitin	Antagonism vs pseudomonas	+ +
Primaquine	Chloroquine, dapsone, INH, probenecid, quinine, sulfonamides, TMP/SMX, others	↑ risk of hemolysis in G6PD-deficient patients	+ +

Protease Inhibitors—Anti-HIV Drugs. (*Atazan* = atazanavir; *Fosampren* = fosamprenavir; *Indin* = indinavir; *Lopin* = lopinavir; *Nelfin* = nelfinavir; *Riton* =ritonavir; *Saquin* = saquinavir; *Tipran* = tipranavir). For interactions with antiretrovirals, *see Table 22B & C*
Only a partial list—check package insert
Also see http://aidsinfo.nih.gov

Atazan	Fosampren	Indin	Lopin	Nelfin	Riton	Saquin	Tipran	OTHER DRUG (B)	EFFECT	SIGNIF.
								Analgesics:		
						+	+	1. Alfentanil, fentanyl, hydrocodone, tramadol	↑ levels of B	+
	+				+		+	2. Codeine, hydromorphone, morphine, methadone	↓ levels of B	+
+	+	+	+	+	+	+	+	**Anti-arrhythmics: amiodarone, lidocaine, mexiletine, flecainide**	↑ levels of B; **do not co-administer**	+ +
+	+	+	+	+	+			**Anticonvulsants: carbamazepine, clonazepam, phenytoin, phenobarbital**	↓ levels of A, ↑ levels of B	+ +
+	+	+				+		Antidepressants, all tricyclic	↑ levels of B	+ +
+						+	+	Antidepressants, all other	↑ levels of B; do not use pimozide	+ +
					+			**Antihistamine:** Loratadine	↑ levels of B	+ +
	+							Atovaquone	↓ levels of B	+
+	+	+	+	+	+	+	+	**Benzodiazepines, e.g., diazepam, midazolam, triazolam**	↑ **levels of B—do not use**	+ +
					+			Beta blockers: Metoprolol, pindolol, propranolol, timolol	↑ levels of B	+
+	+	+	+	+	+	+	+	Calcium channel blockers (all)	↑ levels of B	+ +
+			+	+	+	+	+	Clarithro, erythro	↑ levels of B if renal impairment	+
+		+	+	+			+	Contraceptives, oral	↓ levels of B	+ +
	+			+	+		+	Corticosteroids: prednisone, dexamethasone	↓ levels of A, ↑ levels of B	+
+	+	+	+	+	+	+	+	Cyclosporine	↑ levels of B, monitor levels	+
+	+			+	+	+	+	Ergot derivatives	↑ **levels of B—do not use**	+ +
	+	+		+	+	+		Erythromycin, clarithromycin	↑ levels of A & B	+
		+				+		Grapefruit juice (>200 ml/day)	↓ indinavir ↑ saquinavir levels	+ +
+	+	+	+	+	+	+		H2 receptor antagonists	↓ levels of A	+ +
+	+	+	+	+	+	+	+	**HMG-CoA reductase inhibitors (statins): lovastatin, simvastatin**	↑ **levels of B—do not use**	+ +
+								Irinotecan	↑ **levels of B—do not use**	+ +
	+	+	+		+	+	+	Ketoconazole, itraconazole, ? vori	↑ levels of A, ↑ levels of B	+
	+			+			+	Metronidazole	Poss. disulfiram reaction, alcohol	+
+	+	+	+	+	+			Pimozide	↑ **levels of B—do not use**	+ +
+	+	+	+	+	+			Proton pump inhibitors	↓ levels of A	+ +
+	+	+	+	+	+	+	+	Rifampin, rifabutin	↓ levels of A, ↑ levels of B **(avoid)**	+ + **(avoid)**
+	+	+	+	+	+	+	+	Sildenafil (Viagra), tadalafil, vardenafil	Varies, some ↑ & some ↓ levels of B	+ +
+	+	+	+	+	+	+	+	**St. John's wort**	↓ **levels of A—do not use**	+ +
+								Tenofovir	↓ levels of B—add ritonavir	+ +
		+	+		+			Theophylline	↓ levels of B	+
+	+		+		+		+	Warfarin	↑ levels of B	+

150

TABLE 22 (5)

ANTI-INFECTIVE AGENT (A)	OTHER DRUG (B)	EFFECT	SIGNIFICANCE/CERTAINTY
Pyrazinamide	INH, rifampin	May ↑ risk of hepatotoxicity	±
Pyrimethamine	Lorazepam	↑ risk of hepatotoxicity	+
	Sulfonamides, TMP/SMX	↑ risk of marrow suppression	+
	Zidovudine	↑ risk of marrow suppression	+
Quinine	Digoxin	↑ digoxin levels; ↑ toxicity	++
	Mefloquine	↑ arrhythmias	+
	Oral anticoagulants	↑ prothrombin time	++
Quinupristin-dalfopristin (Synercid)	Anti-HIV drugs: NNRTIs & PIs	↑ levels of B	++
	Antineoplastic: vincristine, docetaxel, paclitaxel	↑ levels of B	++
	Calcium channel blockers	↑ levels of B	++
	Carbamazepine	↑ levels of B	++
	Cyclosporine, tacrolimus	↑ levels of B	++
	Lidocaine	↑ levels of B	++
	Methylprednisolone	↑ levels of B	++
	Midazolam, diazepam	↑ levels of B	++
	Statins	↑ levels of B	++
Ribavirin	Didanosine	↑ levels of B → toxicity—**avoid**	++
	Stavudine	↓ levels of B	++
	Zidovudine	↓ levels of B	++
Rifamycins (rifampin, rifabutin) See footnote for less severe or less common interactions[1] Ref.: ArIM 162:985, 2002	Al OH, ketoconazole, PZA	↓ levels of A	+
	Atovaquone	↑ levels of A, ↓ levels of B	+
	Beta adrenergic blockers (metoprolol, propranolol)	↓ effect of B	+
	Clarithromycin	↑ levels of A, ↓ levels of B	++
	Corticosteroids	↑ replacement requirement of B	++
	Cyclosporine	↓ effect of B	++
	Delavirdine	**↑ levels of A, ↓ levels of B—avoid**	++
	Digoxin	↓ levels of B	++
	Disopyramide	↓ levels of B	++
	Fluconazole	↑ levels of A[1]	+
	Amprenavir, indinavir, nelfinavir, ritonavir	↑ levels of A (↓ dose of A), ↓ levels of B	++
	INH	Converts INH to toxic hydrazine	++
	Itraconazole[2], ketoconazole	↓ levels of B, ↑ levels of A[2]	++
	Methadone	↓ serum levels (withdrawal)	+
	Nevirapine	**↓ levels of B—avoid**	++
	Oral anticoagulants	Suboptimal anticoagulation	++
	Oral contraceptives	↓ effectiveness; spotting, pregnancy	+
	Phenytoin	↓ levels of B	+
	Protease inhibitors	**↑ levels of A, ↓ levels of B—CAUTION**	++
	Quinidine	↓ effect of B	+
	Sulfonylureas	↓ hypoglycemic effect	+
	Tacrolimus	↓ levels of B	++
	Theophylline	↓ levels of B	+
	TMP/SMX	↑ levels of A	+
	Tocainide	↓ effect of B	+
Rimantadine	See Amantadine		
Ritonavir	See protease inhibitors and Table 22B & C		
Saquinavir	See protease inhibitors and Table 22B & C		
Stavudine	Dapsone, INH	May ↑ risk of peripheral neuropathy	±
	Ribavirin	↓ levels of A—**avoid**	++
	Zidovudine	Mutual interference—do not combine	++
Sulfonamides	Cyclosporine	↓ cyclosporine levels	+
	Methotrexate	↑ antifolate activity	+
	Oral anticoagulants	↑ prothrombin time; bleeding	+
	Phenobarbital, rifampin	↓ levels of A	+
	Phenytoin	↑ levels of B; nystagmus, ataxia	+
	Sulfonylureas	↑ hypoglycemic effect	+
Telithromycin (Ketek)	Carbamazine	↓ levels of A	++
	Digoxin	↑ levels of B—do digoxin levels	++
	Ergot alkaloids	**↑ levels of B—avoid**	++
	Itraconazole; ketoconazole	↑ levels of A; no dose change	+
	Metoprolol	↑ levels of B	++
	Midazolam	↑ levels of B	++
	Oral anticoagulants	↑ prothrombin time	+
	Phenobarb, phenytoin	↓ levels of A	++
	Pimozide	**↑ levels of B; QT prolongation—AVOID**	++

[1] The following is a partial list of drugs with rifampin-induced ↑ metabolism and hence lower than anticipated serum levels: ACE inhibitors, dapsone, diazepam, digoxin, diltiazem, doxycycline, fluconazole, fluvastatin, haloperidol, nifedipine, progestins, triazolam, tricyclics, voriconazole, zidovudine
[2] Up to 4 weeks may be required after RIF discontinued to achieve detectable serum itra levels; ↑ levels associated with uveitis or polymyolysis

TABLE 22 (6)

ANTI-INFECTIVE AGENT (A)	OTHER DRUG (B)	EFFECT	SIGNIFICANCE/ CERTAINTY
elithromycin (*ontinued*)	Rifampin	↓ **levels of A—avoid**	+ +
	Simvastatin	↑ levels of B (↑ risk of myopathy)	+ +
	Sotalol	↓ levels of B	+ +
	Theophylline	↑ levels of B	+ +
enofovir	Atazanavir	↓ levels of B—add ritonavir	+ +
	Didanosine (ddl)	↑ **levels of B (reduce dose)**	+ +
erbinafine	Cimetidine	↑ levels of A	+
	Phenobarbital, rifampin	↓ levels of A	+
etracyclines	*See Doxycycline, plus:*		
	Atovaquone	↓ levels of B	+
	Digoxin	↑ toxicity of B (may persist several months—up to 10% pts)	+ +
	Methoxyflurane	↑ toxicity; polyuria, renal failure	+
	Sucralfate	↓ absorption of A (separate by ≥2 hrs)	+
hiabendazole	Theophyllines	↑ serum theophylline, nausea	+
igecycline	Oral contraceptives	↓ levels of B	+ +
inidazole (Tindamax)	*See Metronidazole—similar entity, expect similar interactions*		
obramycin	*See Aminoglycosides*		
rimethoprim	Amantadine, dapsone, digoxin, methotrexate, procainamide, zidovudine	↑ serum levels of B	+ +
	Potassium-sparing diuretics	↑ serum K^+	+ +
	Thiazide diuretics	↓ serum Na^+	+
rimethoprim-Sulfa- aethoxazole	Azathioprine	Reports of leukopenia	+
	Cyclosporine	↓ levels of B, ↑ serum creatinine	+
	Loperamide	↑ levels of B	+
	Methotrexate	Enhanced marrow suppression	+ +
	Oral contraceptives, pimozide, and 6-mercaptopurine	↓ effect of B	+
	Phenytoin	↑ levels of B	+
	Rifampin	↑ levels of B	+
	Warfarin	↑ activity of B	+
ancomycin	Aminoglycosides	↑ frequency of nephrotoxicity	+ +
alcitabine (ddC) (HIVID)	Valproic acid, pentamidine (IV), alcohol, lamivudine	↑ pancreatitis risk	+
	Cisplatin, INH, metronidazole, vincristine, nitrofurantoin, d4T, dapsone	↑ risk of peripheral neuropathy	+
idovudine (ZDV) (Retrovir)	Atovaquone, fluconazole, metha- done	↑ levels of A	+
	Clarithromycin	↓ levels of A	±
	Indomethacin	↑ levels of ZDV toxic metabolite	+
	Nelfinavir	↓ levels of A	+ +
	Probenecid, TMP/SMX	↑ levels of A	+
	Ribavirin	↓ **levels of A—avoid**	+ +
	Rifampin/rifabutin	↓ levels of A	+ +
	Stavudine	**Interference—DO NOT COMBINE!**	+ +

TABLE 22B: DRUG-DRUG INTERACTIONS BETWEEN PROTEASE INHIBITORS
(Adapted from Guidelines for the Use of Antiretroviral Agents in HIV-Infected Adults & Adolescents; see www.aidsinfo.nih.gov)

NAME (Abbreviation, Trade Name)	Atazanavir (ATV, Reyataz)	Fosamprenavir (FOS-APV, Lexiva)	Indinavir (IDV, Crixivan)	Lopinavir/Ritonavir (LP/R, Kaletra)	Nelfinavir (NFV, Viracept)	Ritonavir (RTV, Norvir)	Saquinavir (SQV, Invirase)	Tipranavir (TPV, Aptivus)
Atazanavir (ATV, Reyataz)			Do not co-administer; risk of additive ↑ in indirect bilirubin	RTV 100 mg ↑ ATV AUC 238%		ATV/RTV 300/100 mg q24h	Combination not recommended	No data
Fosamprenavir (FOS-APV, Lexiva)				Rx-naïve: LP/R no dose change. Rx-experienced: LP/R 600/150 mg bid		200 mg RTV q24h + FOS-APV 1400 mg q24h	Insufficient data	Do not combine
Indinavir (IDV, Crixivan)	Do not co-administer; risk of additive ↑ in bilirubin			IDV AUC ↑. IDV dose 600 mg bid	↑ IDV & NFV levels. Dose: IDV 1200 mg bid, NFV 1250 mg bid	Dose: IDV/RTV bid as 800/100 mg or 800/200 mg	SQV levels ↑ 4-7 fold. Dose: Insufficient data	Do not combine
Lopinavir/Ritonavir (LP/R, Kaletra)	RTV 100 mg ↑ ATV AUC 238%	Rx-naïve: LP/R no dose change. Rx-experienced: LP/R 600/150 mg bid	IDV AUC ↑. IDV dose 600 mg bid		Rx-naïve: LP/R no dose change. Rx-experienced: LP/R 600/150 mg bid	LP is co-formulated with RTV	SQV levels ↑. Dose: SQV 1000 mg bid; LP/R standard	Do not combine
Nelfinavir (NFV, Viracept)			↑ IDV & NFV levels. Dose: IDV 1200 mg bid, NFV 1250 mg bid	Rx-naïve: LP/R no dose change. Rx-experienced: LP/R 600/150 mg bid		Dose: RTV 400 mg bid + NFV 500-750 mg bid	SQV levels ↑. Dose: SQV 800 mg tid or 1200 mg bid	Do not combine
Ritonavir (RTV, Norvir)	ATV/RTV 300/100 mg q24h	200 mg RTV q24h + FOS-APV 1400 mg q24h	Dose: IDV/RTV bid as 800/100 mg or 800/200 mg	LP is co-formulated with RTV	Dose: RTV 400 mg + NFV 500-750 mg bid		Dose: 1000 mg SQV/100 mg RTV bid or 400/400 mg bid	TPV 500 mg bid + RTV 200 mg bid
Saquinavir (SQV, Invirase)	Combination not recommended	Insufficient data	SQV levels ↑ 4-7 fold. Dose: Insufficient data	SQV levels ↑. Dose: SQV 800 mg bid; LP/R standard	Dose: NFV standard. SQV 800 mg tid or 1200 mg bid	Dose: 1000 mg SQV/100 mg RTV bid or 400/400 mg bid		Do not combine
Tipranavir (TPV, Aptivus)	No data	Do not combine	Do not combine	Do not combine	Do not combine	TPV 500 mg bid + RTV 200 mg bid	Do not combine	

TABLE 22C: DRUG-DRUG INTERACTIONS BETWEEN NON-NUCLEOSIDE REVERSE TRANSCRIPTASE INHIBITORS (NNRTIs) AND PROTEASE INHIBITORS.
(Adapted from Guidelines for the Use of Antiretroviral Agents in HIV-Infected Adults & Adolescents; see www.aidsinfo.nih.gov)

NAME (Abbreviation, Trade Name)	Atazanavir (ATV, Reyataz)	Fosamprenavir (FOS-APV, Lexiva)	Indinavir (IDV, Crixivan)	Lopinavir/Ritonavir (LP/R, Kaletra)	Nelfinavir (NFV, Viracept)	Ritonavir (RTV, Norvir)	Saquinavir (SQV, Invirase)	Tipranavir (TPV, Aptivus)
Delavirdine (DLV, Rescriptor)	No data	Co-administration not recommended	IDV levels ↑ 40%. Dose: IDV 600 mg q8h; DLV standard	Expect LP levels to ↑. No dose data	NFV levels ↑ 2X; DLV levels ↓ 50%. Dose: No data	Levels of RTV ↑ 70%. Dose: DLV standard, RTV no data	SQV levels ↑ 5X. Dose: SQV 800 mg tid, DLV standard	No data
Efavirenz (EFZ, Sustiva)	ATV AUC ↓ 74%. Dose: ↑ EFZ standard; ATA/RTV 300/100 mg q24h with food	FOS-APV levels ↓. Dose: EFZ standard; FOS-APV 1400 mg + RTV 300 mg q24h or 700 mg FOS-APV + 100 mg RTV bid	Levels: IDV ↓ 31%. Dose: IDV 1000 mg q8h; EFV standard	Rx-naïve: LP/R no dose change. Rx-experienced: LP/R 600/150 mg bid	Standard doses	Standard doses	Level: SQV ↓ 62%. Dose: SQV softgel 400 mg + RTV 400 mg bid	No data
Nevirapine (NVP, Viramune)	No data	No data	IDV levels ↓ 28%. Dose: IDV 1000 mg q8h or combine with RTV; NVP standard	Rx-naïve: LP/R no dose change. Rx-experienced: LP/R 600/150 mg bid	Standard doses	Standard doses	Dose: SQV softgel + RTV 400/400 mg both bid	No data

TABLE 23: LIST OF GENERIC AND COMMON TRADE NAMES

GENERIC NAME: TRADE NAMES	GENERIC NAME: TRADE NAMES	GENERIC NAME: TRADE NAMES
Abacavir: Ziagen	Drotrecogin alfa: Xigris	Nitazoxanide: Alinia
Acyclovir: Zovirax	Efavirenz: Sustiva	Nitrofurantoin: Macrobid, Macrodantin
Adefovir: Hepsera	Emtricitabine: Emtriva	Nystatin: Mycostatin
Albendazole: Albenza	Emtricitabine + tenofovir: Truvada	Ofloxacin: Floxin
Amantadine: Symmetrel	Enfuvirtide (T-20): Fuzeon	Oseltamivir: Tamiflu
Amikacin: Amikin	Entecavir: Baraclude	Oxacillin: Prostaphlin
Amoxicillin: Amoxil, Polymox	Ertapenem: Invanz	Palivizumab: Synagis
Amox./clav.: Augmentin, Augmentin ES-600; Augmentin XR	Erythromycin(s): Ilotycin	Paromomycin: Humatin
Amphotericin B: Fungizone	*Ethyl succinate:* Pediamycin	Pentamidine: NebuPent, Pentam 300
Ampho B-liposomal: AmBisome	*Glucoheptonate:* Erythrocin	Piperacillin: Pipracil
Ampho B-cholesteryl complex: Amphotec	*Estolate:* Ilosone	Piperacillin/tazobactam: Zosyn
Ampho B-lipid complex: Abelcet	Erythro/sulfisoxazole: Pediazole	Piperazine: Antepar
Ampicillin: Omnipen, Polycillin	Ethambutol: Myambutol	Podophyllotoxin: Condylox
Ampicillin/sulbactam: Unasyn	Ethionamide: Trecator	Posaconazole: Noxafil
Atazanavir: Reyataz	Famciclovir: Famvir	Praziquantel: Biltricide
Atovaquone: Mepron	Fluconazole: Diflucan	Primaquine: Primachine
Atovaquone + proguanil: Malarone	Flucytosine: Ancobon	Proguanil: Paludrine
Azithromycin: Zithromax	Fosamprenavir: Lexiva	Pyrantel pamoate: Antiminth
Azithromycin ER: Zmax	Foscarnet: Foscavir	Pyrimethamine: Daraprim
Aztreonam: Azactam	Fosfomycin: Monurol	Pyrimethamine/sulfadoxine: Fansidar
Caspofungin: Cancidas	Ganciclovir: Cytovene	Quinupristin/dalfopristin: Synercid
Cefaclor: Ceclor, Ceclor CD	Gatifloxacin: Tequin	Ribavirin: Virazole, Rebetol
Cefadroxil: Duricef	Gemifloxacin: Factive	Rifabutin: Mycobutin
Cefazolin: Ancef, Kefzol	Gentamicin: Garamycin	Rifampin: Rifadin, Rimactane
Cefdinir: Omnicef	Griseofulvin: Fulvicin	Rifapentine: Priftin
Cefditoren pivoxil: Spectracef	Halofantrine: Halfan	Rifaximin: Xifaxan
Cefepime: Maxipime	Idoxuridine: Dendrid, Stoxil	Rimantadine: Flumadine
Cefixime^NUS: Suprax	INH + RIF: Rifamate	Ritonavir: Norvir
Cefoperazone-sulbactam: Sulperazon^NUS	INH + RIF + PZA: Rifater	Saquinavir: Invirase, Fortovase
Cefotaxime: Claforan	Interferon alfa: Roferon-A, Intron A	Spectinomycin: Trobicin
Cefotetan: Cefotan	Interferon, pegylated: PEG-Intron, Pegasys	Stavudine: Zerit
Cefoxitin: Mefoxin	Interferon + ribavirin: Rebetron	Stibogluconate: Pentostam
Cefpodoxime proxetil: Vantin	Imipenem + cilastatin: Primaxin	Silver sulfadiazine: Silvadene
Cefprozil: Cefzil	Imiquimod: Aldara	Sulfamethoxazole: Gantanol
Ceftazidime: Fortaz, Tazicef, Tazidime	Indinavir: Crixivan	Sulfasalazine: Azulfidine
Ceftibuten: Cedax	Itraconazole: Sporanox	Sulfisoxazole: Gantrisin
Ceftizoxime: Cefizox	Iodoquinol: Yodoxin	Telithromycin: Ketek
Ceftriaxone: Rocephin	Ivermectin: Stromectol	Tenofovir: Viread
Cefuroxime: Zinacef, Kefurox, Ceftin	Kanamycin: Kantrex	Terbinafine: Lamisil
Cephalexin: Keflex	Ketoconazole: Nizoral	Thalidomide: Thalomid
Cephradine: Anspor, Velosef	Lamivudine: Epivir, Epivir-HBV	Thiabendazole: Mintezol
Chloroquine: Aralen	Lamivudine + abacavir: Epzicom	Ticarcillin: Ticar
Cidofovir: Vistide	Levofloxacin: Levaquin	Tigecycline: Tygacil
Ciprofloxacin: Cipro, Cipro XR	Linezolid: Zyvox	Tinidazole: Tindamax
Clarithromycin: Biaxin, Biaxin XL	Lomefloxacin: Maxaquin	Tipranavir: Aptivus
Clindamycin: Cleocin	Lopinavir/ritonavir: Kaletra	Tobramycin: Nebcin
Clofazimine: Lamprene	Loracarbef: Lorabid	Tretinoin: Retin A
Clotrimazole: Lotrimin, Mycelex	Mafenide: Sulfamylon	Trifluridine: Viroptic
Cloxacillin: Tegopen	Mebendazole: Vermox	Trimethoprim: Proloprim, Trimpex
Colistimethate: Coly-Mycin M	Mefloquine: Lariam	Trimethoprim/sulfamethoxazole: Bactrim, Septra
Cycloserine: Seromycin	Meropenem: Merrem	Valacyclovir: Valtrex
Daptomycin: Cubicin	Mesalamine: Asacol, Pentasa	Valganciclovir: Valcyte
Delavirdine: Rescriptor	Methenamine: Hiprex, Mandelamine	Vancomycin: Vancocin
Dicloxacillin: Dynapen	Metronidazole: Flagyl	Voriconazole: Vfend
Didanosine: Videx	Micafungin: Mycamine	Zalcitabine: HIVID
Diethylcarbamazine: Hetrazan	Minocycline: Minocin	Zanamivir: Relenza
Diloxanide furoate: Furamide	Moxifloxacin: Avelox	Zidovudine (ZDV): Retrovir
Dirithromycin: Dynabac	Mupirocin: Bactroban	Zidovudine + 3TC: Combivir
Doxycycline: Vibramycin	Nafcillin: Unipen	Zidovudine + 3TC + abacavir: Trizivir
	Nelfinavir: Viracept	
	Nevirapine: Viramune	

TABLE 23 (2)
LIST OF COMMON TRADE AND GENERIC NAMES

TRADE NAME: GENERIC NAME	TRADE NAME: GENERIC NAME	TRADE NAME: GENERIC NAME
Abelcet: Ampho B-lipid complex	Garamycin: Gentamicin	Retin A: Tretinoin
Albenza: Albendazole	Halfan: Halofantrine	Retrovir: Zidovudine (ZDV)
Aldara: Imiquimod	Hepsera: Adefovir	Reyataz: Atazanavir
Alinia: Nitazoxanide	Herplex: Idoxuridine	Rifadin: Rifampin
AmBisome: Ampho B-liposomal	Hiprex: Methenamine hippurate	Rifamate: INH + RIF
Amikin: Amikacin	HIVID: Zalcitabine	Rifater: INH + RIF + PZA
Amoxil: Amoxicillin	Humatin: Paromomycin	Rimactane: Rifampin
Amphotec: Ampho B-cholesteryl complex	Ilosone: Erythromycin estolate	Rocephin: Ceftriaxone
Ancef: Cefazolin	Ilotycin: Erythromycin	Roferon-A: Interferon alfa
Ancobon: Flucytosine	Intron A: Interferon alfa	Septra: Trimethoprim/sulfa
Anspor: Cephradine	Invanz: Ertapenem	Seromycin: Cycloserine
Antepar: Piperazine	Invirase: Saquinavir	Silvadene: Silver sulfadiazine
Antiminth: Pyrantel pamoate	Kantrex: Kanamycin	Spectracef: Cefditoren pivoxil
Aptivus: Tipranavir	Kaletra: Lopinavir/ritonavir	Sporanox: Itraconazole
Aralen: Chloroquine	Keflex: Cephalexin	Stoxil: Idoxuridine
Asacol: Mesalamine	Kefurox: Cefuroxime	Stromectol: Ivermectin
Augmentin, Augmentin ES-600 Augmentin XR: Amox./clav.	Ketek: Telithromycin	Sulfamylon: Mafenide
Avelox: Moxifloxacin	Lamisil: Terbinafine	Sulperazon[NUS]: Cefoperazone-sulbactam
Azactam: Aztreonam	Lamprene: Clofazimine	Suprax: Cefixime[NUS]
Azulfidine: Sulfasalazine	Lariam: Mefloquine	Sustiva: Efavirenz
Bactroban: Mupirocin	Levaquin: Levofloxacin	Symmetrel: Amantadine
Bactrim: Trimethoprim/sulfamethoxazole	Lexiva: Fosamprenavir	Synagis: Palivizumab
Baraclude: Entecavir	Lorabid: Loracarbef	Synercid: Quinupristin/dalfopristin
Biaxin, Biaxin XL: Clarithromycin	Macrodantin, Macrobid: Nitrofurantoin	Tamiflu: Oseltamivir
Biltricide: Praziquantel	Malarone: Atovaquone + proguanil	Tazicef: Ceftazidime
Cancidas: Caspofungin	Mandelamine: Methenamine mandel.	Tegopen: Cloxacillin
Ceclor, Ceclor CD: Cefaclor	Maxaquin: Lomefloxacin	Tequin: Gatifloxacin
Cedax: Ceftibuten	Maxipime: Cefepime	Thalomid: Thalidomide
Cefizox: Ceftizoxime	Mefoxin: Cefoxitin	Ticar: Ticarcillin
Cefotan: Cefotetan	Mepron: Atovaquone	Timentin: Ticarcillin-clavulanic acid
Ceftin: Cefuroxime axetil	Merrem: Meropenem	Tinactin: Tolnaftate
Cefzil: Cefprozil	Minocin: Minocycline	Tindamax: Tinidazole
Cipro, Cipro XR: Ciprofloxacin & extended release	Mintezol: Thiabendazole	Trecator SC: Ethionamide
Claforan: Cefotaxime	Monocid: Cefonicid	Trizivir: Abacavir + ZDV + 3TC
Coly-Mycin M: Colistimethate	Monurol: Fosfomycin	Trobicin: Spectinomycin
Combivir: ZDV + 3TC	Myambutol: Ethambutol	Truvada: Emtricitabine + tenofovir
Crixivan: Indinavir	Mycamine: Micafungin	Tygacil: Tigecycline
Cubicin: Daptomycin	Mycobutin: Rifabutin	Unasyn: Ampicillin/sulbactam
Cytovene: Ganciclovir	Mycostatin: Nystatin	Unipen: Nafcillin
Daraprim: Pyrimethamine	Nafcil: Nafcillin	Valcyte: Valganciclovir
Diflucan: Fluconazole	Nebcin: Tobramycin	Valtrex: Valacyclovir
Duricef: Cefadroxil	NebuPent: Pentamidine	Vancocin: Vancomycin
Dynapen: Dicloxacillin	Nizoral: Ketoconazole	Vantin: Cefpodoxime proxetil
Emtriva: Emtricitabine	Norvir: Ritonavir	Velosef: Cephradine
Epivir, Epivir-HBV: Lamivudine	Noxafil: Posaconazole	Vermox: Mebendazole
Epzicom: Lamivudine + abacavir	Omnicef: Cefdinir	Vfend: Voriconazole
Factive: Gemifloxacin	Omnipen: Ampicillin	Vibramycin: Doxycycline
Famvir: Famciclovir	Pediamycin: Erythro. ethyl succinate	Videx: Didanosine
Fansidar: Pyrimethamine + sulfadoxine	Pediazole: Erythro. ethyl succinate + sulfisoxazole	Viracept: Nelfinavir
Flagyl: Metronidazole	Pegasys, PEG-Intron: Interferon, pegylated	Viramune: Nevirapine
Floxin: Ofloxacin	Pentam 300: Pentamidine	Virazole: Ribavirin
Flumadine: Rimantadine	Pentasa: Mesalamine	Viread: Tenofovir
Fortaz: Ceftazidime	Pipracil: Piperacillin	Vistide: Cidofovir
Fortovase: Saquinavir	Polycillin: Ampicillin	Xifaxan: Rifaximin
Fulvicin: Griseofulvin	Polymox: Amoxicillin	Xigris: Drotrecogin alfa
Fungizone: Amphotericin B	Priftin: Rifapentine	Yodoxin: Iodoquinol
Furadantin: Nitrofurantoin	Primaxin: Imipenem + cilastatin	Zerit: Stavudine
Fuzeon: Enfuvirtide (T-20)	Proloprim: Trimethoprim	Ziagen: Abacavir
Gantanol: Sulfamethoxazole	Prostaphlin: Oxacillin	Zinacef: Cefuroxime
Gantrisin: Sulfisoxazole	Rebetol: Ribavirin	Zithromax: Azithromycin
	Rebetron: Interferon + ribavirin	Zmax: Azithromycin ER
	Relenza: Zanamivir	Zovirax: Acyclovir
	Rescriptor: Delavirdine	Zosyn: Piperacillin/tazobactam
		Zyvox: Linezolid

INDEX TO MAJOR ENTITIES

Bold numbers indicate major considerations. Recommendations in Table 1 not indexed; antibiotic selection often depends on modifying circumstances and alternative agents.

158